Child Abuse and Neglect

Challenges and Opportunities

Child Abuse and Neglect

Challenges and Opportunities

RN Srivastava
Pediatrician
Past President, Indian Academy of Pediatrics
Adviser Indian Child Abuse and Neglect and Child Labour Group
New Delhi, India

Rajeev Seth
Pediatrician
Chairman, Indian Child Abuse and Neglect and Child Labour
New Delhi, India
Council or International Society for Prevention of Child Abuse and Neglect

Joan van Niekerk
Manager training and Advocacy
Childline, South Africa
President elect, International Society for Prevention of Child Abuse and Neglect

Foreword
Jenny Gray
President
International Society for Prevention of Child Abuse and Neglect

JAYPEE BROTHERS MEDICAL PUBLISHERS (P) LTD

New Delhi • London • Philadelphia • Panama

Jaypee Brothers Medical Publishers (P) Ltd

Headquarters

Jaypee Brothers Medical Publishers (P) Ltd
4838/24, Ansari Road, Daryaganj
New Delhi 110 002, India
Phone: +91-11-43574357
Fax: +91-11-43574314
Email: jaypee@jaypeebrothers.com

Overseas Offices

J.P. Medical Ltd
83 Victoria Street, London
SW1H 0HW (UK)
Phone: +44-2031708910
Fax: +02-03-0086180
Email: info@jpmedpub.com

Jaypee-Highlights Medical Publishers Inc.
City of Knowledge, Bld. 237, Clayton
Panama City, Panama
Phone: + 507-301-0496
Fax: + 507-301-0499
Email: cservice@jphmedical.com

Jaypee Brothers Medical Publishers Ltd
The Bourse
111 South Independence Mall East
Suite 835, Philadelphia, PA 19106, USA
Phone: + 267-519-9789
Email: joe.rusko@jaypeebrothers.com

Jaypee Brothers Medical Publishers (P) Ltd
17/1-B Babar Road, Block-B, Shaymali
Mohammadpur, Dhaka-1207
Bangladesh
Mobile: +08801912003485
Email: jaypeedhaka@gmail.com

Jaypee Brothers Medical Publishers (P) Ltd
Shorakhute, Kathmandu
Nepal
Phone: +00977-9841528578
Email: jaypee.nepal@gmail.com

Website: www.jaypeebrothers.com
Website: www.jaypeedigital.com

Inquiries for bulk sales may be solicited at: jaypee@jaypeebrothers.com

This book has been published in good faith that the contents provided by the contributors contained herein are original, and is intended for educational purposes only. While every effort is made to ensure accuracy of information, the publisher and the editors specifically disclaim any damage, liability, or loss incurred, directly or indirectly, from the use or application of any of the contents of this work. If not specifically stated, all figures and tables are courtesy of the editors. Where appropriate, the readers should consult with a specialist or contact the manufacturer of the drug or device.

Child Abuse and Neglect: Challenges and Opportunities

First Edition: **2013**

ISBN : 978-93-5090-449-7

Printed at Rajkamal Electric Press, Plot No. 2, Phase-IV, Kundli, Haryana.

Contributors

Adam M Tomison
Director and Chief Executive,
Australian Institute of Criminology
Adjunct Professor,
Australian Catholic University
Councillor, International Society for Prevention of
Child Abuse and Neglect
Canberra, Australia

Aisha Mehnaz
Professor of Pediatrics,
Chairperson KONPAL,
Focal person for Pakistan Pediatric Association's
Child Rights Group,
Karachi, Sindh,
Pakistan
aishamehnaz@hotmail.com

Anjali Saxena
Pediatrician, Max Super Specialty Hospital
Delhi
anjali067@yahoo.com

Anne Lindboe
Pediatrician, Ombudsman for Children
Helsinki, Norway
Anne.Lindboe@barneombudet.no

Bernard Gerbaka
President, Lebanese Institute of Child Rights,
and the Lebanese Union for Child Protection,
Vice President, University of Child and Youth
Observatory in Lebanon
Beyrouth, Lebanon
berger@idm.net.lb

Chhaya Prasad
Director,
Child Development Clinic,
Regional Institute for Mentally Handicapped,
Chandigarh, India
Chhaya_sam@yahoo.co.in

Devendra Sareen
Professor of Pediatrics,
Maharana Bhupal Government Hospital,
Udaipur, Rajasthan, India
drsareen@yahoo.com

Emma Williams
Seniar Research Fellow, The Northern Institute,
Charles Darwin University, Canberra, Australia

Jenny Gray
President, International Society for Prevention of
Child Abuse and Neglect
London, UK
jennyagray@ntlworld.com

Jerry Thomas
Director, Bosco Institute, Lite Plus, Jorhat,
Assam, India
jerryotom@gmail.com

Joan van Niekerk
Clinical Social Worker
Manager Training and Advocay,
Childline President elect,
International Society for Prevention of
Child Abuse and Neglect,
Pretoria, South Africa

Kaya Manzel
Membership Assistant, International Society for
Prevention of Child Abuse and Neglect
Aurora, USA
membership@ispcan.org

Martin Finkel
Professor of Pediatrics. Director,
Child Abuse Research Institute (CARES) University
of Medicine and Dentistry of New Jersey
School of Osteopathic Medicine
New Jersey, USA
finkelm@umdnj.org

Mary J Marret
Associate Professor of Pediatrics,
University of Malaya,
Kuala Lumpur, Malaysia
marret@um.edu.my

Mehek Naeem
Member, Central Executive Council,
(PAHACHHAN)

Michael Ungar
Resilience Research Center,
Dalhousie University, Halifax, Canada
Michael.unger@dal.ca

Naeem Zafar
Associate Professor of Pediatrics,
Chief Executive officer,
PAHCHHAN, Lohore, Pakistan
drnzafar@hotmail.com

Nina Agrawal
Child Abuse Pediatrician, Audrey Hepburn
Children's House, Hackensack University Medical
Center, New Jersey, USA
nina.agrawal07@gmail.com

PM Nair
Indian Police Service, Government of India,
Adjunct Professor (Anti-Human Trafficking)
School of Law,
Indira Gandhi National Open University,
New Delhi
nairpm@hotmail.com

Peter Newell
Co-ordinator, Global Initiative to end
All Corporal Punishment of Children
London, UK
peter@endcorporalpunishment.org

RK Gorea
Professor of Forensic Medicine,
Rama Medical College,
Kanpur, Uttar Pradesh, India
gorea_r@yahoo.com

RN Srivastava
Pediatrician, Past President
Indian Academy of Pediatrics,
Adviser, Indian Child Abuse and Neglect and
Child Labour Group, New Delhi, India
drrnsri@gmail.com

Rajeev Seth
Pediatrician, Chairman Indian Child Abuse and
Child Neglect and Child Labour Group
Councillor, International Society for Prevention of
Child Abuse and Neglect, New Delhi, India
sethrajeev@gmail.com

Ranbir Singh
Vice Chancellor, National Law University,
Delhi
singhranbir@yahoo.com

Razia Ismail Abbasi
Director, India Alliance for Child Rights,
New Delhi, India
iacr@gmail.com

Reidar Hjermann
Clinical Psychologist,
Past Ombudsman for Children
Helsinki, Norway
rh@hjermann.no

Renu Singh
Educational Psychologist, Director, Young Lives
University of Oxford,
Senior Adviser,
Save the Children, New Delhi, India
renusab@gmail.com

Richard Roylance
Councilor, International Society for Prevention of
Child Abuse and Neglect
Brisbane, Australia
rroylance1@mac.com

Shanti Raman
Pediatrician, Medical Director Child Protection,
Sydney and South Western Sydney Local Health
Districts and University of New South Wales,
Sydney, Australia
s.raman@unsw.edu.au

Sibnath Deb
Professor of Applied Psychology, Pondicherry
University, Puducherry, India
sibnath23@gmail.com

Sue Foley
Councilor, International Society for Prevention of
Child Abuse and neglect
Sydney, Australia
sue.foley@health.nsw.gov.au

Swati Bhave
Pediatrician, Past President, Indian Academy
of Pediatrics ,Executive Director, Association of
Adolescent and Child Care in India,
Mumbai, Maharashtra, India
sybhave@gmail.com

Tufail Mohammed
Member, Child Rights and Abuse Committee,
Pakistan Pediatric Association, Councilor,
International Society for Prevention of
Child Abuse and Neglect
tufailm@brain.net.pk

Vandana Prasad
Community Pediatrician, National Covenor,
Public Health Resource Network,
New Delhi, India
chuakhat@yahoo.com

Ved Kumari
Professor of Law, Delhi University, Delhi, India
vedkumari@gmail.com

Foreword

Everyone has a responsibility to protect the world's children—families, communities, societies and governments. They are our future but also our present. We are all part of a family and together we can make a difference to the daily lives of children and support them to achieve their potential and become competent, well-functioning adults.

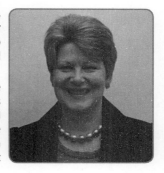

Sadly, we know that too many children in every country across the world experience abuse, neglect and violence. Maltreatment occurs across all social strata in families, schools and other institutional settings as well as on the streets and behind closed doors. New forms of exploitation are occurring through, e.g. IT advances. We are constantly being challenged on how best to protect children from harm and just as importantly to prevent it from occurring in the first place.

This book originated from the 9th Asia-Pacific Regional ISPCAN Conference which took place in New Delhi in October 2011. It was an inspiring event in which children actively participated. These chapters have grown out of the presentations at the conference. They are intended to support all those working in the field of abuse and neglect, be they in governments, NGOs or local community-based organizations, to implement evidence-based policies and practices.

It is fitting that this publication is following on from an ISPCAN Conference which took place just under 60 years after Drs Henry Kempe and Brandt Steele's seminal paper, 'The Battered Child Syndrome'. Henry Kempe is the founder of the International Society for the Prevention of Child Abuse and Neglect (ISPCAN). He passionately believed in professionals from all disciplines working together to both protect and prevent children from being abused or neglected. He also believed that this was the right of each child. I hope that everyone reading this book will use it to further the cause of a world where children are truly valued, nurtured and protected into adulthood.

Jenny Gray
President
International Society for
Prevention of Child Abuse and Neglect
December 2012

Preface

We are very pleased to bring out *"Child Abuse and Neglect: Challenges and Opportunities"*. The increasing prevalence and incidence of diverse forms of child abuse and neglect across the globe presents serious challenges. Additionally, large populations of children are at substantial risk from adverse effects of extreme poverty, illiteracy and uncontrolled family size, resulting in provision of very little care to children during the early formative years. Although child rights are universal, the problems and the magnitude of neglect, abuse and exploitation vary in different countries. In recent years, international and national organizations have very actively addressed these issues and most governments have initiated appropriate measures to tackle the menace of child abuse and neglect (CAN). There is a great need to bring out clinical advancements in this field and peer-reviewed literature for ongoing education of all concerned multidisciplinary professionals.

The decision to bring out this book was made during the 9th ISPCAN Asia-Pacific Conference on Child Abuse and Neglect at New Delhi in October 2011. The conference was very well attended, and a galaxy of experts from both developed and developing countries presented and discussed their views on various problems of CAN. This book contains an expanded and edited version of their up-to-date views and those of some other contributors, each having several professional years of scholarship and experience. Effective care and advocacy for these children should flow from our up-to-date knowledge and evidence-based clinical practice.

In the introduction, Srivastava and Jenny Gray mention the challenges and opportunities of CAN in the national and global context. Physical abuse is discussed by Agrawal and Gorea, the latter gives the medico-legal aspects in India. Various issues of corporal punishment in the Middle East and North African regions are discussed by Bernard Gerbaka. Child sexual abuse is an extremely common and serious problem across the globe. Its international perspective is presented by Roylance, Foley and Manzel and the Indian situation by Bhave. Finkel discusses the medical and forensic aspects of child sexual abuse and its management. Child trafficking and child labor constitute most repugnant violations of child rights, which are widely prevalent in several countries. Nair and Seth present the issues involved. The problems of child abuse and neglect are often ignored during disaster situations. Zafar and Naeem describe their experience with these issues during massive earthquake and floods in Pakistan and Tufail Mohammed emphasizes the need for preparedness.

Child neglect has been variably defined, but it has wider dimensions depending upon socioeconomic and educational status in different countries and different communities. These are considered by Mehnaz. Renu Singh draws attention to neglect of children with disabilities.

The issues of child protection and prevention of abuse and neglect, including elements of protection systems, assigning responsibility and public health approach have been discussed by Joan van Niekerk, Seth, Prasad, and Unger. Tomison describes his experience with monitoring and evaluating community-based interventions. There is now global support for eliminating all forms of violent punishment to children. Newell reviews the present status.

Judicial aspects of child abuse and neglect are discussed by Singh and the challenges of juvenile justice by Ved Kumari. Adverse social and cultural factors influence child maltreatment in South Asia. These are highlighted by Raman, Marret and Prasad and Deb, who also describes the current legal measures in India. Media has a very important role in providing information and influencing public opinion, which can result in attitudinal changes. Sarin et al discuss these issues.

The need for participation of children in policy and decision making is being realized. Children must be listened to and learnt from. Hjermann and Lindboe present their experience of interaction with them. Abbasi comments on APCCAN and the ensuing Delhi Declaration.

The present book thus encompasses discussion of diverse and complex issues related to child abuse and neglect, focusing on the enormous challenges as well as the growing efforts to tackle them. The presentations by eminent experts follow varied formats and individualized expressions upon their experience and convictions. The statements do not necessarily reflect the views or policies of the International Society for Child Abuse and Neglect or the Indian Child Abuse and Neglect and Child Labor Group, although a large consensus exists.

We sincerely hope this book would be read with interest and critique and be of help, invaluable resource and reference guide for all those working for the larger interests of child welfare including pediatricians, mental health professionals, psychologists, educationists, teachers, students of child rights, law, policy and programs, International and Government agencies, Legislators, policy makers, Child Rights activists and Non-Government Organizations, and even parents.

We are indebted to the dedicated and expert contributors for their hard work, knowledge and good judgment.

We are grateful to M/s Jaypee Brothers Medical Publishers, New Delhi, India for their help in the publication of this book.

RN Srivastava
Rajeev Seth
Joan van Niekerk

Contents

Section 1 Introduction

Section 2 Extent, Forms of Child Abuse and Neglect

Section 3 Protection and Prevention

Section 1

Introduction

Child Abuse and Neglect: Challenges and Opportunities

RN Srivastava

Introduction

The concerns over abuse and neglect of children have received global attention over the more than past three decades. There is increasing recognition of the extent of physical and sexual abuse of children as well as their exploitation in various ways. A large number of national and international organizations have addressed various issues and several countries have undertaken measures to tackle the problems and protect children from harm.

Child abuse

Child abuse includes all forms of physical or emotional ill-treatment, sexual abuse and exploitation, which results in actual or potential harm to child's health, survival and development. Abusive acts may cause or have high potential of causing harm to physical, mental, spiritual, moral and social development of the child. However, abuse is not an "all or none" phenomenon. There is a wide range of abusive acts varying from emotional abuse to corporal "punishment" and serious physical injury to grave sexual offences and child trafficking and exploitation.

Various forms of physical abuse are more easily recognized. Domestic child abuse and that in schools is often not reported, and in many societies considered as childhood hazards. Child rearing practices and methods of administering disciplinary measures widely vary in different cultures. Thus rigid definitions of abuse may not be uniformly applicable.

The issues of child sexual abuse have been extensively examined and their forms, extent, immediate and long term adverse effects recognized. The government of India has recently adopted stringent judicial measures to protect children from sexual offences. The practice of corporal punishment, long entrenched in social systems in most societies, is now firmly regarded as a reprehensible practice and global initiatives are being taken towards eliminating all forms of physical/corporal violence to children.

Emotional abuse is defined as a failure to provide a developmentally appropriate, supportive environment to enable stable and full range of emotional and social competence commensurate with the child's potentials. Thus restriction of movement, patterns of belittling, denigration, threatening, scaring, discriminating, ridiculing or other forms of non-physical forms of hostile or rejecting treatment are considered abusive. *These acts must be reasonably within the control of parents and viewed in the context of society in which the child lives.* The perception of what constitutes emotional abuse may vary in different societies and although broad and inclusive norms are desirable, the diversity of child rearing practices should be understood.

Neglect

Neglect implies failure to provide for the development of child in all spheres: health, education, nutrition, emotional development, shelter and safe living conditions.[1] *It includes failure to properly supervise and protect children from harm* as much as possible. A simplified proposed definition is "child neglect occurs when a child's basic needs are not actually met, resulting in actual or potential harm. Basic needs include food, clothing health care, supervision, protection, nurturance, love and a home. A broader view inclusive of societal neglect has been suggested: "Any act of commission or omission by individuals, institutions, government or society, together with their resultant conditions, which deprive children of equal rights and liberties, and/or interfere with their optimal development constitute by definition, abusive or neglectful acts or conditions".

Although *abuse* is a willful and intentional act, neglect also can be due to *ignorance* or *inability* of the parents or care providers to meet the child's requirements, for various reasons. In developing countries denial of health care, nutrition and education to children are the most serious forms of neglect.

The patterns and extent of child abuse and neglect (CAN) vary greatly in different countries. There also are regional, socioeconomic and cultural factors that influence child welfare and CAN. Thus, while the problems are truly global, the solutions might not be universally applicable and would necessarily have to be evolved locally.

Prevalence of child abuse

Physical abuse of children is very common and often fatal. Violence takes place in homes, schools, communities, streets, institutions and work places. Globally, 500 million to 1.5 billion children are estimated to experience violence every year and 73–150 million girls are subjected to sexual abuse. A widely quoted study in India involving 12,000 children reported that two-thirds were beaten by parents or teachers. Fifty-two percent admitted to some form of sexual abuse.[2] There are disturbing reports of male child sexual exploitation at a number of pilgrim tourism sites.[3]

Challenges and difficulties in developing countries

The chief underlying causes of CAN, and indeed all aspects of child development and welfare, include poverty, lack of education and large family size. There are about 440 million children (below the age of 18 years) in India. About 27 million children are born every year in India, a majority in the underprivileged where the parents cannot provide adequate care. Thus, health care and early developmental requirements are denied. Children who ought to be in schools are employed in various forms of work or in the streets and are risk for child abuse. There is a sizable migrant population where children remain deprived of education and health care. Long-standing adverse sociocultural traditions and practices such as corporal punishment, discrimination against girls, child marriages and employment of children are extremely resistant to change.

Poverty: Poverty must be regarded as societal neglect. The constraints it imposes adversely impact the child's health and development, especially in early years. Infant and under 5–year malnutrition is very common and minor illnesses go mostly untreated. Mortality rates are high in poor populations. There is a lack of a stimulatory environment. Various adverse factors result in poor learning and cognitive development. The link between poverty and child maltreatment has also been recognized in economically advanced countries: in USA the rate of neglect is reported to be 7 times higher in lowest income families compared to others.

Urban migration: Migration to large cities from impoverished villages is a serious problem in developing countries. The migrants live in overcrowded communities with few amenities and are often homeless. There may be about 18 million streetchildren of whom 60% are adolescents. These children are mostly out of school and indulge in menial work, organized begging, rag picking and are subjected to abuse. Substance addiction and sexually transmitted diseases are very common in these children.[4] Because of a lack of understanding and information about educational and health care facilities that are provided by the government free of cost are not utilized.

Children at work: About 20–50 million children in India are reported to be in the work force. They are often employed in hazardous work (carpet making, production of firework articles, glass blowing) and are paid low wages. They are abused and deprived of education. A large number of children are work in "non-organized sector" (roadside eateries, repair shops, sweeping, cleaning, helping adult workers) and many are employed as domestic help. Abuse and maltreatment are very common in theses children and they remain deprived of proper health care and education.

Societal attitudes

Adverse attitudes of adults towards children form a major barrier towards prevention of CAN. The lack of concern is reflected in abuse of children employed as domestic help and in various sundry jobs. Children on the streets and begging elicit no reaction from adults. Religious leaders in South Asia and neighbouring countries have a very large following and wield considerable influence. However, they seldom talk about problems of children or other social evils, seemingly not wishing to be regarded as social reformers.

Opportunities

Children in developing countries face serious problems that comparatively may be of little importance in economically advanced countries. Unless the root cause viz. poverty and illiteracy are addressed and the families empowered CAN will be very difficult to control. Each country will need to identify and prioritize the most pressing problems and institute appropriate measures to tackle them. *Clear, attainable and measurable goals should be set.*

An increasing awareness of the gravity of CAN among the civil society, various agencies working for child welfare and child rights, international agencies and governments offers an opportunity to control this scourge affecting millions of children. A large number of Non-Government Organizations (NGOs) are strongly voicing for child rights and prevention of CAN.

International efforts

Several United Nations (UN) and World Health Organizations (WHO) initiatives have been taken. A UN declaration at 21st special session in 2002, signed by 192 countries, clearly specifies that children must be protected against any acts of violence, abuse, exploitation and discrimination. In 2011, the Committee on the Rights of the Child in its General Comment 13 recommended the child's right to *protection from all forms of corporal punishment*. The International Society for Prevention of Child Abuse and Neglect (ISPCAN) was established in 1977.[5] It has very actively worked to create awareness and conduct training programmes in many countries. The South Asian Initiative to end Violence Against Children (SAIVEC) was started in 2010.[6] Its constituents include governments, regional coordinating groups, and NGOs. It aims at looking into how to prevent and respond to violence and building a protective environment.

Initiatives in india

The government has planned to substantially enhance allocation of resources for health care and education and all round development of underprivileged communities. These measures would greatly impact on various issues related to CAN. Neighbouring countries in South East Asia and several others in South East Asia face problems similar to India and some have instituted appropriate steps to control CAN.

Integrated child development scheme: One of the earlier, country-wide programmes aimed at welfare, especially nutrition of children, is to be strengthened.

Rural development: Primary and essential health care and schooling are being given much needed attention. A large proportion of child labour is in the agricultural sector, which leads to educational neglect. Concerns over sanitation, safe water and vector control are being addressed. Rural employment is being ensured.

Right to education: Primary education up to the age of 14 years has been made a child's right and free of cost. The school infrastructure is to be improved, mid day meals provided and modern teaching methods are to be introduced.

National rural health mission: An ambitious, well planned programme has been launched to provide health care especially to women and children. Health education and information is to be imparted by Accredited Social Health Activists (*ASHAs*).

Child protection

An Integrated Child Protection Scheme has been launched, aimed to institutionalize essential services, strengthen structures, enhance capacity at all levels, create a database and knowledge base for child protection services. Child protection at family and community level is to be encouraged and appropriate intersectoral responses ensured. *The guiding principles recognize that child protection is a primary responsibility of the family, supported by community, government and civil society.*

The National Commission for Protection of Child Rights was established by the government in 2007. It has a wide mandate and considerable powers. Child welfare committees and telephonic help lines (childlines) have been started where reports of child abuse or a child likely, or threatened to be harmed can be made and help sought.

Judicial measures

Judicial mechanisms have been closely examined in recent years. The government has adopted a number of socio-legal measures to tackle child abuse and ensure child protection.[7,8] Some of these include the Juvenile Justice Act, Prohibition of Child Marriage, and the recently adopted protection of children from sexual offences. Corporal punishment has been prohibited in schools.

Media and CAN

Media has emerged as an extremely powerful and pervasive tool. Although sensational reporting appears to be the norm, there are many instances, where the media has played an informative and constructive role.[9] It has enormous potential to influence the masses and needs to be used in a judicious manner to disseminate appropriate information about child welfare and CAN. Messages from leading figures in show business, sportspersons and religious leaders can be very influential.

Efforts of non-government organizations

A very large number of national and international NGOs are actively involved in tackling various aspects of CAN. They are providing information, training and rehabilitative facilities and playing a crucial role in advocacy for child rights and influencing the policymakers in the government.

Empowering children

It is increasingly being realised that children must be listened to. They must raise their voice and express their concerns. In educated and enlightened families a dialogic and *non-violent* approach needs to be adopted towards child rearing, which would gradually become the societal norm. Children should be allowed to say what they want to say and not what the parents or teachers want. Their contribution to the making of culture should be recognized and they should not be seen as passive recipients of social thoughts and practices.

Conclusion

Child abuse and neglect encompass a wide range of neglect, maltreatment and exploitation of children. Violence against children occurs in all societies although the patterns and extent vary. In developing countries denial of health care and education to a very large number of children in poor, illiterate communities must be regarded as most serious forms of neglect. Sociocultural and attitudinal factors are major constraints to prevention of CAN. Each country needs to identify the more serious problems, define the root causes and take appropriate measures to tackle them. Global awareness and action and governmental efforts in many countries, strong advocacy by world bodies, international and national societies, a host of NGOs and civil society provide an opportunity to contain the scourge of CAN.

References

1. Mehnaz A. Child neglect : wider dimensions. In: Child Abuse and Neglect: challenges and opportunities. Jaypee Brothers Medical Publishers Ltd, New Delhi, 2013: 100–109.
2. Ministry of Women and Child Development, Government of India. Study on child abuse in India. Available from wcd.nic.in/childabuse.pdf.
3. ECPAT. Unholy nexus: male child sexual exploitation in pilgrim tourism sites in India. www.equitabletourism.org
4. Hornor G. Child sexual abuse: consequences and implications. *J Pediatr Health Care*. 2010; 24:358–64.
5. International Society for Prevention of Child Abuse and Neglect. www.ispcan.org

6. South Asian Initiative to end violence against children.

7. Deb S. Socio-legal measures for protection of child rights in India. In: Child abuse and neglect: challenges and opportunities. Jaypee Brothers Medical Publishers Ltd, New Delhi, 2013: 191–206.

8. Singh R. Enforcing justice through law and governance in the context of child abuse. In: Child abuse and neglect: challenges and opportunities. Jaypee Brothers Medical Publishers Ltd., New Delhi 2013: 173–181.

9. Sarin D. Media and child protection. In Child Abuse and Neglect: challenges and opportunities. Jaypee Brothers Medical Publishers Ltd, New Delhi, 2013: 219–225.

2

Child Protection: Child Abuse and Neglect: Global Perspectives

Jenny Gray

Introduction

In 1962, over sixty years ago, Drs Henry Kempe and Brandt Steele published their seminal paper, *The Battered Child Syndrome,* which raised awareness and exposed the reality of child abuse. More recently, the United Nations Secretary General commissioned a study to provide a detailed picture of the nature, extent, causes and consequences of violence in five main settings including the family, schools and institutions. Professor Pinheiro, in his 2006 *Report for the UN Study on Violence against Children,* found that violence was prevalent in all settings and 'knows no bounds of geography, class, politics, race or culture'. He echoed Kempe's vision for a society free from violence against children and was clear that 'no violence against children is justifiable; all violence against children is preventable' (Pinheiro 2006, p.5).

How common is child maltreatment?

Despite there being an increasing level of general agreement about what constitutes child maltreatment, it is very difficult to gain accurate national data on the numbers of children being abused or neglected. Much is not reported. There are also cultural and societal differences about what is regarded as abuse and neglect, which may change over time.

A recent International Society for the Prevention of Child Abuse and Neglect (ISPCAN) survey (Dubowitz, 2012) found that overall in 54% of the respondents' countries, a government agency maintained an official count of the numbers of cases of child abuse or neglect which were reported to a statutory body. The regional range was from 100% in Oceania to 50% in Europe with 56% in Asia, and from 68% in high income countries and 25% from low income countries having such a system. We know however that the existence of official statistics does not give us data on the true extent of child abuse on a country. For example, recent research in the UK (Radford et al. 2011) found that the level of child maltreatment reported by young people aged 11–17 years in their study was 11 times higher than that reported in the government's statistics. This supports the generally held view that cases reported to statutory agencies represent only the tip of the iceberg and that the majority of incidents of child maltreatment remain unreported even in countries with well developed child protection systems. It is therefore virtually impossible to measure the true extent of violence against children globally.

The data on physical violence compiled for the UN Secretary General's Study on Violence against Children (2006) estimated that between 500 million and 1.5 billion children experience violence annually. Just over 10 years ago studies from many countries in all regions of the world suggested that up to 80–98% of children suffer physical punishment in their own homes, with a third or more experiencing severe punishment resulting from the use of implements (World Health Organisation, 2001). More recent data from 33 low and middle income families, covering about 10% of the world's population of children, estimated that 3 out of 4 children experience violent discipline in their own home (Multiple Indicator Cluster Surveys and Demographic and Health Surveys 2005–2006). Establishing reliable data on the number of children who have been subjected to sexual abuse and sexual exploitation is particularly challenging because of the clandestine nature of this type of abuse (UNICEF, 2009). However, there are some data showing that significant proportions of adolescent girls report having been victims of sexual violence. These ranged from 21% in Uganda and in the Democratic Republic of Congo to 5% in both the Phillipines and India (Demographic and Health Surveys, 2005–2006). The most recent 2012 report from UNICEF which examined the situation of children growing up in urban settings (some 79% of the world's children) found that 'denials of children's right to survival, health, nutrition, education and protection are widespread'.

What constitutes child maltreatment?

Although violence against children has not been eradicated, interestingly there is a high degree of commonality between regions and countries about what constitutes child maltreatment in relation to certain types of abuse or neglect. This consensus is continuing to grow over time. A recent survey undertaken by ISPCAN (Dubowitz, 2012) identified the most common behaviours which respondents from all but three of the 69 participating countries considered to be child abuse and neglect. These were: physical abuse by parents or caregivers; and sexual abuse, defined as incest, sexual touching or pornography. Other behaviours mentioned by 80% of all respondents as constituting maltreatment include failure to provide adequate food, clothing or shelter; abandonment by a parent or caretaker; commercial sexual exploitation; exposing a child to pornography; child prostitution; children living on the street; physical beating of a child by any adult; forcing a child to beg; child labour under age 12 years and abuse or neglect occurring within foster care, educational settings, and detention facilities.

One of the behaviours least often mentioned as being child abuse is physical discipline, with only 53% of respondents reporting it is considered abusive in their country. By region, the proportions ranged from 100% in Oceania (i.e. Australia and New Zealand) to 44% in both Asia and Africa. Dubowitz (2012) suggests that despite physical discipline being potentially harmful to children's development it remains a normative practice in many countries.

The survey also showed that there were clear differences in perspectives according to the country's income level. In general low income countries were more likely not to consider some experiences as maltreatment, even severe ones such as abandoning and prostituting a child. Dubowitz (2012) speculates that there may be cultural or semantic differences in determining whether such serious circumstances are labelled maltreatment. He also hypothesises that in high and some middle income countries with greater resources and support for families and children there is 'clear and strong disapproval' of such practices, whereas there may be 'less outrage or a sense of futility' in counties with few resources.

The UN convention on the rights of the child

The UN Convention on the Rights of the Child (CRC) sets internationally agreed expectations and standards in relation to children's wellbeing and rights. The CRC provides each signatory country with the foundation on which to build a system to keep its children safe from harm and to support their optimal upbringing within their family, wherever possible. In addition, international or regional treaties or protocols may set out what is expected to happen in a specific area. For example, the *Optional Protocol on the Convention of the Rights of the Child on the sale of children, child prostitution and child pornography* which criminalises all forms of sexual exploitation of children and emphasises support to children who are victims.

Article 19 of the CRC relates specifically to the protection of children from all forms of violence, the provision of services to children and their caregivers and to the prevention of violence.

> ### UN Convention on the Rights of the Child, Article 19
>
> 1. State parties shall take all appropriate legislative, administrative, social and educational measures to protect the child from all forms of physical or mental violence, injury or abuse, neglect or negligent treatment, maltreatment or exploitation, including sexual abuse, whereas in the care of parent(s), legal guardian(s), or any other person who has the care of the child.
>
> 2. Such protective measures should, as appropriate, include effective procedures for the establishment of social programmes to provide necessary support for the child and for those who have care of the child, as well as for other forms of prevention and for identification, reporting, referral, investigation, treatment and follow-up of instances of child maltreatment described heretofore, and, as appropriate for judicial involvemen.

The *General Comment No 13: The Right of the Child to Freedom from All Forms of Violence,* adopted by the UN Committee on the Rights of the Child in February, 2011, aims to assist the implementation of Article 19 by providing 'clear interpretations, greater detail and supportive guidance' to all those working with and for children. The General Comment No 13 is particularly directed at governments which have ratified the CRC, other stakeholders such as professionals, international and national non-government agencies and advocates, including children and young people (Bennett et al. 2012).

The document takes a child rights approach to care giving and protection, broadening the traditional narrow emphasis on protecting the child from loss of life and immediate harm to also securing optimal outcomes for the child's wellbeing and development through into adulthood. It provides a conceptual framework which emphasises that 'child protection must begin with proactive primary prevention' of all forms of violence as well as explicitly prohibiting them (Bennett et al. 2012).

In any civilised society *everyone* has a responsibility to:

- Protect children from harm
- Respond to all forms of violence
- Promote children's wellbeing; and
- Ensure the right of each child to be free from all forms of violence.

Children's healthy development

Each child is unique, but all children's development is sequential—that is they gain competence in certain developmental tasks such as progressing from crawling to walking, babbling to talking, or from concrete to abstract thinking and are able to function more adequately as a result of these changes (Mussen et al. 1990, p.4). The development of children is influenced by many factors, including internal factors such as temperament, and internal factors such as input from parents and other, so that as children grow up their circumstances will interact with their intrinsic capabilities (Algate 2006, p.33). It is therefore important to take a developmental and ecological approach to understanding the child within his or her family and community environment.

Children's developmental tasks and competencies can be considered in three age periods: infancy to pre-school, middle childhood and adolescence. Children's early years are characterized by rapid brain development which is shaped by the quality of the attachment relationship they form with their primary caregiver (usually the mother). As they grow older, they develop more autonomy and begin to 'develop a sense of who they are, what other people feel and learn to direct their attention and recognise and control their own emotions and behaviour' (Daniel 2006, p.190). Middle childhood is often thought of as a relatively quiet period but the development of self in the context of a wide range of social relationships, is crucial to making a successful transition to adolescence and later adulthood (Schofield 2006, p.196). This is the stage when children develop the ability to think logically and to work things out for themselves—skills needed throughout life. The developmental tasks of adolescence centre on forming a coherent sense of self-identity and forming close friendships with their peer group as well as academic achievement. It can also be a time of questioning one's family belief systems and of rebelling. The physical changes associated with puberty are generally seen to be the starting point for adolescence, with the end point being marked by the individual achieving full maturity (Bailey 2006, p. 208).

The impact of environment and experiences on children's brain development

Recent developments in neuroscience are continuing to help us understand the impact of the environment and experiences on children's brain development. This is greatest during the first three years of life, but particularly so during the first year of an infant's life when the brain is developing most rapidly. There are specific periods, often referred to as *sensitive periods*, when the child's brain is more strongly affected by a certain type of experience and other times, known as *critical periods* when the impact of experience on development can be irreversible. Early interactions between a 'caregiver and baby play a significant role in how a child develops the capacity to respond appropriately to stressful circumstances and the ability to regulate their own negative emotions if and when these occur, such as following an injection, an injury or on the first day at school' (Brown and Ward, 2012).

Parental problems such as mental illness, domestic violence, drug and alcohol misuse and learning disabilities can have a major impact on parent's capacity to respond to their children's needs and to be able to change and adapt the way in which they parent as their children grow and develop over time (Cleaver et al. 2011). A parent with a major drug problem is not going to be able to think about their children's needs and similarly whereas a parent may be able to cope with a younger child. They may not be able to respond to the needs of their children as they grow up. Quite properly there is a huge emphasis on the importance of early intervention during an infants first few years of life but we also understand that the needs of vulnerable adolescents may be overlooked as shown in a recent UK study on adolescents who are being neglected (Rees et al. 2010).

Brown and Ward (2012, p. 47) have set out the impact of abuse and neglect on children's development:

- Exposure to domestic violence and/or parental substance misuse *in utero* can have a long-term negative impact on the unborn child.
- High quality care can determine the extent to which children who are genetically predisposed to mental illness or learning disability, or who are exposed to abusive or neglectful parental behaviours, are affected.
- Chronic exposure to trauma through aggressive, hostile or neglectful parenting can lead to stress system deregulation. Exposure to toxic stress in early childhood can cause permanent damage to the brain and have severe and long-term consequences for all aspects of future learning, behaviour and health.
- Neglected children may experience chronic exposure to toxic stress as their needs fail to be met. This is compounded by a lack of stimulation and social deprivation.
- Severe global neglect (i.e. severe neglect in more than one domain) during the first three years of life stunts the growth of the brain.
- Children who have been sexually abused may experience sleep problems, bedwetting or soiling, problems with school work or missing school, and risk-taking behaviour in adolescence including multiple sexual relationships.
- Adolescents who have experienced abusive or neglectful parenting in childhood are more likely to engage in risk-taking behaviours such as substance misuse and criminal activity.
- Adults who have been physically abused in childhood show poorer physical and intellectual development, more difficult and aggressive behaviour, poorer social relationships and are more frequently arrested for violent crimes than their peers.

Consequences of child maltreatment

Although physical and sexual abuse are recognised as having a major long-term effect on children's developmental progress, emotional abuse and neglect also have far reaching and serious consequences for children (Barlow and Schroder 2010; Daniel et al. 2011; Farmer and Lutman 2012; Rees et al. 2010).

The consequences of child maltreatment can last throughout a person's life, affecting their ability to work, to form supportive adult relationships and to successful parent their own children thus perpetuating the cycle of privation. The costs of abuse and neglect to society are high—not only in human terms but also in economic ones as, e.g. a high proportion of the users of mental health services and people who are incarcerated have suffered childhood maltreatment.

A framework for intervention

This detrimental long-term impact of maltreatment on children's lives is not inevitable. Research has shown that children can recover from abuse or other negative experiences, but it is more difficult for those who have been seriously abused and their recovery is dependant on the interventions of significant adults and the positive ecology of their environment (Aldgate 2006, p.33). It is therefore important to see intervention as a public health issue, with prevention at its heart as programmes that prevent the occurrence of abuse and neglect are likely to be more effective than those aiming to address its consequences. A three level model is a common way of conceptualising a model of prevention (Krug et al. 2002; WHO Europe, 2007). In this model primary prevention encompasses universal approaches aimed at the whole population in order to reduce the incidence of maltreatment; secondary prevention encompasses targeted approaches to those families where there is a greater likelihood of abuse or neglect and the families need more support; and, tertiary prevention relates to specialist services designed to prevent further re-victimization and impairment to the child's health and development where maltreatment has been identified.

Figure 1 below presents on the left hand side a way of illustrating the provision of preventive interventions prior to the occurrence of maltreatment, and distinguishes between universal (primary) and targeted (secondary) interventions. The right hand side maps interventions (tertiary) intended for use after maltreatment has occurred.

These include those which are designed to prevent the recurrence of maltreatment and those which are designed to prevent the long-term impairment of children's health and development.

Davies and Ward (2011) in their overview of 15 research projects commissioned as part of the UK Government's Safeguarding Children Research Programme used this intervention framework for organizing the findings from these studies. Their findings are set out below.

Universal interventions

Two population based approaches were identified which have been shown through rigorous eva-luation to be effective. The first was the introduction in 1979 in Sweden of legislation that banned all forms of physical chastisement including smacking. By 1994 only a third of middle school children reported receiving physical punishment from a parent, and most was in its mildest forms (arm grabbing or mild slaps). Only 3% had received a harsh slap and 1% had been hit with an object. For 11 years after the introduction of the ban, no child died of suspected physical abuse.

The second is the Triple P—Positive Parenting Programme. It is a multi-level parenting support strategy which aims to prevent severe behavioural, emotional and developmental problems in children by enhancing the knowledge, skills and confidence in their parents (Sanders, 2008). It has been evaluated in the US, found to be effective (Prinz et al. 2009), and is currently being evaluated in Glasgow, Scotland.

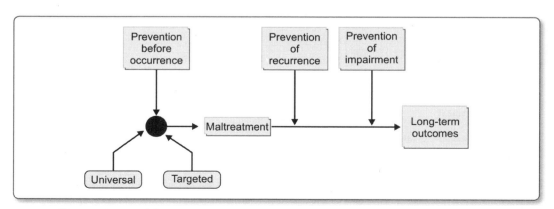

Figure 1: Framework for intervention and prevention of child maltreatment (MacMillan et al. 2009)

Targeted interventions

The most effective targeted intervention approaches appeared to be home visiting schemes and multi-component interventions used in parent training (Barlow et al. 2006). The Nurse Family Partnership which was developed in the US has been the subject of rigorous evaluations where it is shown to have lasting impacts, including reducing children's injuries and adolescent anti-social behaviour (Olds et al. 1994, 1998 and 1998). The programme is known as the Family Nurse Partnership in the UK. It has been the subject of a formative evaluation with promising indications and is currently being evaluated in a randomised control trial which is due to report in 2013.

The Triple P-Positive Parenting Programme also has modules which can also be used as a targeted intervention to families where there is an increased likelihood of maltreatment. In addition, the Webster-Stratton Incredible Years programme has also been shown to be effective in reducing problems associated with maltreatment (Webster-Stratton and Reid 2010).

Specialist Interventions

Davies and Ward (2010) reviewed a range of interventions and identified several which were likely to benefit children who had been abused or neglected and their families. They identified:

Programmes for parents

- Parents under pressure which is effective for substance misusing parents and may be helpful for other parents (Dawe and Harnett, 2007);
- The Enhanced Triple P-Positive Parenting Programme for addressing adults' own experiences of poor parenting and the psychological consequences of abuse (Sanders et al. 2004; Prinz et al. 2009);
- Cognitive Behavioural Therapy which can be effective in reducing emotionally abusive parenting, particularly where individual sessions are combined with group based sessions (Iwaniec, 1997).

Programmes for parents and children

- Preschooler-Parent Psychotherapy improves maternal and child representations where

there is a known history of abuse in the family (Toth et al. 2002).
- Interaction Guidance may be effective in improving the parent-child relationships in infants with faltering growth, but further evaluation would be valuable (Benoit et al. 2001).
- Parent-Child Interaction Therapy is a cognitive behavioural model that has been shown to be effective in reducing physical abuse (Chaffin et al. 2004).

Programmes for families

- Multi-Systemic Therapy for Child Abuse and Neglect reduces the likelihood and mitigation of the consequences of the physical abuse of adolescents (Svenson et al. 2010).

Programmes for children

- Therapeutic Preschool for children aged 1–24 months, who have been maltreated or are at risk of being maltreated, has a significant and lasting impact on parenting and child behaviour (Moore et al. 1998);
- Peer-Led Social Skills Training for 3–5 year olds with a history of maltreatment who are socially withdrawn (Fantuzzo et al. 1996);
- Multidimensional Treatment Foster Care for maltreated children in the public care system. A range of programmes have been designed for adolescents, older children and preschoolers (Fisher et al. 2005; Fisher and Kim 2007).

UK experience has shown that evidence-based programmes developed in one country and used in another may need to be adapted to fit with differing legislative requirements as well as cultural and linguistic differences (Wiggins et al. 2012). This can be achieved at the same time as maintaining the integrity of the programme but may require careful piloting and evaluation to achieve successful implementation of these new programmes and the same good outcomes for children and families.

Conclusion

When we look back over 60 years it is easy to wonder if anything has improved to prevent children from suffering harm but there is cause to be optimistic. Our understanding what types of behaviours and experiences are abusive and of the impact on children of different forms of abuse and neglect has increased dramatically and it continues to do so. The views of children who have suffered maltreatment and of their families inform our practice developments. Our knowledge base will continue to grow with the combination of advances in neuroscience and knowledge gained from practice with children and families.

Leading change in this area is particularly challenging. It may be difficult to get communities and politicians to recognise that abuse and neglect is occurring and recurring. The value of collaborative working—at all levels—is not always recognised as being cost effective and supporting good outcomes for children. We are now much clearer about what is required to protect our children and the *General Comment No 13: The right of the child to freedom from all forms of violence* provides a template for action. We owe it to our children to work well with our colleagues—in governments, organisations and local communities—and offer the best possible services to prevent child maltreatment and to protect children from suffering harm.

Bibliography

1. Aldgate J. *Children, Development and Ecology*. In: J. Aldgate (Ed). The Developing World of the Child (pp. 17–34). London: Jessica Kingsley Publishers.

2. Aldgate, J, Jones, DPH, Rose, W and Jeffery, C. *The Developing World of the Child*. London: Jessica Kingsley Publishers, 2006.

3. Bailey, S. *Adolescence and Beyond: Twelve Years Onwards*. In: J Aldgate, (Ed), *The Developing World of the Child*, 2006: 208–285. London: Jessica Kingsley Publishers.

4. Barlow, J, and Schrader-McMillan A. *Safeguarding Children from Emotional Maltreatment: What Works?* London: Jessica Kingsley Publishers, 2010.

5. Barlow, J., Simkiss, D., & Stewart-Brown, S. Interventions to prevent or ameliorate child physical abuse and neglect: Findings from a systematic review. *Journal of Children's Services,* 2006; 1:6–28.

6. Bennett, S., Hart, S., & Wernham, M. (2012). *The UN Convention on the Rights of the Child General Comment 13: Towards enlightenment and progress for global child protecton*. In H. Dubowitz (Ed.), *World Perspectives on Child Abuse. Tenth Edition* (pp. 120–123). ISPCAN: Denver.

7. Benoit, D., Madigan, S., Lecce, S., Shea, B., & Goldberg, S. Atypical maternal behaviour toward feeding-disordered infants before and after intervention. *Infant Mental Health Journal,* 2001; 22(6): 611–626.

8. Brown, R., & Ward, H. (2012). *Decision-making within a child's timeframe. An overview of current research evidence for family justice professionals concerning child development and the impact of maltreatment. Working Paper 16*. London: Childhood Wellbeing Research Centre. https://www.education.gov.uk/publications/eOrderingDownload/CWRC-00117-2012.pdf. Accessed 22 November 2012.

9. Chaffin, M., Silovsky, J.F., Funderburk, B., Valle, L.A., Brestan, E.V., Balachova, T., et al. Parent-child interaction therapy with physically abusive parents: Efficacy for reducing future abuse reports. *Journal of Consulting and Clinical Psychology,* 2004; 72(3): 500–10.

10. Ieaver, H., Unell, I., & Aldgate, J. (2011). *Children's Needs – Parenting Capacity. Child Abuse: Parental mental illness, learning disability, substance misuse, and domestic violence. 2nd Edition*. London: The Stationery Office. https://www.education.gov.uk/publications/eOrderingDownload/Childrens%20Needs%20Parenting%20Capacity.pdf. Accessed on 22 November.

11. Daniel, B. (2006). *Early Childhood: Zero to Four Years*. In J. Aldgate, (Eds.), *The Developing World of the Child* (pp. 186-195). London: Jessica Kingsley Publishers.

12. Daniel, B., Taylor, J., & Scott, J. (2011). *Recognizing and Helping the Neglected Child: Evidence-Based Practice*. London: Jessica Kingsley Publishers.

13. Davies, C., & Ward, H. (2011). *Safeguarding Children Across Services: Messages from Research on Identifying and Responding to Child Maltreatment*. London: Jessica Kingsley Publishers. https://www.education.gov.uk/publications/eOrderingDownload/DFE-RR164.pdf. Accessed 22 November 2012.

14. Dubowitz, H., (Ed) (2012) *World Perspectives on Child Abuse. Tenth Edition*. ISPCAN: Denver.

15. Fantuzzo, J., Sutton-Smith, B., Atkins, M., Meyers, R., Stevenson, H., Coolahan, K., et al. Community-based resilient peer treatment of withdrawn maltreated preschool children. *Journal of Consulting and Clinical Psychology,* 1996; 64:1377–1386.

16. Farmer, E., & Lutman, E. (2012). *Effective Working with Neglected Children and their Families: Linking Interventions with Long-term Outcomes*. London: Jessica Kingsley Publishers.

17. Fisher, P.A., & Kim, H.K. Intervention effects on foster preschoolers' attachment-related behaviours

from a randomized trial. *Prevention Science, 2007;* 8:161–170.

18. Fisher, P.A., Burraston, B., & Pears, K. The early intervention foster care program: Permanent placement outcomes from a randomized trial. *Child Maltreatment,* 2005; 10:61–71.

19. Harnett, P., & Dawe, S. Reducing child abuse potential for child abuse among families: Implications for assessment and treatment. *Brief Treatment and Crisis Intervention,* 2008; 8:226–235.

20. Iwaniec, D. Evaluating parent training for emotionally abusive and neglectful parents: Comparing individual versus individual and group intervention. *Research in Social Work Practice,* 1997; 7(3):329–349.

21. Kempe, H., & Steele, B.F. The Battered Child Syndrome. *Journal of the American Medical Association,* 1962; 181:17–24.

22. Krug. E.G., Dahlberg, L.L., Mercy, J.A., Zwi, A.B., and Lozano R. (Ed).(2002) *World report on violence and health.* Geneva: World Health Organization.

23. MacMillan H.L., Wathen C.N., Barlow, J., Fergusson, D.M., Leventhal, J.M., Taussig, H.N. Interventions to prevent child maltreatment and associated impairment. *Lancet,* 2009; 373:250–266.

24. Moore, E., Armsden, G., & Gogerty, P.L. A twelve-year follow up study of maltreated and at-risk children who received early therapeutic child care. *Child Maltreatment,* 1998; 3:3–16.

25. Mussen, P., Conger, J.J., Kagan, J., & Huston, A.C. (1990). Child Development and Personality. 7th Edn. New York: Harper Collins.

26. Office of the United Nations High Commissioner for Human Rights. (2000). *Optional Protocol on the Convention of the Rights of the Child on the sale of children, child prostitution and child pornography.* www2.ohchr/English/law/crc-sale.htm. Accessed On 22 November 2012.

27. Olds, D., Eckenrode, J., Henderson, C.R., Kitzman, H., Powers, J., Cole, R., et al. Long-term effects of home visitation on maternal life course and child abuse and neglect: 15-year follow up of a randomized trail. *Journal of the American Medical Association,* 1997; 278:637–643.

28. Olds, D., Henderson, C. R., Cole, R. C., Eckenrode, J., Kitzman, H., Luckey, D., et al. Long-term effects of home visitation on children's criminal and anti social behaviour: 15-year follow up of a randomized trail. *Journal of the American Medical Association,* 1998; 280(14):1238–1244.

29. Olds, D. L., Henderson, C.R., & Kitzman, H. Does prenatal and infancy nurse home visitation have enduring effects on qualities of parental caregiving and child health at 25 to 50 months of life? *Pediatrics,* 1994; 93:89–98.

30. Olds, D.L., Robinson, J., O'Brien, R., Luckey, D.W., Pettitt, L.M., Henderson, C.R., et al. Home visiting by nurses and by paraprofessionals: A randomized controlled trial. *Pediatrics,* 2002; 11(3):486–496.

31. Pinheiro, P.S. (2006). *Report of the Independent expert for the United Nations study on violence against children.* New York, NY: United Nations (UN) General Assembly.

32. Prinz, R.J., Sanders, M.R., Shapiro, C.J., Whitaker, D.J., & Lutzker, J.R. Population–based prevention of child maltreatment: The US Triple P system population trial. *Prevention Science,* 2009; 10(1):1–12.

33. Radford, L., Corral, S., Bradley, C., Fisher, H., Bassett, C., Howat, N., et al. (2011). *Child Abuse and Neglect in the UK today.* London: NSPCC. http://www.nspcc.org.uk/inform/research/findings/child_abuse_neglect_research_PDF_wdf84181.pdf. Accessed 22 November 2012.

34. Rees, G., Stein, M., Hicks, L., & Gorin, S. (2011). *Adolescent Neglect: Research, Policy and Practice.* London: Jessica Kingsley Publishers.

35. Sanders, M. R. The Triple P-Positive Parenting Programme: A public health approach to parenting support. *Journal of Family Psychology,* 2008; 22: 506–517.

36. Sanders, M.R., Pidgeon, A.M., Gravestock, F., Connors, M.D., Brown, S., & Young, R.W. Does parental attributional retraining and anger management enhance the effects of the Triple P - Positive Parenting Program with parents at risk of child maltreatment? *Behavioural Therapy,* 2004; 35:513–35.

37. Schofield, G. (2008). *Middle Childhood: Five to Eleven Years.* In J. Aldgate, (Eds.), *The Developing World of the Child* (pp.196–207). London: Jessica Kingsley Publishers.

38. Swenson, C., Schaeffer, C., Henggeler, S., Faldowski, R., & Mayhew, A. Multi-systemic therapy for child abuse and neglect: A randomised controlled effectiveness trial. *Journal of Family Psychology,* 2010; 24:497–507.

39. Toth, S.L., Rogosch, F.A., Cicchetti, D., & Manly, J.T. The efficacy of toddler–parent psychotherapy to reorganise attachment in the young offspring of mothers with major depressive disorder: A randomised preventive trial. *Journal of Consulting and Clinical Psychology,* 2006; 74:6.

40. UNICEF. (2009). *A Report Card on Child Protection.* UNICEF, New York.

41. UNICEF. (2011). *Child Protection from Violence, Exploitation and Abuse: a statistical snapshot.* UNICEF, New York.

42.   UNICEF. (2012). *The State of the World's Children: Children in an Urban World*. UNICEF, New York. http://www.unicef.org/pubications/index_61789.hmtl. Accessed 22 November 2012. https://www.education.gov.uk/publications/RSG/publicationDetail/Page1/DFE-RR245. Accessed 22 November 2012.

43.   United Nations Committee on the Rights of the Child. (2011). *General Comment No 13: The right of the child to freedom from all forms of violence*. http://www2.ohchr.org/english/bodies/crc/comments.htm. Accessed 22 November 2012.

44.   Webster-Stratton, C., & Reid, J. Adapting the Incredible Years, and evidence-based parenting programme, for families involved in the child welfare system. *Journal of Children's Services,* 2010; 5(1):25–42.

45.   Wiggins, M., Austerberg, H., & Ward, H. (2012) Implementing Evidence-based programmes: key issues for success. Research Report DfE – RR245. London: Department for Education.

46.   World Health Organisation. Regional Office for Europe. (2007). Preventing child maltreatment in Europe: a public health approach. Policy briefing. Copenhagen: World Health Organisation. http://www.euro.who.int/__data/assets/pdf_file/0012/98778/E90618.pdf. Accessed 22 November 2012.

Section 2

Extent, Forms of Child Abuse and Neglect

3

Child Physical Abuse

Nina Agrawal

Introduction

Child physical abuse, as defined by the World Health Organization, is that which results in actual or potential harm from an interaction or lack of an interaction, which is reasonably within the control of a parent or person in a position of responsibility, power, or trust.[1] Twenty-five to fifty percent of the world's children report being physically abused.[2] Global studies suggest that up to 80–98% of children suffer physical punishment in their homes, with a third or more experiencing severe physical punishment from the use of implements.[3]

Physical abuse can produce various types of injuries. Interpretation of injuries as inflicted or accidental is a complex and systematic process. Injuries needs to be considered within the context of multiple key factors including the explanation provided, the child's developmental capabilities, and a comprehensive medical evaluation. These factors, when taken collectively, can help the professional determine the need for referral and investigation. Optimal assessment requires a collaborative approach among medical professionals, social services, law enforcement, and other professionals who come in contact with children.

This chapter seeks to provide the professional with guidance on the assessment of possible child physical abuse, when to be concerned about physical abuse, and when to pursue further evaluation. Common examples of inflicted skin injuries and fractures will be presented.

Assessment

A *detailed explanation* of the injury is the most important part of the assessment of possible physical abuse. An explanation should be obtained from the caregiver and the verbal child, separately, and in a non-judgmental manner. Questions should include *"What happened?", "Where did it happen?", "When did it happen?",* and *"Who was there when it happened?".* Open ended questions such as *"Tell me what happened."* should be used and responses should be documented verbatim in quotes whenever possible. The child should be asked questions in a developmentally appropriate manner. Absent, vague, or a changing explanation and inconsistent explanations provided by various caregivers are some factors which may raise the suspicion for inflicted trauma.

The child's *developmental capabilities*, specifically gross motor skills, are critical when considering the plausibility of the explanation provided. Abuse must be considered in an infant who is not independently mobile and has signs of trauma. When children begin to walk, they are more susceptible to accidental injuries of all types.

A thorough *medical evaluation* is essential in the differentiation of inflicted trauma from accidental trauma and non-traumatic medical conditions. The child should be fully disrobed. Suspicious injuries may be concealed by clothing. The medical professional should document skin injuries by written descriptions, drawings, and/or photodocumentation with a measuring reference whenever possible. A follow-up medical examination may be helpful in distinguishing trauma from a medical condition mimicking trauma. Bruises, burns, and fractures will change and heal over a certain period of time while many medical conditions may persist.

Bruises

A bruise is bleeding beneath intact skin due to blunt impact trauma.[4] Bruises are the most commonly seen skin injury in physical abuse and accidental trauma in children.[5]

As in all assessments of possible physical abuse, a detailed explanation of the injury, identification of the child's developmental capabilities, and a thorough medical evaluation are essential in the differentiation of inflicted from accidental trauma. In addition to *what, where, when,* and *who was there* when the injury occurred, characteristics of the impacted surface or object should be identified. The developmental status is important especially in infants. Accidental bruises are very rare in children less than 6 months of age and increase significantly at approximately 9 months of age when children begin to walk.[6,7]

The medical evaluation should include documentation of the color, shape, size, and location of skin findings. The two most important characteristics used to interpret bruises are location and pattern. Locations on the body that are more likely to be associated with inflicted trauma are the face, ears, neck, genitalia, buttocks, trunk, upper arms, and upper legs. Locations on the body commonly affected in accidental trauma are near bony prominences, involve the front of the body, and include the shins, knees, chin, forehead, elbows, and ankles.[6, 8]

The presence of a patterned mark can indicate the implement used to inflict the injury. A slap injury may result in an outline of the hand when blood vessels break between the fingers and blood is pushed away from the point of impact. Loop marks are usually worse at their extreme ends because the far end of the flexible cord travels at a faster rate of speed.[8] A stick may result in linear bruises. Hitting the ear and buttocks may result in characteristic bruising at anatomic lines of stress. A blow to the ear may leave bruising at the top of the external part of the ear. Striking the buttocks can result in vertical marks at the inner margins of the buttocks.[9]

The professional may be asked to comment on the timing of an injury. However, it should be noted that bruises cannot accurately be dated based on color or other features of appearance. Bruises of identical age and etiology on the same person may appear differently and change colors at different times. Healing of bruises is highly variable and dependent on multiple factors including the amount of force applied, the location of the injury, skin color, and the child's age. Regarding location, skin around the eyes is loose, thin, and bruises more easily than thicker skin on the bottom of the hands or the feet. Regarding skin color, paler skin will exhibit bruises more easily than darker skin.[10]

The medical evaluation should include a thorough consideration of medical conditions which may mimic inflicted bruises. The medical professional should ask about symptoms of a bleeding disorder including bruising easily, nose bleeds, gum bleeding, heavy menstrual periods, and excessive bleeding after surgery such as circumcision or dental procedures. The presence of a family history of bleeding disorders should be determined. Diagnostic studies may be indicated to further evaluate the possibility of a bleeding disorder or other medical conditions. Medical conditions which may mimic inflicted bruises include dermal melanosis, hemangiomas, erythema multiforme, allergic contact dermatitis, Henoch–Schönlein purpura (umlaut on o), Ehlers–Danlos syndrome, hemophilia, idiopathic thrombocytopenic purpura, Von Willebrand disease, vitamin K deficiency, hemolytic uremic syndrome, and phytophotodermatitis.[8, 11] It should be noted that the presence of a medical condition does not exclude the possibility of abuse.

Burns

A burn is a skin injury caused by heat.[12] Common sources of heat are hot liquids, hot objects, flame, and chemicals.

A detailed explanation of the injury from the caregiver and child, when possible, is essential in the differentiation of an inflicted from an accidental burn. Particular attention should be devoted to obtaining a description of the setting in which the injury reportedly occurred. Scene investigations by child protective services and law enforcement can gather crucial details that are useful in the assessment of a possibly inflicted burn. These details may include identification of the temperature of tap water, the height of the stove from the floor, the ease of turning faucets, and food residue found on clothing or at the scene.

The developmental capabilities of the child are important. The child's position at the time of injury and ability to independently contact the burn source needs to be determined. It may be helpful to have the caregiver demonstrate how the injury occurred.

The medical evaluation should include documentation of the depth, distribution, and extent of the burn. Burn depth is categorized as superficial partial thickness, deep partial thickness, and full thickness. All depth categories can be found in both inflicted and accidental burns. Superficial partial thickness burns manifest as redness and pain without blisters. A common cause of accidental superficial partial thickness burns is prolonged exposure to sunlight, commonly referred to as sunburn. A deep partial thickness burn will exhibit blisters and be painful. Contact with hot liquids and hot objects are a common cause of deep partial thickness burns in children. A full thickness burn will appear leathery, pale, dry, and be insensitive to touch. Oily or thick substances can cause full thickness burns, because they stick to the body and hold heat for longer periods of time.[8] The variability in burn depth should also be assessed. A burn of uniform depth is concerning for inflicted trauma.

The distribution or locations of the burn should be identified. Intentional scald burns typically involve the feet, legs, hands, and buttocks. Symmetrical burns on both sides of the body are also a concern for inflicted trauma. In contrast, accidental scald burns tend to occur on the face, head, neck, palms, and front of the body when children reach up and pull a hot liquid down onto their body. An assessment of the burned skin in relationship to the spared areas of skin can be helpful in determining the position of the child at the time of the burn.

The presence of a pattern burn should be determined. Intentional burns usually have clear lines of demarcation between burned and unburned skin. A stocking or glove like pattern may be seen in an immersion burn involving the hands or feet, This is to be differentiated from an accidental scald burn where the hot liquid may leave splash marks or a trickle-down pattern with an irregular shaped border. What the child was wearing at the time of the injury should be determined as this can affect the burn shape. A hot object intentionally held against the skin will typically result in a well demarcated and, possibly, a clear imprint of the object. An example is an inflicted cigarette burn which is usually well circumscribed and of uniform full thickness depth. This is in contrast to an accidental cigarette burn which will have a less well-defined margin and possibly a brushed appearance due to ashes. Additional examples of objects used in abusive contact burns are household appliances, cooking utensils, and branding tools.

A thorough search for other inflicted injuries should be conducted in any child who presents with a burn. Diagnostic studies for children less than 2 years of age with a suspicious burn should include a skeletal survey to evaluate the possibility of abusive fractures. As in all medical evaluations, the possibility of a non-traumatic cause should be considered. Common mimics of inflicted burn injuries are eczema, diaper dermatitis from ingested irritants, contact dermatitis, impetigo, tinea corporis, and cultural practices.[11]

Fractures

A fracture is a breaking of a bone. No fracture type is diagnostic for abuse. In order to determine the likelihood that a fracture is the result of inflicted trauma, the professional must carefully consider the injury in relationship to the child's developmental capabilities, the explanation provided, and a thorough medical evaluation including appropriate radiographic imaging.

A comprehensive and detailed explanation should be elicited from the caregiver and child, when possible, to help identify the mechanism of injury. The explanation should encompass the events preceding the injury until the time the child presented for medical care. Questions that may elucidate this information include: "*What was the initial position of the child?*", "*What was the child doing?*", "*Did the child exhibit pain at any time?*", "*What prompted the caregiver to seek medical care for the child?*" If the explanation of the fracture involves a fall, questions may include "*What was the distance of the fall?*", "*Did the child hit any objects during the fall?*", "*What was the final landing position of the child?*", "*What was the landing surface?*", "*Was the surface wet or slippery*"?, and *"What did the child do and how did the child behave after the fall?"*.

The child's developmental capabilities are critical especially in fractures involving infants. Fractures of the arms and legs are of low suspicion for abuse in the ambulating child, but are of higher suspicion in the infant who is not yet able to walk.[13] It should be noted that the possibility of abuse cannot be excluded based solely on the child's developmental capabilities. The injury must also be consistent with the details of the explanation provided. Accidental spiral tibial or lower leg fractures occur in toddlers often due to a twisting mechanism while running. However, if the caregiver reports the child was able to walk without difficulty after the fracture occurred, this would not be considered a plausible history and abuse must be considered.

A thorough medical evaluation is of paramount importance in assessing for additional injuries and medical conditions mimicking abusive injuries. Recent fractures may be identified on physical examination as soft tissue swelling over the fracture site, deformity of the involved limb, or decreased mobility of the affected extremity. Healing fractures especially over the ribs may be identified on physical examination as palpable masses resulting from callus formation. It should be noted that the absence of bruises near a fracture involving the extremities and ribs is not uncommon.[14]

While no fracture type is diagnostic of abuse, fractures which are highly specific for abuse are classic metaphyseal lesions, rib fractures (especially posterior), scapular fractures, spinous process fractures, and sternal fractures. Classic metaphyseal lesions can occur when an infant is twisted or pulled by an extremity as well as by acceleration and decelerational forces when an infant is shaken resulting in shearing of the metaphyses.[15] Posterior rib fractures typically results from an adult grasping the child around the chest and forcibly compressing the anterior or front of the chest against the posterior or back of the chest. While rib fractures may present with non-specific symptoms, most are detected by radiograph.[16] When metaphyseal lesions and posterior rib fractures are identified, a thorough evaluation for intracranial injury as a result of abusive head trauma should be performed.

Fractures of moderate specificity for abuse are multiple fractures, especially bilateral, fractures of different ages, fractures of the hands and feet, complex skull fractures, epiphyseal separations, and vertebral body fractures. Fractures of low specificity for abuse are clavicular fractures, long bone shaft fractures, linear skull fractures, and subperiosteal new bone formation.[15] The index of suspicion for inflicted trauma may decrease or increase as the fracture is considered within the context of the child's developmental capabilities, the explanation provided, and a thorough search for other injuries.

When an injury suspicious for non-accidental trauma is identified in a child less than 2 year olds, a skeletal survey should be performed. A skeletal survey is a series of radiographic images that encompasses the entire skeleton. A "babygram" which is a single view of the entire skeleton is not recommended.[17] A skeletal survey should include two or more views of the axial skeleton and at least one frontal view of the appendicular skeleton. In addition, right and left posterior oblique views of the entire rib cage should be taken.[18] The skeletal survey may reveal additional fractures especially classic metaphyseal lesions. The skeletal survey is also helpful in assessing the overall status of the skeleton and any signs of bone fragility which may predispose the child to fractures. A follow up skeletal survey in 2 weeks may be warranted to identify acute fractures, especially of the ribs and digits that were not visualized on the initial films due to lack of callus formation. Follow-up skeletal survey has been found to identify a significant number of additional injuries.[19] Bone injuries may be dated based on visualization of callus formation on radiographs. It should be noted that skull fractures cannot be dated as there is no callus formation in skull bone.

In any child who presents with an unexplained fracture, it is important to consider medical and genetic conditions which may cause bone fragility and fractures in response to minor trauma. These medical conditions include osteogenesis imperfecta, osteopenia of prematurity, rickets, osteomyelitis, copper deficiency, and demineralization from paralysis of a limb. Rarer conditions include Menkes syndrome, scurvy, osteopetrosis, congenital syphilitic periostitis, and metabolic and kidney disease leading to calcium wasting.[20] However, the presence of a medical condition does not exclude the possibility of co-existing abuse.

Conclusion

The professional must consider whether the injury or injuries are consistent with the explanation provided and the developmental capabilities of the child. If there is concern for abuse, referral to a pediatrician experienced in the evaluation and management of child abuse is recommended. Increased and accurate identification of physical abuse can significantly improve the safety, health, and well being of children.

References

1. World Health Organization Report of the Consultation on Child Abuse Prevention, 1999. http://apps.who.int/iris/handle/10665/65900.

2. World Health Organization Media Center Child Maltreatment Fact Sheet, 2010. http://www.who.int/mediacentre/factsheets/fs150/en/index.html.

3. Report of the independent expert for the United Nations study on violence against children, 2006. http://daccess-dds-ny.un.org/doc/UNDOC/GEN/N06/491/05/PDF/N0649105.pdf?OpenElement.

4. Harris T, Flaherty E. Bruises and Skin Lesions. In: Jenny C (ed). Child Abuse and Neglect: Diagnosis, Treatment, and Evidence. Saunders, Missouri, 2011.

5. Roberton DM, Barbor P, Hull D Unusual Injury? Recent injury in normal children and children with suspected non-accidental injury. BMJ, 1982; 285:1399–1401.

6. Labbe (Labbe with accent) J, Caouete G. Recent skin injuries in normal children. Pediatrics 2001; 108:271–276. doi: 10.1542/peds.108.2.271.

7. Sugar N, Taylor J, Feldman K. Bruises in Infants and Toddlers: Those Who Don't Cruise Rarely Bruise. Arch Pediatr Adolesc Med, 1999; 153:399–403. doi:10-1001/pubs.Pediatr Adolesc Med.-ISSN-1072-4710-153-4-poa8307.

8. Jenny C, Reece R. Cutaneous Manifestations of Child Abuse. In: Reece R, Christian C (Eds). Child Abuse: Medical Diagnosis and Management, 3rd edn. American Academy of Pediatrics, 2009.

9. Feldman K. Patterned Abusive Bruises of the Buttocks and the Pinnae. Pediatrics, 1992; 90:633–636.

10. Stephenson T, Bialis Y. Estimation of the age of bruising. Arch Dis Child 1996, 74: 53–55. doi: 10.1136/adc.74.1.53.

11. Makoroff KL, McGraw MM. Skin Conditions Confused with Child Abuse. In: Jenny C (ed). Child Abuse and Neglect: Diagnosis, Treatment, and Evidence. Saunders, Missouri, 2011.

12. Stedman's Medical Dictionary Williams & Wilkins, Baltimore, 1987.

13. Kemp AM, Dunstan F, Harrison S, Morris S, Mann M, Rolfe K. Patterns of skeletal fractures in child abuse: systematic review. BMJ, 2008: 337:a1518. doi: 10.1136/bmj.a1518.

14. Peters ML, Starling SP, Barnes-Eley ML, Heisler KW. The Presence of Bruising Associated with Fractures. Arch Pediatr Adolesc Med, 2008; 162:877–881.

15. Kleinmann P Skeletal Trauma: General Considerations. In: Kleinmann P(Ed) Diagnostic Imaging of Child Abuse, 2nd edn. Mosby, Missouri, 1998.

16. Cooperman D, Merten D. Skeletal Manifestations of Child Abuse. In: Reece R, Christian C (Ed). Child Abuse: Medical Diagnosis and Management, 3rd edn. American Academy of Pediatrics, 2009.

17. American Academy of Pediatrics Section on Radiology. Diagnostic imaging of child abuse. Pediatrics 2000; 105:1345–8.

18. American College of Radiology ACR–SPR Practice Guideline for Skeletal Surveys in Children, 2011 http://www.acr.org/~/media/9BDCDBEE99B84E87BAAC2B1695BC07B6.pdf.

19. Zimmerman S, Makoroff K, Care M, et al. Utility of follow-up skeletal surveys in suspected child physical abuse evaluations. Child Abuse Negl, 2005; 29:1075–83. http://dx.doi.org/10.1016/j.bbr.2011.03.031.

20. Jenny CJ and the Committee on Child Abuse and Neglect. Evaluating infants and young children with multiple fractures. Pediatrics, 2006; 118:1299–303. doi: 10.1542/peds.2006–1795.

4

Medicolegal Aspects of Child Abuse in India

RK Gorea

Introduction

Child abuse or maltreatment constitutes all forms of physical and/or emotional ill-treatment, sexual abuse, neglect or negligent treatment or commercial or other exploitation, resulting in actual or potential harm to the child's health, survival, development or dignity, in the context of a relationship of responsibility, trust or power (WHO Report, 1999)

From time to time Indian government has taken steps to protect the rights of children and to prevent child abuse. The National Policy for the children was drafted and agreed upon in 1974 which states, "it shall be the policy of the State to provide adequate services to children, both before and after birth and through the period of growth, to ensure their full physical, mental and social development. It further stresses that the State shall progressively increase the scope of such services so that, within a reasonable time, all children in the country enjoy optimum conditions for their balanced growth (NPCC, 2001)". Later on it ratified the United Nations Convention on Rights of the Child in 1992 and then decided to form a statutory body National Commission for Children for prevention of child abuses and neglect.

Majority of children in India have faced some kind of abuse in their life. Some of these crimes have been well identified and laws have been enacted against them. There are adverse sociocultural practices like child marriages, which have been prohibited by law. However, society often does not oppose these evils and therefore the authorities find it difficult implement such laws.

There are some recent laws against some accepted practices like ragging in educational institutions, which remains a common practice, but the laws are showing some effect. Voices are being raised against corporal punishment in schools, and some courts have given their decisions against such practice. However, some parents, school management staff and people in the society at large support corporal punishment to schoolchildren.

A large number of children become victims of child abuse. There are crimes which are punishable as per Indian Penal Code (IPC) whereas others are punishable under special and local laws Subordinate local law (SLL).

Forms of abuse

Female infanticide

Infanticide is defined as a killing of a child 0–1 year of age as opposed to feticide, which is aborting a fetus (Gorea 2010). A serious problem in India is female feticide after determining the sex of the fetus. For several years the practice of female feticide went unchecked due to which male to female population ratio got disturbed. The 2001 census (National Commission for Women, 2008) reveals that such disparity is greater among children of age newborn to 6 years, in some States as Punjab (793 girls to 1000 boys), Haryana (820 girls to 1000 boys), Chandigarh (845 girls to 1000 boys), Himachal Pradesh (897 girls to 1000 boys), and Delhi (865 girls to 1000 boys). According to 2011 census there are 940 females against 1000 males in India (http://censusindia.gov.in, 2011).

The 2011 census shows 7.1 million fewer girls than boys aged under the age of seven, up from 6 million in 2001 and from 4.2 million in 1991. The sex ratio in the age group is now 915 girls to 1000 boys, the lowest since records began in 1961 (Laurence, 2011).

In India there is no special law regarding infanticide, which is covered by Section 302 of IPC like any other murder. Feticide is covered by Sections 315 and 316 of the IPC.

The root cause for the female feticide is the practice of dowry system at the time of marriage. People are afraid to have the female babies because when grown up females will have to married and dowry will be demanded. If sufficient dowry is not given, it sometimes leads to "dowry deaths". It is unfortunate that the practice of female infanticide still continues. To tackle it there should be awareness campaigns of equal rights of the both genders by the governments. Stringent punishment must be given to those responsible for female feticide. Dowry system must be abolished. The Dowry Prohibition Act 1961 has not been very effective, as social evils cannot be eradicated by legal measures.

Child battering

The practice of various forms of corporal punishment is very common in India and almost a social norm. The parents consider it their right to threaten use abusive language, slap and beat the child if he does not behave according to their wishes. The Police also does not take such practice into cognizance as it is considered appropriate for the benefit of the children, and necessary to prevent them from getting into bad habits. Physical abuse just does not happen inside the home but also at public places. There are no suitable laws to stop such child abuse in India.

Murder of children

Children are killed for a variety of reasons. They form easy targets for taking revenge from their parents. Murder is covered under section 302 IPC. Sometimes sacrifices of children are offered to God in India with the help of tantriks (witch doctors) to seek blessing of God for getting a child by the childless parents, or to obtain more earthly things.

Body piercings, branding

Many children are subjected to and branding body piercings by various pointed objects to please the Gods and many times they go in processions with body piercings and often adults accompany them. Mostly the piercings are done in the cheeks and the tongue. Governments do not intervene considering this practice as a religious matter of the people.

Abandonment of child

Sometimes unwanted children, mostly girls are abandoned. The parents are often very poor and have other children. This act is covered under section 317 of IPC. However, it is very difficult to apprehend the parents and bring them to the book.

Child labor

Poverty leads many parents to send their children to work, to supplement the family income. Children work at a variety of occupations such as domestic help, in small food shops, help to vendors, in automobile workshops, firecracker manufacturing, carpet weaving, and match stick industries and in several other industries. Though there is Child Labor (Prohibition and Regulation) Act, 1986 but some provisions of this act fixes the age of child as 14–16 years as compared to age of child as 18 years as decided by WHO. The Act has not been very effective and a large number of children remain in the work force.

Work in hazardous environment

Children work in industries in an environment that can be injurious to their health and growth. They are prone to many accidents as they are immature to understand and apprehend the dangers. Tuberculosis and other respiratory diseases are particularly common in these children.

Child Labor Prohibition and Regulation Act

Legislative Action Plan: Enacted in 1986. It focus on general developmental programmes for benefiting child labor and there is project based plan of action. The Act prohibits employment of children in certain specified hazardous occupations and processes and regulates the working conditions in others.

Physical abuse

Physical abuse is evidenced by abrasions, bruises, small lacerations, burns and scalds. There may be single or repeated incidents. It is very common and more often seen in boys (Sharma, 2005). Physical abuse is covered by Section 323–326, 307, 308 of Indian Penal Code.

Sexual abuse

In child sexual abuse the activity being intended to gratify or satisfy the needs of the other person. This may include but is not limited to inducement or coercion of a child to engage in any unlawful sexual activity; exploitative use of a child in prostitution or other unlawful sexual practices, pornographic performances and production of pornographic material.

In India girls are more prone to sexual abuse (Sharma et al, 2005). One in four girls and one in eight boys are reportedly sexually abused before the age of 18 years (Healthychildren.org). Children in the age group of 14–16 years were more prone to sexual abuse (Sharma et al, 2005). These offences may involve natural or unnatural sexual acts and sexual perversions. Rape, incest, sodomy are frequently seen sexual abuses and cases of oral sex, sadism and exhibitionism are also reported. There are no special laws and training of the investigating officers to deal with these crimes on children and these offences are covered as the offences in the adults under Section 376 and 377 IPC. It is essential to have specially trained officials to handle cases of child sex abuse too minimize the trauma to the victims.

Child prostitution, sex tourism, and child pornography

The term normally refers to prostitution by a minor, or person under the local age of majority. Section 373 IPC deals with buying of girls and 372 IPC deals with selling of girls for prostitution. children often are lured or forced for pornographic acts. Many children are prostituted over the Internet with the use of webcams to facilitate this abuse, and child. People may travel to foreign countries to indulge in child prostitution to avoid laws in their own country of residence. A customer may negotiate an exchange directly with a child prostitute in order to receive sexual gratification, or through an intermediary who controls or oversees the prostitute's activities for profit. The provision of children for sexual purposes may also be an object of exchange between adults. Child trafficking and commercial sexual exploitation (CSE) are egregious crimes, extreme forms of child maltreatment, and major violations of children's human rights (Rafferty, 2008).

Corporal punishment in schools

Corporal punishment is quite prevalent and is mostly considered an accepted norm in the various schools of India. Teachers take it in good faith for the betterment of children. They are often unaware regarding the consequences which a teacher may have to face if the parents resort to legal action against them.

Corporal punishment is rarely reported and it goes as an accepted practice by teachers, students and parents. A division bench of Delhi High Court commented "Brutal treatment of children can never inculcate discipline in them - obedience exacted by striking fear of punishment can make the child adopt the same tactics when he grows up for getting what he wants" (Tribune, 2000). Many such cases of corporal punishment leading to serious injuries and psychological damage and even deaths have been observed (Gorea et al, 2011).

Ragging

Ragging is any disorderly conduct, whether by words spoken or written, or by an Act which has the effect of teasing, treating or handling with rudeness any student, indulging in rowdy or undisciplined activities which cause or are likely to cause annoyance, hardship or psychological harm or to raise fear or apprehension thereof in a fresher or a junior student and which has the effect of causing or generating a sense of shame or embarrassment so as to adversely affect the psyche of a fresher or a junior student (Chopra, 2009).

Ragging differs in different institutions varies from befooling, downgrading and degrading them, physical punishment, sexual exploitations and emotional harassments. Persons have committed suicides being frustrated and feeling helpless over such incidents. Raghavan committee report was released in July 2007 to stop the ragging (noragging. com, 2009). University Grant Commission has issued regulations on the curbing of problem of ragging in higher educational institutions in 2009 (http://news.outlookindia.com, 2009). Though majority of students did not like ragging but still it continues.

Disgraceful treatment to disabled children

Children with disability have often to bear the taunts of fellow children and they have to live with it. They have to often go to schools where there are no special arrangements for them, and they have to face difficulties. Children with disabilities are four times more likely to face physical violence and sexual violence (Jones et al. 2012). This is due to stigma, discrimination and ignorance about disability. Mostly there is lack of social support for such children and those taking care of them. These children need support of the society and the government.

Child marriages

Child marriages were quite prevalent in the last two centuries in India but child marriages have been banned since a long time in India by Child Marriage Restraint Act of 1929. This act helped to reduce the menace of child marriages but did not completely ended it as is shown by the Statistics indicate that 125 cases were reported in 2005; 99 cases in 2006 and 96 cases in 2007 were prosecuted.

Honor killings

When girls do not marry according to the wishes of the family members they may be killed to maintain "family honour" by the family members. Usually this happens when they marry where the elders do approve of the marriage due to different social status or different religions or castes of the two families. *Khaps* (village panchayats) usually) give the verdict for honour killings. Supreme Court Panel has suggested that there in need to rein in the *Khaps* to stop them for giving decisions for honour killings (Sinha, 2012). Usually such couples are grown up but sometimes one of the partners may not have attained the majority.

Procuring minors, kidnapping and abduction of children

4384 cases of kidnapping and abduction of children have been reported in India in the year 2011 (http://ncrb.nic.in, 2011). These cases are covered under section 363–366 and 371–373 of IPC. 51 were booked under section 366A IPC for procurement of minor girls. Usually minors are procured for sexual activities. Kidnappings are done mainly for ransom or blackmailing.

Suicides pacts involving children

Sometimes the adults commit suicides and many times they force the children to commit suicide with them or kill them before committing suicide. Mostly deaths in such cases are by drowning. Author committed postmortem examination in one such case where father mother and two children dried of drowning. Sixty-one cases of abetment of suicide by children have been reported in India in the year 2011 (http://ncrb.nic. in, 2011) under 305 IPC.

Mechanisms for protection of child rights in India

There are several existing Laws and Acts and constitutional guarantees to protect the children from child abuses and neglect.

Constitutional guarantees

Through various articles enshrined in the Fundamental Rights and the Directive Principles of State Policy, lays down that: The State shall provide free and compulsory education to all children of the age 6–14 years. (Article 21-A);Children shall be given opportunities and facilities to develop in a healthy manner and in conditions of freedom and dignity and that childhood and youth shall be protected against moral and material abandonment (Article 39-f);

- International conventions and declarations
- National policies and legislations addressing child rights

- Juvenile Justice (Care and Protection) Act, 2000 (amended, 2006)
- The Immoral Traffic (Prevention) Act, 1956
- The Commissions for the Protection of Child Rights Act, 2005
- Pre-Natal Diagnostic Technique (PNDT) Act and regulations and prevention of misuse
- Child Labor (Prevention and Regulation) Act, 1986.

Indian Penal Code (IPC)

- Murder (Section 302 IPC)
- Foeticide (Sections 315 and 316)
- Infanticide (Section 302)
- Abetment to Suicide: Abetment to commit suicide of minor (Section 305)
- Exposure and Abandonment: Crime against children by parents or others to expose or to leave them with the intention of abandonment (Section 317)
- Procurement of minor girls by inducement or by force to seduce or have illicit intercourse (Section 366-A)
- Selling of girls for prostitution (Section 372)
- Buying of girls for prostitution (Section 373)
- Kidnapping and abduction
- Kidnapping for exporting (Section 360)
- Kidnapping from lawful guardianship (Section 361)
- Kidnapping for ransom (Section 364A)
- Kidnapping for camel racing, etc. (Section 363)
- Kidnapping for begging (Section 363-A)
- Kidnapping to compel for marriage (Section 366)
- Kidnapping for slavery, etc. (Section 367)
- Kidnapping for stealing from its person: under 10 years of age only (Section 369)
- Rape Section 376 IPC
- Unnatural sexual offences 377 IPC.

The Commissions for the Protection of Child Rights Act, 2005

The Act provides for the Constitution of a National and State Commissions for protection of Child Rights in Every State and Union Territory (http://www.ncpcr.gov.in, 2005). The functions and powers of the National and State Commissions will be to:

- Examine and review the legal safeguards provided by or under any law for the protection

of child rights and recommend measures for their effective implementation
- Prepare and present annual and periodic reports upon the working of these safeguards
- Inquire into violations of child rights and recommend initiation of proceedings where necessary
- Undertake periodic review of policies, programmes and other activities related to child rights in reference to the treaties and other international instruments
- Spread awareness about child rights among various sections of society
- Children's Courts for speedy trial of offences against children or of violation of child rights.
- State Governments and UT Administrations to appoint a special public prosecutor for every Children's Court
- Apart from these laws mainly concerning children, there are a host of related social legislations and criminal laws which have some beneficial provisions for the care, protection and rehabilitation of children. The laws relating to commerce, industry and trade have some provisions for children, but they hardly provide any protection or cater to their developmental needs.

This commission was set up in the year 2007 to look into all these aspects.

Despite the above mentioned legislations, there are still major gaps in the legal provisions relating to child abuse in myriad situations, particularly in cases of trafficking, sexual and forced labour, child pornography, sex tourism and sexual assault on male children. The Ministry of Women and Child Development has formulating a comprehensive legislation on offences against children.

In India there is Child Helpline (Phone No.1098). There is Society for Prevention of Injuries and Corporal Punishment SPIC to orient the teachers and school managements and make students aware about corporal punishments and ragging (forensicwayout.com/SPIC, 2012; http://www.spic.org.in/, 2012)). There are several NGOs and child welfare committees to help the children and prevent child abuses and neglect.

Medicolegal aspects

In India forensic medicine experts, police persons, pediatricians and nurses first come into contact with the victims of child abuse and neglect. Out of these police persons, pediatricians and nurses have very little knowledge about handling of cases of child abuse and neglect and forensic medicine experts have knowledge but may or may not have experience in such matters. Trained and experienced persons should be available to handle cases of child abuse and neglect to avoid losing of evidence, poor documentation and traumatic experience of inept handling in such cases on victims. "Poor management after disclosure can increase psychological damage (Aggarwal et al, 2010). When treating case of child abuse pediatricians should believe, support, reassure, treat and ensure rehabilitation of victims of child abuse, keeping the best interest of the child as the primary goal (Aggarwal et al, 2010).

In India different Acts and Laws have no uniform age of a child. Railways Act, Juvenile justice Act and Child Labor Act have different ages for children. It should be made uniform as per the recommendations of UNCRC, 1989 which is "every human being below the age of 18 years unless, under the law applicable to the child, majority is attained earlier". Determination of these different ages is also a tedious process and the offenders use these loopholes to protect themselves on the technical grounds.

Detailed process and follow-up in case of child abuse by pediatricians is well described by Aggarwal et al, 2010. Forensic nurses can play an important role in providing support to this process. However, forensic nursing science is yet to develop in India though awareness in the medical and nursing fraternity has been brought by Indo Pacific Academy of Forensic Nursing Sciences INPAFNUS (http://bestforensicnurse.com, 2011). In cases of sexual assault forensic medicine experts and gynecologists can play a vital role.

Conclusions

The problems of child abuse and neglect persist despite governmental efforts to tackle them. Several forms of abuse such as corporal punishment in schools, institutions and homes need to be addressed with advocacy, explanation and information. Poverty and illiteracy are the root causes of many forms of CAN. The families must be empowered and informed. Adverse societal attitudes are slow and difficult to change. The difficult and complex issues of child labour in many unorganized sector need special laws, which must be properly and adequately enforced. We need to create a society where male and female children have equal rights to survival, health care, education, protection and dignity.

Bibliography

1. Aggarwal K, Dalwai S, Galagali P, et al. Recommendations on Recognition and Response to Child Abuse and Neglect in the Indian Setting Indian Pediatr 2010; 47: 493–504.

2. Child Abuse and Neglect Prevention. http://www.rand.org/pubs/working_papers/2009/RAND_WR632.pdf Accessed on 13 July 2012.

3. Chopra M. Ragging in Educational Institutions: a Human rights Perspective, 2009. http://www.legalserviceindia.com/articles/ragging.htm accessed on Oct 29, 2009.

4. Convention on the Rights of the Child. United Nations Children's Fund. Delhi, 2004.

5. Crimes in India 2011 compendium. National crimes record bureau Ministry of Home affairs. New Delhi http://ncrb.gov.in accessed on July 5, 2012:p III, 89–98.

6. Gorea A, Gorea L, Gorea RK, Arora A. Holistic approach to prevent injuries and corporal punishments in schools. Egyptian J Forensic Sciences 2011; 1: 25–29.

7. Gorea L, Gorea A, Gorea RK, et al. Individual, community, institutional responsibility in prevention of ragging of students in educational institutions. VCFL Sciences J 2012; 2(2):58–64.

8. Gorea RK. A case of mummification reported as spiritual coma In Textbook of Forensic Medicine & Toxicology, Krishan V. Elsevier Publishers, 2005.

9. Gorea RK. Sociocultural Crimes: A Forensic Approach in Forensic Nursing Science, 2nd edn. Lynch VA and Duval JB, Elsevier Mosby, 2010.

10. HC Bans. Corporal Punishment for School Children: The Tribune, Vol. 120, No. 333. City Ed. Chandigarh, Dec 2, 2000, p.1

11. Healthychildren.org. Safety & Prevention. What to know about child abuse. http://www.healthychildren.org/English/safety-prevention/at-home/Pages/What-to-Know-about-Child-Abuse.aspx accessed on May 11, 2012.

12. http://bestforensicnurse.com accessed on Feb, 2011.

13. http://censusindia.gov.in/2011-prov-results/indiaatglance.html accessed on July 15, 2012.

14. http://forensicwayout.com/SPIC/tabid/127/Default.aspx accessed on July 17, 2012.

15. http://ncrb.nic.in/CD-CII2011/cii-2011/Table%206.2.pdfaccessed on July 11, 2012.

16. http://noragging.com/index.php/Table/Resources/Laws/ visited on Oct. 30, 2009.

17. http://www.cdphe.state.co.us/ps/cctf/canmanual/CurrentTopicsinChildMaltx2.pdf> Accessed on June 14, 2012.

18. http://www.ncpcr.gov.in/Acts/National_Commission_for_Protection_of_Child_Rights_Act_2005.pdf accessed on July 15, 2012.

19. http://www.spic.org.in/ accessed on July 17, 2012.

20. Jones L, Bellis MA, Wood S, Hughes K, McCoy E, Eckley L, Bates G, Mikton C, Shakespeare T, Alana Prevalence and risk of violence against children with disabilities: a systematic review and meta-analysis of observational studies. The Lancet, Early Online Publication, 12 July 2012 doi:10.1016/S0140-6736(12)60692-8

21. Laurence, Jeremy. The Independent. 2011. The full extent of India's 'gendercide' http://www.independent.co.uk/news/world/asia/the-full-extent-of-indias-gendercide-2288585.htmlaccessed on July 15, 2012.

22. Managing Child Abuse- A Handbook for Medical Officers. SEA/Injuries/6. World Health Organization-Regional Office for South East Asia, New Delhi. 2004.

23. National Commission for Women. (2008). http://ncw.nic.in/PNDT%20conference.pdf accessed on Dec. 27, 2008.

24. National Commission for Women. (2008). http://ncw.nic.in/PNDT%20conference.pdf accessed on Dec. 27, 2008.

25. National Crime Records Bureau(2007a). Crime against women. http://ncrb.nic.in/cii2007/cii-2007/CHAP5.pdf accessed on Dec 20, 2008.

26. National policy and charter for the children 2001, Ministry of human Resource Development, Government of India.

27. ncrb.nic.in (2007c). Crime against children. Viewed at http://ncrb.nic.in/cii2007/cii-2007/CHAP6.pdf on Dec 20, 2008.

28. Rafferty Y. The Impact of Trafficking on Children: Psychological and Social Policy Perspectives Child Development Perspectives, 2(1):13–18.

29. Report of the Consultation on Child Abuse Prevention, 29-31 March 1999, WHO, Geneva. Geneva, World Health Organization, 1999 (document WHO/HSC/PVI/99.1). Available from http://whqlibdoc.who.int/hq/1999/aaa00302.pdf. Accessed on 13 July, 2012.

30. Sharma BR, Harish D, Bangar S, Gupta M. Violation of children's rights: can forensic medicine help? JIAFM, 2005; 27(3):139–144.

31. Subba SH, Sadip S, Senthilkumaran S , Menezes RG. Battered child syndrome: Is India in dire straits? Egyptian J Forensic Sciences 2011; 1:111–113.

32. Taboos. (2008a) viewed at http://channel.nationalgeographic.com/series/taboo#tab-Videos/05411_00 on Dec. 27, 2008.

5

Corporal Punishment in the Middle East and North Africa Region

Bernard Gerbaka

"We worry what a child will become tomorrow, yet we forget he/she is someone today"
(Stacia Staucher)

Introduction

More than twenty years, the UN Convention on the Rights of the Child (UNCRC) came into force (1990); it was ratified by all states in the Middle East and North Africa and Gulf (MENAG) region[1]. Since then, the Committee on the Rights of the Child made it clear that compliance requires prohibition of corporal punishment. The Committee recommended that states parties prohibit corporal punishment in the home and other settings, making such recommendations to 162 states, including all in the MENAG region.

The Committee clarified the obligation of states to end corporal punishment of children through prohibition in law and other measures in General Comment No. 8 (2006) on "The right of the child to protection from corporal punishment and other cruel or degrading forms of punishment (Articles 19; 28, para. 2; and 37, inter alia)". The Committee adopted a comprehensive definition of corporal punishment making the stand that there can be no justification for laws that condone any degree or form of corporal punishment in childrearing.

Also, the Committee stated that teachings condoning or promoting corporal punishment do not provide a justification for the failure of states to prohibit and eliminate it:

"Some raise faith-based justifications for corporal punishment, suggesting that certain interpretations of religious texts not only justify its use, but provide a duty to use it. Freedom of religious belief is upheld for everyone in the International Covenant on Civil and Political Rights (Article 18), but practice of a religion or belief must be consistent with respect for others' human dignity and physical integrity. Freedom to practice one's religion or belief may be legitimately limited in order to protect the fundamental rights and freedoms of others. In certain States, the Committee has found that children, in some cases from a very young age, in other cases from the time that they are judged to have reached puberty, may be sentenced to punishments of extreme violence, including stoning and amputation, prescribed under certain interpretations of religious law. Such punishments plainly violate the Convention and other international human rights standards, as has been highlighted also by the Human Rights Committee and the Committee against Torture, and must be prohibited" (para. 29).

In the same year as the General Comment was adopted, the general report and recommendations of the UN Study on Violence against Children (VAC) were presented to the UN General Assembly 3. The Study highlighted the huge extent to which children are subjected to corporal punishment in their homes and other settings in all regions and recommended urgent law reform for the prohibition.

Defining corporal punishment (CP)

"The Committee defines 'corporal' or 'physical' punishment as any punishment in which physical force is used and intended to cause some degree of pain or discomfort, however light. Most involves hitting ('smacking', 'slapping', 'spanking') children, with the hand or with an implement–a whip, stick, belt, shoe, wooden spoon, etc. But it can also involve, e.g. kicking, shaking or throwing children, scratching, pinching, biting, pulling hair or boxing ears, forcing children to stay in uncomfortable positions, burning, scalding or forced ingestion (e.g. washing children's mouths out with soap or forcing them to swallow hot spices). In the view of the Committee, corporal punishment is invariably degrading. In addition, there are other non-physical forms of punishment that are also cruel and degrading and thus incompatible with the convention. These include, e.g. punishment that belittles, humiliates, denigrates, scapegoats, threatens, scares or ridicules the child." (General Comment No. 8, para. 11)

Other human rights instruments

The treaty monitoring bodies of other international human rights instruments—many of which have been ratified by states in the region — have interpreted them as requiring prohibition of corporal punishment. For example, recommendations to prohibit corporal punishment of children have been made by the Human Rights Committee, the Committee against Torture, the Committee on Economic, Social and Cultural Rights and the Committee on the Elimination of Discrimination Against Women.

In the Arab region

Although CP is lawful in most MENAG states, violent punishment of children is recognised as a violation of human rights and there is accumulating research into its dangers on one side, and accelerating progress globally toward prohibition of it on the other. Globally, 25 states have achieved complete prohibition in 2011 and at least another 22 are committed to achieve this goal soon after.

Among the key recommendations of the UN Secretary-General's Study on Violence Against Children was the prohibition of all violence, including all types of corporal punishment. The Special Representative to the Secretary-General, Marta Santos Pais, sees prohibition as a high priority in her leadership of the follow-up process.

The Convention on the Rights of the Child (CRC), which celebrated its 20th anniversary on 20 November 2009, has been ratified by all States in the Middle East and North Africa region. The Convention requires State parties to protect children from "all forms of physical and mental violence" while in the care of parent (s), legal guardians or any other person who has the care of the child. The Committee on the Rights of the Child, monitoring the compliance of states with the CRC, has made clear that "violence" includes physical punishment and in its landmark General Comment No. 8 on "the right of the child to protection from corporal punishment and other cruel or degrading forms of punishment", defines corporal or physical punishment as "any punishment in which physical force is used and intended to cause some degree of pain or discomfort, however light". The Committee notes that prohibiting and eliminating all corporal punishment is not only an immediate obligation of States, "It is also a key strategy for reducing and preventing all forms of violence in societies".

The UN study on violence against children [UNVAC] examined the phenomenon of violence against children [VAC] in the MENAG Region, its different forms, its causes, and its impact on children, in order to identify the necessary measures to eradicate this problem. These measures could range from implementing national legislations and protection services to awareness programs that include children themselves, such as teaching children to protect themselves from exposure to violence [recommendation of the UN General Assembly in its resolution no. 57/190].

The Committee on the Rights of the Child (CRC) has ensured that the UNVAC should lead to the development of intervention strategies that aim at protecting children from all forms of violence, with a view to effectively provide protection and prevention [A/56/488]. In addition to the CRC, other human rights instruments require protection of children from corporal punishment. The Arab Charter of Human Rights, like all international instruments, is rooted in respect for the human dignity of all; it prohibits all cruel, degrading or humiliating treatment (Article 8), upholds equality under the law and equal protection without discrimination (Article 11). And article 33 refers to the protection of all members of the family "and the prohibition of all forms of violence or abuse in the relations among its members, and particularly against women and children".

The Cairo Declaration, adopted by participants in the November 2009 conference on the Convention on the Rights of the Child and Islamic Jurisprudence, urged all Organization of the Islamic Conference (OIC) Member States to prohibit all corporal punishment and other cruel or degrading forms of punishment or treatment of children, in all settings including within schools and within the family, linking law reform with the promotion of positive, non-violent forms of discipline. The conference was organized by the Ministry of State for Family and Population of Egypt and co-sponsored by the OIC and UNICEF.

In 2010, the League of Arab states, the Global Initiative to End All Corporal Punishment of Children, Save the Children Sweden and civil society organizations in these states, conveyed to promote the protection of children and their right to grow up without physical or mental violence.

Legislation discrepancies and pitfalls

All countries of the Middle East and North Africa region have endorsed the CRC. Some countries did not make any reservations, while others have made reservations regarding provisions that were taken to be incompatible with Islamic jurisprudence. Seventeen countries (with Djibouti, Somalia, Comoros, Palestine, Mauritania) have signed or endorsed the optional protocol regarding child trafficking, child prostitution and child pornography, 1 has signed the optional protocol on torture, 15 have either signed or endorsed the optional protocol on children in armed conflicts (with Djibouti, Somalia, Palestine).

Universal Periodic Review (UPR)

The UPR is a review every four years of UN member states' human rights records by the Human Rights Council. It was established in 2006 and enables each state to describe the actions they have taken to fulfill their international human rights obligations. Recommendations are made which the state responds to and which will be followed up at future sessions. Members of the Council regularly raise the issue of corporal punishment of children during the reviews and recommendations

are timely made to prohibit it in the home and/or other settings. Until 2011, such recommendations have been made to almost 100 states, including the MENAG region.

Recommendations by treaty monitoring bodies to states in the MENAG region

As the Committee on the Rights of the Child has expressed concern at corporal punishment of children in the region and repeatedly recommended its prohibition and elimination, Countries from the MENAG region have expressed relevant interest and concern. Table 1 provides an overview of these recommendations and indicates whether the recommendation focused on a particular setting or covered the home and all settings.

The UNCRC and other international treaties are legal instruments. States that ratify them have a legal obligation under international human rights law to comply with their provisions, and this includes ensuring that all corporal punishment of children is prohibited in all settings, including the home.

Many of the instruments provide mechanisms for increasing pressure on states that fail to meet their obligations. These can be in the form of communications/complaints mechanisms, which allow individual victims or groups of victims to submit a complaint to the committee that monitors implementation of the convention concerning alleged violations of rights under the convention. They normally require that all efforts to resolve the matter within the state have been tried and have failed.

Another mechanism for pursuing persistent rights violations is a procedure in which the committee monitoring the convention makes inquiries into the situation in a state regarding specific rights in the convention, outside of the normal reporting procedure. Furthermore, the Optional Protocol to the Convention against Torture provides for a system of regular visits to places where people are deprived of their liberty "in order to prevent torture and other cruel, inhuman or degrading treatment or punishment" (Article 1). An Optional Protocol providing a communication procedure for the Convention on the Rights of the Child was adopted by the UN Human Rights Council and the General Assembly in 2011.

TABLE 1: Legal Status of Corporal Punishment Prohibition to Children					
	Home	Education	Justice (Sentence)	Justice (Discipline)	Alternative care
Algeria	NO	YES	YES	?	NO
Bahrain	NO	YES	?	?	?
Djibouti	NO	YES[1]	?	NO	?
Egypt	NO	YES	YES	YES[2]	NO
Iran	NO	YES	NO	NO	NO
Iraq	NO	YES	YES	?	?
Jordan	NO	YES	YES	YES	YES[3]
Kuwait	NO	YES	YES[4]	NO	?
Lebanon	NO	NO[5]	YES	YES	NO
Libyan Arab Jamahiriya	NO	YES	NO	?	?
Morocco	NO	NO[6]	YES	YES	NO
Oman	NO	YES	?	NO	NO
Palestine	NO	NO[7]	YES[8]	NO	NO
Qatar	NO	NO[9]	NO[10]	?	NO
Saudi Arabia	NO	YES	NO	NO	NO
Sudan	NO	NO	NO	NO	NO
Syrian Arab Republic	NO	NO[11]	YES	?	NO
Tunisia	NO	NO[12]	YES	YES	NO
United Arab Emirates	NO	YES	NO	NO	NO
Western Sahara	NO	?	?	?	?
Yemen	NO	YES	NO	NO	NO

[1] Information unconfirmed
[2] Prohibited in prisons, but possibly not in social welfare institutions
[3] Information unconfirmed
[4] But corporal punishment possibly reintroduced under plans to amend Penal Code to comply with Islamic law
[5] Prohibited by Ministerial direction
[6] Prohibited by Ministerial direction
[7] Prohibited by Ministerial direction
[8] But possibly lawful under Shari'a
[9] Prohibited by Ministerial Decree
[10] But possibly prohibited by recent legal reform
[11] But Ministry of Education advises against use
[12] Prohibited by Ministerial Circular

Global and regional progress toward prohibition

Worldwide, the pace at which states have realized and acted upon the human rights imperative to give legal protection to children from all forms of corporal punishment has accelerated since Sweden became the first country to achieve full prohibition in 1979 (Fig. 1).

With the achievement of South Sudan's independence in 2011, there are now 30 states in which it is against the law to assault children in the name of discipline or punishment in the family home and all other settings. In the majority of states corporal punishment in the family is still lawful, but parliaments are increasingly passing laws, which protect children from corporal punishment in schools (120 states), penal institutions

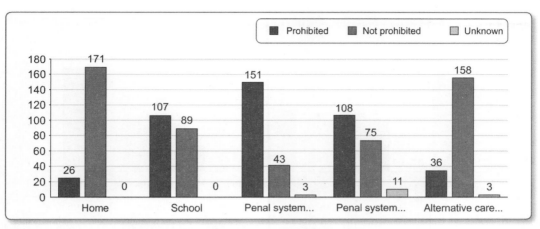

Figure 1 Corporal punishment globally.

(113 states) and alternative care settings (37 states). In the majority of states worldwide (152) corporal punishment cannot lawfully be imposed on children and young people as a sentence for crime.

Collectively, states in the MENAG region have a remarkable and long-standing commitment to implementing the recommendations of the UN Study on Violence against Children, including the prohibition and elimination of corporal punishment in all settings (Fig. 2). However, the current turmoil in some arab states is a significant obstacle to the implementation and the reform of such laws.

There is some coordinated action at the MENAG level to promote law reform, and there are currently a number of social movements addressing corporal punishment and domestic violence. However, for the most part these commitments and activities have not yet led to the enactment of laws prohibiting corporal punishment in all settings of children's lives.

Regional commitments, action and opportunities: The MENAG league of Arab state (LAS) initiative

Corporal punishment—and other cruel or degrading treatment, which involves violence and physical abuse, or threat from any form of beating—is still a social concept in terms of domestic issues and harsh education measures, relevant with violence, at the international level, and in the Arab region.

Within this framework, Jordan, UAE, Tunisia, Algeria, Oman, Qatar, Lebanon, Egypt, Morocco, Yemen have developed a series of laws and procedures that prohibit corporal punishment in schools, but implementation still lacks. The LAS held a meeting in Beirut, 2009, to bring forward tools for legal frames and implementation processes within the arab region. Peter Newell and Representative of the UN Secretary General on Violence against Children, Marta Santos Pais, attended. The details of law reform were discussed in depth and representatives from Government and key civil society organizations from each MENAG. Member State developed a National Action Plan to achieve prohibition of corporal punishment in all settings. Governments committed to speeding up law reform and it was decided that in all eight MENAG member states, civil society organizations, including children, would work closely with their Government representative to implement the action plans, with technical support from the 8.

The report of the workshop and the national action plans can be downloaded at www.las.info

The following reports identify opportunities for law reform to achieve prohibition of corporal punishment in most states in the region. Given Governments' long-standing commitment to prohibition, the support of UN agencies, national and international non-government organizations and the strong regional coordination, states in MENAG are well placed to take advantage of such opportunities

The reports summarize for each MENAG state the relevant human rights instruments they have

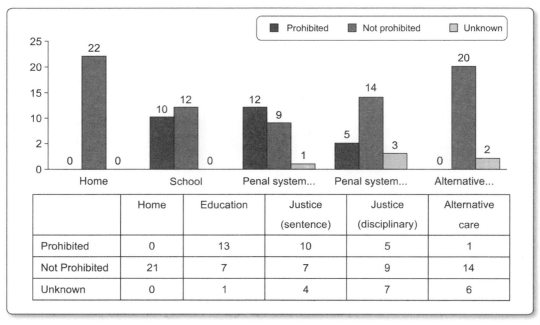

	Home	Education	Justice (sentence)	Justice (disciplinary)	Alternative care
Prohibited	0	13	10	5	1
Not Prohibited	21	7	7	9	14
Unknown	0	1	4	7	6

Figure 2 Corporal punishment in the MENAG region.

ratified and the communications/complaints mechanisms and inquiry procedures that are applicable in that state.

Banning violence

Some States in the MENAG region developed educational models for rehabilitation and reintegration on one side, and prohibit violence against children in all settings, including corporal punishment and harmful traditional practices and torture. Laws however vary from one country to another: countries like Jordan, UAE, Tunisia, Algeria, Sudan, Oman, Qatar, Libya, Egypt, Morocco, and Yemen, made remarkable progress in editing appropriate legal texts with higher standards for the protection of children from all forms of violence, while other countries such as Syria set task forces to reduce violence. Other countries prepared a draft law to offer a specific protection of children from all forms of violence, like Lebanon.

In reality, corporal punishment is a mainly visible and common means of discipline to children in most Arab countries. Severe physical abuse is often easily recognized; however, cases of fatal or severe shaken babies and alleged or factitious disorders (Münchausen by proxy) as well as unidentified sudden infant deaths are reasons of concern; on the

other hand, allegations of CAN have been raised in situations of family dislocation and cause important disruption in the child well-being and deviations in court decisions. Also, close to 95% of children with problems in behavior are at risk of physical means of discipline, which leaves a broad grey band to be interpreted by individuals, based on their knowledge on one side, and cultural background and beliefs on the other. Risk factors for child maltreatment also include: poverty, scattered families and poor skills in conflict management. In some countries, political violence and politicization of children are fertile fields for VAC and child violence.

In school settings, corporal punishment is a visible and common means of discipline to children.

It includes corporal punishment at schools or threat to use any form of physical violence in addition to humiliation, ridicule, verbal abuse or neglect. Physical punishment continues to prevail in schools, even in states who legislated against such violence (e.g. Egypt, Morocco, Algeria) and states which have not provided clear legal provisions that ban physical punishments at school such as Iraq, Kuwait, Lebanon and Yemen, where such measures are accepted as disciplinary tools, in spite of a strong professional and NGOs movement toward banning permissive relevant laws.

Other forms of violence include: Bullying, violence against teachers, physical fight, and deterioration of school performance, school drop-out, drug dealing, peer violence or alcohol abuse. Severe physical abuse is rare in such environments; anecdotal cases are however reported.

Conclusion

The stand against Corporal Punishment includes provision of all corporal punishment and other cruel or degrading forms of punishment or treatment of children, in all settings including within schools and within the family, linking law reform with social exercise, including the promotion of positive, non-violent forms of discipline. Country reports describe existing legislation relevant to corporal punishment in each state, research that has been carried out on the issue, recommendations from treaty monitoring bodies and steps that have been taken toward law reform to achieve prohibition. It is vital that the pursuit of law reform is based on a thorough understanding of what prohibition means—crucially that all forms of corporal punishment are prohibited, however light, and that prohibition applies to children wherever they are, without exception. All legal defenses for the use of corporal punishment must be repealed. Prohibition is achieved when children have the same legal protection from assault that adults have long benefitted from.

In cases of persistent failure to enact prohibition, use can be made of the Convention on the Rights of the Child and other international human rights instruments as legal instruments which place an obligation on Governments to effect law reform and of the various human rights mechanisms which exist to pursue violations of children's human rights.

Examples of explicit prohibition:

- "Children are entitled to care, security and a good upbringing. Children are to be treated with respect for their person and individuality and may not be subjected to corporal punishment or any other humiliating treatment." (*Sweden, Parenthood and Guardianship Code, amended 1979, Article 1*)
- "Physical punishment of the child by the parents, as well as other inhuman or degrading treatment or punishments are prohibited." (*Ukraine, Family Code, 2003, Article 150*)

"Every person has the right to freedom and security of the person, which includes the right not to be ... subjected to corporal punishment...." (*Kenya, Draft Constitution, 2010, Article 29*).

Cairo declaration

Cairo declaration clearly requested to ban all forms of violence against children. Child protection from all forms of violence, and

- To urgently review and reform legislation to ensure prohibition of violence against children and to link law reform with promotion of positive, non-violent forms of discipline
- To give particular attention to combat harmful practices, including FGM, child marriage, crimes committed in the name of honor, use of children as camel jockeys, child trafficking, child domestic service and other forms of child labor
- To establish a high level focal point to coordinate all actions to prevent and combat violence against children, and promote the development of a well-resourced national strategy on violence against children, engaging with civil society, including children and young people
- To provide protection for children under occupation, and in times of war
- For those who violate the CRC by killing children or subject them to imprisonment, corporal and/or psychological torture, to be made accountable and brought to court
- To target poverty alleviation
- To facilitate the establishment of a children's forum to promote the contribution of children to the process of follow-up to the UN Study on Violence against Children and to keep children informed about developments in this area.

In 2013, the American Academy of Pediatrics edited the following:

Whereas,   the American Academy of Pediatrics is committed to the physical, mental and social health and well-being of all children; and

Whereas,   despite its common acceptance, and even advocacy for its use, spanking has been demonstrated to be no more effective than other approaches for managing undesired behavior in children; and

Whereas, because of the known dangers and negative consequences of spanking as demonstrated by many scientific studies; and,

Whereas, there are good alternatives to spanking; and,

Whereas, because the Academy strongly opposes striking a child for any reason yet provides an inconsistent message by saying "The Academy does not recommend"; therefore be it,

RESOLVED, that the Academy formally adopts a policy which emphatically rejects the use of spanking as an appropriate form of discipline, and instead promotes good alternative forms of discipline.

REFER TO: 2013 Annual Leadership Forum"

Pediatricians in MENAG can lobby for the implementation of such policy in their professional practice! They may promote non-violent education! They can integrate such positions in their curriculum! Many areas are available for them and other health professionals in this regard. Children in the US are as valuable as children in the MENAG region. We can show our care and our stand.

Acknowledgements

Jamila Bia, Barbara Bonner, Howard Dubowitz, Majid Eleissa, Adib Essali, Danya Glaser, Aida Gorbel, Hani Jahshan, Mona Kamel, Hassan Kassim, Abdelouadoud Kharbouch, Fadheela Al-Mahroos, Marcellina Mian, Elie Mikhael, Maha Al-Muneef, Robert Newell, Desmond Runyan, Randa Yousef.

Resources and references

1. Abolishing corporal punishment of children. Questions and answers (2007). Council of Europe Publishing.

2. Al-Mahroos,F. et al., "Child abuse: Bahrain's experience", Child Abuse & Neglect February 2005; 29(2):187–193

3. Barakat, Mouta and Iman Ezz, (2003), Violence Towards Child Survey study in the -Basic Schooling Education in Syria, UNICEF – Damascus

4. Cairo Declaration on the Convention (CRC) and Islamic Jurisprudence, Cairo-November 23rd and 24th 2009

5. Committee on the Rights of the Child. (2006). *General Comment No. 8 (2006): The right of the child to protection from corporal punishment and/or cruel or degrading forms of punishment (articles 1, 28(2), and 37, inter alia)* (CRC/C/GC/8). Geneva, Switzerland: United Nations. Downloaded August 21, 2006, from http://www.ohchr.org/english/bodies/crc/docs/co/CRC.C.GC.8.pdf

6. Committee on the Rights of the Child www2.ohchr.org/english/bodies/crc/comments.htm

7. Countries'reports to the CRC, (1997-2003) Concluding Observations of the Committee: Algeria, Iraq, Kuwait, Yemen, Jordan, Saudi Arabia, Egypt, Oman, Qatar, Bahrain, Emirates, Israel, Lebanon, Tunisia, Libya, Morocco, Sudan, Syria

8. Durrant, J. (2006). *Changing the landscape for children: Corporal punishment and family policy in Sweden*. Paper presented at the Australian Institute of Family Studies, Melbourne, VIC. from <www.aifs.gov.au/institute/seminars/2006/durrant.pdf

9. Ending corporal punishment of children: A handbook for working with and within religious communities (2011), Global Initiative, Save the Children Sweden and Churches'Network for Non-violence

10. Ending legalized violence against children: Global report 2010, Global Initiative and Save the Children Sweden Global Initiative e-newsletter, info@endcorporalpunishment.org

11. General Comment No. 8 on the right of the child to protection from corporal punishment and other cruel or degrading forms of punishment (articles 19, 28(2) and 37, inter alia) (2006), Committee on the Rights of the Child Campaigns Manual: Ending corporal punishment and other cruel and degrading punishment of children through law reform and social change (2010), Global Initiative and Save the Children Sweden

12. Gerbaka.B, Awada.S, Mikhael.E: The reply of the Lebanese state on the UN questionnaire on VAC, 2004

13. Gerbaka.B: BUILDING A MULTISECTORAL TASKFORCE IN LEBANON FOR THE PREVENTION OF CHILD ABUSE AND NEGLECT; Public Health Approaches to Child Maltreatment: Prevention as a Priority; TOWN AND COUNTRY RESORT & CONVENTION CENTER, SAN DIEGO, CA; JANUARY. 23, 2006

14. Gerbaka.B : The prevention of child abuse and neglect [CAN] is a long-standing teamwork, relies on a regional expertise and needs an international cooperation; TOWN AND COUNTRY RESORT & CONVENTION CENTER, SAN DIEGO, CA. January 26, 2006

15. Gershoff, E.T. (2008). *Report on Physical Punishment in the United States: What Research Tells Us About Its Effects on Children*. Columbus, OH: Center for Effective Discipline.

16. Global Initiative to End All Corporal Punishment of Children www.endcorporalpunishment.org

17. Haj-Yahia, M., et. al (2002), The Incidence of Adolescent Maltreatment in Arab Society and Some of Its Psychological Effects, Journal of Family Issues, 23/8

18. http://arabnews.com/saudiarabia/women_day/article306363.ece?comments=all

19. http://www.amnesty.org/en/news-and-updates/report/evidence-bahraini-security-forces%E2%80%99-brutality-revealed-2011-03-16

20. http://www.amnesty.org/en/news-and-updates/un-urged-put-human-rights-first-middle-east-2011-03-15

21. http://www.crin.org/resources/infodetail.asp?id=24403

22. http://www.dailystar.com.lb/article.asp?edition_id=1&categ_id=5&article_id=126514#axzz1IZ5JIZoV

23. http://www.middle-east-online.com/english/?id=45083

24. http://www.unicef.org/infobycountry/yemen_57968.html

25. http://www.yementimes.com/defaultdet.aspx?SUB_ID=35838

26. International Bureau for Children's Rights (IBCR), MENA newsletters, March 2009 – October 2012

27. Prohibiting all corporal punishment of children: Frequently Asked Questions (also available in a child-friendly version) (2009), Global Initiative Prohibiting corporal punishment of children: A guide to legal reform and other measures (2009), Global Initiative

28. Salem-Pickarta, J. (2005), Violence in Schools in the Middle East and North Africa: Features, Causes, Intervention, and Prevention, UNICEF MENAROUnited Nations Secretary-General's Study on Violence against Children (2006)

29. Save the Children- Sweden (2005), Corporal Punishment in Lebanon schools: An SCS Good Practice Report

30. Save the Children Sweden http://resourcecentre.savethechildren.se

31. The International Committee for the Rights of Child meeting, Geneva, June 2006

32. The MENA Regional Consultation on Violence against Children, Cairo, June 2005

33. The UNVAC report on VAC, Paulo Sergio PINHEIRO, 2007

34. United Nations Secretary-General's Study on Violence against Children Adapted for Children and Young People

6

International Perspectives on Child Sexual Abuse

Richard Roylance, Sue Foley,
Kayla Manzel

Introduction

The International Society for Prevention of Child Abuse and Neglect (ISPCAN), founded in 1977, is the pre-eminent non-government multi-disciplinary international membership organization working in the field of child protection. ISPCAN brings together a worldwide cross-section of committed professionals to work toward the global prevention and treatment of child abuse, neglect and exploitation globally. Its mission is to prevent cruelty to children in every nation, in every form: physical abuse, sexual abuse, neglect, street children, child fatalities, child prostitution, sex trafficking, children of war, emotional abuse and child labor, and to support individuals and organizations working to protect children from abuse and neglect worldwide.

This review is an edited distillation from the results of the questionnaire conducted prior to the ISPCAN 'Denver Thinking-Space' 2011, the discussions that took place during the Thinking-Space, feedback from participants after the event, and input from the subsequent APCCAN 2011 Conference workshop in Delhi.

The aim of ISPCAN 'Denver Thinking-Spaces' 2011 was to provide the international community with a 'snap-shot' of high-level clinical and policy advice that is:

- Informed by multi-cultural, multi-lingual and multi-disciplinary input;
- Applicable across language and culture;
- Sensitive to the realities of resources; and
- A practical resource for the use of senior practitioners hoping to influence policy-makers

and senior officials in their own geographical and cultural areas.

35 delegates from 19 countries attended in person, support by an interactive web-cast; and supplemented by input from a workshop run at the APCCAN 2011 Conference in Delhi.

Prior to the event, ISPCAN 'Denver Thinking-Space' participants provided written responses to five questions:

1. What is the formal framework (legislation, agreements, formal and informal understandings, etc.) to manage child sexual abuse cases in your country?
2. What professions, agencies, and/or institutions are responsible for addressing these cases?
3. What are the problems you find most frequently? What are the obstacles or barriers faced in preventing the effective management of these cases? In what ways have these problems been addressed?
4. Are there aspects of the evidence-based/'evaluated' literature about child sexual abuse that you consider to be unhelpful or irrelevant within your region, culture, or language-group? Why? What would you recommend in its place?
5. If you had the power to implement an ideal system, what would the components be?

The detailed responses to these questions will be available on the ISPCAN web-site by September 2012 (www.ispcan.org).

The selection of child sexual abuse and exploitation as the topic for this 'Denver Thinking-Space' 2011 should not be interpreted to imply that this area of child abuse is of more importance than other forms of child abuse and neglect. The predominate focus of this 'Denver Thinking-Space' 2011 on child sexual abuse and exploitation occurring within the home and local community should not be interpreted as diminishing the significance of 'Institutionalized' child sexual abuse such as child trafficking, child prostitution; or organizational nonfeasance, misfeasance or malfeasance; as issues of significant international concern.

Summary of workshop discussions

This paper provides an edited selection from the 'Denver Thinking-Space' 2011 materials focusing on those aspects considered to be of particular interest to the attendees of the APCCAN 2011 Conference in Delhi. There is significantly more material from the 'Denver Thinking-Space' 2011 process that will be available on the ISPCAN web-site from September 2012 (www.ispcan.org). These further materials includes detailed sections on the Legal, Medical and Mental Health aspects of child sexual abuse from an inter-disciplinary, international, and trans-cultural perspective.

Transcultural epidemiology

Child sexual abuse and exploitation (CSA) is not a new phenomenon—it is documented in the written and verbal histories from all cultures. Child sexual abuse and exploitation remains an issue for all peoples of all nations—regardless of race, culture or religion. The ISPCAN journal, *Child Abuse and Neglect* includes many articles about cross cultural incidence of child sexual abuse.

Children are sexually abused and exploited in all the environments in which they are found:

- Their homes;
- Their extended kinship and friendship networks;
- Their 'physical' neighborhoods;
- Their 'virtual' neighborhoods;
- Their 'formal' institutions (e.g., schools and churches); and
- Their 'informal' institutions (e.g., sports and recreational clubs).

Specific definitions of child sexual abuse vary between disciplines, nations and cultural groups; and have further evolved within those groups over time. This is not dissimilar to other fields of human interaction—where significant change has occurred in the globalization of standards of what constitutes acceptable human behavior (such as abolishment of slavery; or the establishment of guidelines for management of physical violence at the national (armed conflict), community (neighborhood violence) or family (interpersonal violence) level.

Despite variation in some aspects of these definitions, there is universal acceptance across national, cultural and religious groups that there are aspects of human sexual interaction (including interactions which are acceptable for sexually and developmentally mature humans—i.e. for 'adults') for which human children are developmentally unprepared; and that these sexual interactions are predominately harmful to children.

There is similar acceptance that human children do develop sexual interests and activities as part of a normal and 'healthy' developmental trajectory to 'adulthood'. However, coercion, intimidation and violence; or the 'sexualization' of the relationships in children's lives which contain innate power imbalances or intimate access (i.e. parents/guardians/teachers/coaches/religious) have been identified as factors likely to divert this normal development process into one harmful to children. Such child sexual abuse and exploitation is universally declared as unacceptable and harmful by national, cultural, and religious groups.

Although child sexual abuse may occur in isolation, it commonly co-exists with other forms of child abuse and neglect (such as child physical abuse, child emotional abuse, child neglect), and shares many of the same risk factors.[1] Interventions aimed at the prevention and treatment of child sexual abuse and exploitation must be designed with this complex interaction in mind.

Global changes in communication technologies are associated with changes in the 'type' and 'degree of risk' for sexual abuse and exploitation to which children may be exposed (e.g. electronic media, electronic social networks, digital imagining and the internet in general,) through entrapment and by exposure to developmentally inappropriate 'sexualized' material. This risk may transcend local community, national, cultural or religious boundaries.

The 'globalization' of world economies and increased ease of travel have led to an increased vulnerability for children to sex trafficking and sex tourism.

As child sexual abuse and child sexual exploitation are not issues that fall solely within the family environment nor solely outside of it, the responsibility for the prevention and treatment of child sexual abuse and child sexual exploitation must be shared between parents/guardians, the community/civil society, the State, and the international community more broadly.[2]

The development of a global, transnational, transcultural, transethnic and transreligious approach to the prevention, identification, and treatment of child abuse and neglect should be of the highest possible priority.

Tradition, change and economic progress:

The concepts of the need to protect children, and that children have a sexual developmental trajectory, are universally held tenets in all of the world's cultures and religions.

Although a particular child-rearing practice may have a long history within a culture (that is, the practice is 'customary' or 'traditional'), this is not sufficient to assert that the practice is neither harmful nor abusive to children. Parents, families, societies, cultures, ethnic and religious groups raise children in a manner that they believe to be beneficial to their children. However, review of practices in the light of a developing evidence-base can allow for the evolution of new and beneficial child protective attitudes and practices within families and society. Based on an evolving foundation of proven effective practices to prevent, identify, investigate and treat suspected child sexual abuse, professionals in different cultures can help individuals and societies rethink and reframe behaviors and evidence-based practices relevant to the care of children.

Although economic 'progress' provides some protection to children from death and morbidity directly associated with poverty, the cultural changes associated with economic progress may not always be in the best interests of children. The social isolation of caregivers for children (often women) that can be associated with economic 'progress' may have adverse side effects, and can

be 'concomitants' of child abuse and neglect, including child sexual abuse. During periods of rapid social changes, all members of a culture are potentially vulnerable, but due to their dependence children are particularly vulnerable at such times.

It is increasingly recognized across all nations and cultures that children are the most important component of 'human capital'. There are strong economic reasons to protect children from sexual abuse if for no other reason.

An ethical argument can be mounted that there is an obligation on those individuals, organizations and societies who hold resources and/or expertise in the prevention, identification, investigation and treatment of child sexual abuse to facilitate the protection of children in less resourced areas across the globe. It is important that this support is sensitive to local national, cultural, ethnic and religious traditions, practices and beliefs— provided that such traditions, practices and beliefs do not lead to child harm. In this regard, the relevant international UN instruments can provide some guidance.

Whatever the local national, cultural, ethnic and religious traditions, if they result in child sexual abuse or exploitation, it is appropriate that they be vigorously challenged.

Definitions

Clinical/Research definitions of child sexual abuse vary in their wordings; and academics and practitioners have struggled with definitions of what is a 'child', what is 'sexual', what is 'abuse', and even what is 'harm'. There is, however, a consistent concept that has arisen from decades of practical clinical experience and research: that children are inherently vulnerable to physical and mental harm when involved in sexualized interactions before they are developmentally mature; and that the risk of these harms is greatly increased by factors such as the concurrent use of threat or force, the degree of physical intrusion, the duration, the degree of subterfuge and coercion. One widely used working definition of sexual abuse is that: 'sexual abuse' involves any sexual activity where consent is not, or cannot be, given. This includes sexual contact that is accomplished by force or threat of force, regardless of the age of the participants; and all sexual contact between an adult and a child, regardless of whether there is deception or whether the child understands the sexual nature of the activity. Sexual contact between a teenager and a younger child can also be abusive if there is a significant disparity in age, development, or size, reducing the younger child capability to refuse. The sexual activity may include sexual penetration, sexual touching, or non-contact sexual acts such as exposure or voyeurism.

Criminal definitions of child sexual abuse are commonly derived from pre-existing criminal laws addressing sexual crimes more generally. As the pervasiveness of child sexual abuse has become apparent, many criminal statutes have been amended and new civil statutes enacted which define child sexual abuse in order to establish accountability and assure treatment when child sexual abuse has occurred. Criminal definitions usually specify different several different forms of sexual abuse, breaking down the behavior into different categories. Thus "sexual intercourse" can include degrees of penetration and different levels of mental intent. "Sexual contact" laws can specify which parts of the body are included and identify activities that are lawfully a legitimate form of child care even though intimate in nature. Similarly "exhibitionism" and "sexual exploitation" are often separately defined in a detailed fashion.

The importance of measurement and analysis

The regular collection of accurate demographic data about child sexual abuse in affluent cultures forced a change in how people in those cultures perceived and responded to the issue of child sexual abuse. This process of collection and meaningful analysis should be entrenched as part of recognized child sexual abuse prevention and treatment systems within all countries and extended globally. The model proposed would be similar in scope and style to other population-level data collection and analysis systems already in existence in many countries such as 'Cancer' or 'Notifiable Disease' Registers. The regular collection of demographic data (e.g., incidence and prevalence) about child sexual abuse is fundamental to any purposeful analysis; and to any strategy to positively effect change.[3]

When data are poorly collected, low 'reported numbers' cannot be taken to reflect a reliable low incidence or low prevalence of the problem. The collection of data alone is insufficient, if that data are of poor quality.

Decision makers within all countries, cultures, ethnic groups and religions need to know the incidence of the different sub-types of child sexual abuse, as well as measuring the adverse consequences of child sexual abuse on their children, their families and their society in order to respond appropriately to the needs of their children, their families and their communities.

Research and evaluation

Research into the etiology, prevention, identification and treatment of child sexual abuse is essential to provide effective interventions.[4]

The development of evidence-based, universally applicable approaches for the prevention, identification and treatment of child sexual abuse is an important strategy. The present literature is predominately generated from affluent countries, and published in English. Although there is reason to believe that much of this research is globally relevant, significant further investment is required to confirm this assumption. It should be noted, that although underlying principles of intervention may be broadly applicable—it is likely that local cultural, language, economic and resource factors will require that some level of modification be undertaken for successful implementation. A commitment to evaluation of these site-specific variations is an important part of this research, implementation and evaluation cycle.

Specifically, there is a need to demonstrate effective interventions in local languages that are culturally congruent and acceptable, practically implementable (both financially and in regard to available expertise), and politically acceptable in circumstances of limited resources.[5]

There are substantial difficulties in researching child sexual abuse, including:

- Challenges in identifying the actual prevalence of child sexual abuse versus incidence reports;
- Challenges in definition, which relate to both diagnosis and to the development of descriptive data on child sexual abuse;
- The importance of avoiding additional harm to victims while respecting their rights;
- The challenge of engaging offenders while protecting their rights;
- The cost of conducting the research and disseminating research outcomes;

- The challenge of meeting scientific requirements for reliability, validity and generalisability of research findings across cultures;
- Challenges related to intra-familiar versus extra-familial child sexual abuse; and
- The stigma that may inhibit disclosure, even where confidentiality is assured.

There is a need to better understand (both qualitatively and quantitatively) the developmental trajectory of 'normal' childhood sexuality (and expected 'normal but atypical variants') to prevent exploitation of normal sexual development.

When child sexual abuse incidence and prevalence figures are based on surveys and other indicators (such as crime records, sexually transmitted diseases or STDs, and pregnancies), researchers can more clearly define what is being counted, and thus describe what they believe the results represent. Research indicates that it is likely that one in ten, or even more, children experience child sexual abuse. [NB: The number of cases can vary by the definition and the methodology used—for example, when more behaviorally specific questions are asked, the higher the rate of child sexual abuse identification.]

When incidence and prevalence studies are based on mandatory reporting laws, the data rely on definitions prescribed by law in the jurisdictions mandating reporting. Such data systems are not common yet, but do provide some advantages in terms of management and research. The use of such databases to compare data between State, National and International jurisdictions remains limited until individual jurisdictions agree to universally consistent data definitions.

Multi-dimensional Perspectives/Philosophies

Child sexual abuse and exploitation can be considered from a number of different (but independently legitimate) perspectives.

Criminal justice issue

Child sexual abuse and exploitation are universally recognized as criminal acts that require some type of legal and correctional response. The role of punishment as a means to prevent future child sexual abuse, and as a response to the harm suffered by the victim, is a corner stone of the legal response. In some systems, a therapeutic response is also attached to the criminal response. Restorative justice may also play a part in this process. In order to mitigate again further 'secondary' harms, legal and investigative services need to keep the rights of the child, in addition to the rights of the accused, in mind. Specific developmental issues in regard to children (cognitive, linguistic and social) need to be accommodated by legal and criminal systems to allow children equal rights and opportunities within these systems. Criminalization and punishment, in isolation from other strategies, provide a limited and incomplete mechanism to prevent, treat and protect children from child sexual abuse.

Child rights issue

Child sexual abuse and exploitation are child rights violations because children have the right to be safe from sexual abuse and exploitation—which may also be associated with other forms of abuse and maltreatment. International meetings and programs have expressed an aspirational consensus regarding the well-being of children that encompasses the problem of child sexual abuse. These include:

- The UN Convention on the Rights of the Child (CRC) and optional protocols;[ii]
- The African Charter on the Rights and Welfare of the Child;[6]
- The role of national government policy and resource allocation to ensure that efforts are made to ensure the creation of a world fit for children;
- The Millennium Development Goals;[7]
- The United Nations Secretary-General's Study on Violence against Children (2006).[8]

Child health and well-being issue

Child sexual abuse and exploitation are a child health and well-being issue because child sexual abuse poses serious physical health and mental health risks for children across their lifespan. In order to improve well-being, people adversely affected by child sexual abuse need timely and effective assessment, treatment, and intervention services. These include medical, mental health, reparative developmental care, non-offending caregiver support and reunification consulting.

Family and community well-being issue

Child sexual abuse and exploitation are well-being issues for families and communities because child sexual abuse erodes trust, reinforces abuse of power, and adversely impacts family relationships.

Public health issue

Child sexual abuse and exploitation are public health issues because of their pervasive natures; the adverse effects upon the health and well-being of individuals (including sexually transmitted infections and unwanted pregnancies), their families and the broader community; and because effective identification, treatment and prevention require interventions at all levels of the community, and across disciplines and systems. An opportunity for sexual offenders and community members affected by child sexual abuse to access effective interventions is an essential part of the public health approach[9].

Risk management issue

Child sexual abuse and exploitation are risk management issues for families, organizations, and the broader community. System measures need to be established to protect children and to manage risks of potential future harm after incidents of sexual abuse have occurred (e.g., screening of possible offenders) in order to ensure the safety of children in organizations, schools and other institutions, as well as to avoid the heavy financial penalties that can accrue from negligent oversight of children's safety.

Related service issue

Child sexual abuse and exploitation are related services issues because child sexual abuse victims are overly represented in healthcare and mental health services, and overly represented in juvenile services and criminal institutions. Therefore, culturally appropriate and effective intervention and prevention strategies need to be developed that are capable of effectively bridging historical organizational conflicts.

Employment and education issue

Child sexual abuse and exploitation are employment and education issues because child sexual abuse adversely affects children in terms of their education and employment options—the effects potentially extending throughout the adult life-cycle, and extending into the next generation.

Professional education issue

Child sexual abuse and exploitation are professional education issues because all professional and ancillary staff involved with children, adults and families require specialized training to maximize effective identification, prevention and intervention capacities.

International issue

Child sexual abuse and child sexual exploitation are international issues with modern changes in transport, information technology and migration creating additional risks for children and require an international approach for the implementation of effective interventions.

Child sexual abuse and exploitation are important issues for:

- Governments
- Law Makers, Law Enforcement and Courts
- Policy Makers
- Communities and Societies—regardless of their specific linguistic, cultural, ethnic, geographical or political characteristics
- Organizations and Institutions: especially schools and religious and recreational organizations
- Prisons and Treatment Facilities for Offenders
- Cultural and Religious Groups
- Practitioners—working with children and their families
- Families
- Individual adults
- Individual children
- Media Organizations
- Organizations with roles in promoting health, well-being, education and justice.

The impact of the types of abuse on children

In undertaking investigations and planning interventions, it is important for jurisdictions to recognize that there is a range of different types of abusive and sexually harmful behaviors toward children, including:

- **Adult males who perpetrate severe forms of sexual abuse** both within and outside the family with evidence of violent, sexually coercive actions against children, peers and adults.

- **Adult male abusers who perpetrate abuse against known children** within the family, extended-family and local community context, who have higher levels of abusive experiences themselves.
- **Sex 'tourists'** who travel from their home country to take advantage of unprotected children in other countries.
- **Internet offenders** who access pornographic material—this can be a solo activity or as part of a complex international network of individuals who are responsible for creating and using pornographic material involving children.[10]
- **Virtual predators**, the majority of whom are adult males, who use the Internet to anonymously stalk and seduce children.
- **Older children and young people**, both boys and girls, who are described as showing 'reactive' patterns of sexually harmful behavior.
- **Older children and young people** who abuse in a coercive fashion against children, peers and adults, both within and outside the family. They have often experienced high levels of maltreatment and adversity, and may have co-morbid disorders such as Attention Deficit and Learning Difficulties.
- **Young people** who are recognized as being responsible for coercive sexual behaviors, or involving younger children in sexually harmful activities. They are young people with high rates of sexual abuse themselves and associated adversity.
- **Adult female sexual abusers** who have been historically less recognized than males, and less well researched. Adult women may offend against children or young people (their own or in their social network) as sole offenders, or in combination with a co-offender.[11]
- **Recognizing family contexts.** There is not a single pattern of family context described that can be recognized as characteristic of the setting for sexually abusive behavior.[12]

The importance of multi-disciplinary teams

Significant variability persists in the response to allegations of child sexual abuse among professional disciplines, national jurisdictions, cultures, and religious groups. Responses to allegations of child sexual abuse within and between these groups is often unpredictable—and dependent upon the existence of informal systems, local expertise and the vagaries of local resource and funding. The establishment of the multi-disciplinary 'Child Protection Teams' marked the beginning of modern success in identifying and responding to child physical abuse. Since child sexual abuse was identified as a systemic issue in the 1970s, it became clear that this model of collaboration between disciplines and agencies is an important systemic response to effectively investigate, manage, treat and prevent child sexual abuse.

Investigations that are coordinated between child protective services, criminal justice agencies, health and forensic services, and treatment services can reduce stress on children, prevent conflicts between the agencies, allow treatment resources to be shared, and allow agencies to support each other, as well as hold each other accountable on behalf of child victims and the public. Over many decades, published research indicates that recommendations generated by Child Protection Teams:

- Increase the likelihood that service for the child or family will be carried out;
- Reduce worker 'burnout' and attrition; and
- Improve collegial relationships between case workers, physicians, law enforcement and lawyers.

Regional Child Protection Consulting Teams provide missing expertise, reduce ambiguity and increase confidence for the local team or local professionals. In up to 30% of cases, appropriate resolution without the consultation would not have occurred.

Essential agencies that should be represented on multi-disciplinary teams include health, public health, child protective services, mental health, civil law, and criminal justice.

The advantage of interdisciplinary work is that it provides a means for sharing knowledge and resources and endorses working together so that complementary approaches can be integrated for the benefit of children, parents and society. This also increases the chances that necessary knowledge will be applied and coordinated responses will occur.

Managing the boundaries between individuals from different disciplines is a key element to the practices and principles or interdisciplinary collaborative work. The contribution of each individual's professional discipline needs to be recognized, perform its appropriate role, and assist with the development of shared skills, which will enhance protections and interventions for children and their families.

As with any complex system, systematized evaluation of the activities of specific professions and agencies against defined outcome measures is essential to define and refine best practice models.

Persons who sexually abuse children

It has been suggested that four 'pre-conditions' must exist for an individual to sexually abuse a child.[13] The abuser must:

- have the motivation to sexually abuse;
- be able to overcome internal inhibitors;
- be able to overcome external inhibitors; and
- be able to overcome the resistance of the child.

Offender characteristics have not proven an especially fruitful avenue for screening or preventing child sexual abuse. Despite popular conceptions, no 'profile' of a child sexual offender has been established with sufficient specificity and/or sensitivity to be of practical use as a screening mechanism.

In all countries, cultures and ethnic and religious groups there has been resistance (both active and passive) to the establishment of systems to prevent, identify and treat child sexual abuse. This resistance has been at the level of individuals; families; and includes professional, educational, sporting and religious agencies—often for complex issues of philosophy, history or tradition. In addition, self-identified groups of individuals who wish to have sexual contact with children, often justify their behavior using strategies to 'normalize' and 'legitimize' their sexually abusive behavior in the eyes of the public and officials.

Criminalization

The fact that child sexual abuse has long been perceived in most countries as a criminal act has meant law enforcement and judicial processes have played a significant role in the initial response to child sexual abuse.

Where a child has been sexually abused by someone outside of the immediate family ('extra-familial' child sexual abuse), especially by someone who has an organizational duty of care; or someone who is involved in trafficking children (or their images) for prostitution or financial gain, there is universal agreement across all nations, cultures and religions that law enforcement and judicial process have a substantial and primary role.

The application of a criminal approach to abuse within the immediate family ('intra-familial' child sexual abuse) has been more controversial. The concept of 'incest' has complex cultural and religious overlays which may result in this type of child sexual abuse being considered as 'different'. Initiation of criminal justice processes following disclosures of 'intra-familial' child sexual abuse may produce outcomes that the child did not anticipate and does not want (e.g., financial disruption of the family; public shaming of the family, punishing and imprisonment of a close family member; marital breakdown). These are less likely to be issues when the abuse is by someone more removed from the child's immediate circle.

Notwithstanding the important role that a criminal response to suspicions of child sexual abuse played when child sexual abuse is first identified as a cultural concern, over time most countries identify that a 'therapeutic' perspective is important to the subsequent health and well-being of affected children and their families. Proponents of this less-punitive approach argue for a distinction between intra-familial and extra-familial child sexual abuse. It is clear that the issue of researching what might constitute effective treatment and rehabilitation systems for persons who sexually abuse children requires further investment. Individuals favoring a therapeutic view also work to understand the origins of sexually abusive behavior in adults or in the sexually harmful behavior of young people.

There is evolving belief that some forms of intra-familial child sexual abuse may be managed at least in part through child protection services, without the active involvement of criminal justice system. The goal is to ensure that a child is protected, treated, and other relevant services provided for the child and family whilst ensuring that the family can provide a safe environment for the child and, when necessary, determining whether the child needs a long-term alternate placement. A court sanctioned 'diversionary system'—managed under similar principles to that used in 'Specialist Drug Courts'—may also have a role in some types of child sexual abuse.

Prevention and treatment

Published research on treatment of abused and neglected children has become more rigorous and more prevalent in the past decade. The research includes studies that report positive treatment results for children who suffer physical abuse, sexual abuse, and/or are neglected. Many types of evidence-based practice are now available, including Trauma-Focused Cognitive Behavioral Therapy and Abuse Focused-Cognitive Behavioral Therapy.[14] It should be noted however, that these interventions have not been evaluated on all ethnic groups, and data from extended follow-up is limited. Such therapeutic approaches hold considerable promise—but we may yet be in a position yet to say with confidence that these interventions are the best ones globally without further research and cultural modification.

A significant minority of cases of child sexual abuse result involve abusive contact between a child and an older minor. An important finding of the past twenty years is that youth who perpetrate child sexual abuse do constitute a threat to other children, that there do exist effective treatment modalities, and that early intervention early is more likely to succeed (and at a lower cost). With appropriate treatment, this group of children who sexually abuse other children has much lower recidivism rates than do untreated minors or adults.

The best way to protect children is to prevent offenders from harming children by targeting risk, provision of an effective intervention, and the prevention of relapse. Counseling of children affected by child sexual abuse is most likely to succeed if it includes all persons in the household.

Essential processes in all cultures and countries

Data collection is an important element in informing societal reaction to the incidence of child sexual abuse and sexual exploitation, regardless of the cultural components of that society. Systems for data collection need to be developed. Once child sexual abuse and sexual exploitation are acknowledged by society, responses to the problem need to be developed - including protective systems, policies and laws, appropriate curriculum & training, and a capacity building process for all professionals concerned.

While acknowledging the national commitments toward the UN Convention on the Rights of the Child in general and Article 19 in particular, national programs need to take into consideration specific factors such as:

- Legal definitions and concepts of child sexual abuse and sexual exploitation;
- Specific types of child sexual abuse and sexual exploitation in some cultures; and
- Differences in implementation capacities in each country and region.

It is noted that the level of development of countries as 'civil societies' is reflected in their commitment to child protection and well-being.

Professionals can play an important role in prevention, training, reporting, rehabilitation and data collection. The involvement of trusted professionals is particularly important in countries where there are gender discrimination issues and where professionals are valued and respected by the society. Children need also to be part of the process in a meaningful way.

It must be noted that other forms of child abuse can be associated with or precede child sexual abuse and sexual exploitation. Therefore, child sexual abuse should be managed as part of a broader child protection system, rather than as an issue fundamentally different that other forms of child abuse.

Supporting best practices in parenting can provide for safe child care earlier in life, provide proper and timely detection of groups at risk (in child and parents). Home visitation is one strategy which has been researched predominately in affluent countries – but has significant promise as a more global intervention.

Principles and practices in the prevention of child sexual abuse

Responsibility for prevention of child sexual abuse is shared by parents, schools, communities, government and the broader society. In seeking to prevent sexual violence against children, it is important to recognize that some risk factors—such as poverty and lack of access to education—must be addressed at policy and practice levels.

Response to situations of conflict, post-conflict and natural disasters must consider evidence that the prevalence of sexual violence and exploitation often increases in contexts of these crises, and respond adequately. Sexual exploitation of children (including 'sex tourism') requires the involvement of all aspects of government, and its prevention cannot be the sole responsibility of child protection services.

Greater emphasis should be placed on primary prevention—preventing violence from ever taking place – as opposed to secondary or tertiary prevention. There is also a need to strengthen the service provision network (e.g. the health care sector needs to be trained to identify and care for cases). Secondary and tertiary prevention should be evidence-based, identifying ways in which victims may be re-victimized and how victims, in turn, can become people who harm others. Evidence-based research is needed regarding the risk and protective factors associated with both perpetration and victimization in order to develop effective preventive strategies. Polyvictimization and the co-occurrence of other forms of abuse must also be acknowledged in the formulation of prevention strategies.

Prevention strategies need to be rigorously evaluated at all levels and take into account the range of social contexts of vulnerable children. Primary prevention of sexual violence may require adaptation to manage the different manifestations of sexual violence, the different groups of high risk individuals and the different groups of vulnerable children and families. Prevention strategies should include a combination of the provision of information (e.g. children's human rights), building skills (e.g. what to do, who to talk to) and provision of resources (for example, 'Hotlines').

Education and training issues—professionals, schools, communities

All victims of child sexual abuse and sexual exploitation and their families have the right to have access to knowledgeable and skilled service providers. Since child sexual abuse and sexual exploitation are ever-evolving fields, children deserve competent practitioners who acknowledge the importance of continuing education.

ISPCAN is a resource for the provision and dissemination of state of the art knowledge and best practice. The dissemination of knowledge may occur through many different strategies, including:

- Regional, national and international conferences;
- Development of a resource library;
- Core discipline specific training to address needs tailored to the developmental stage of a given program, consultation and networking.

The world-community continues to learn about the definition, prevention, assessment, and the treatment of child sexual abuse. As evidenced based understanding of core principles, guidelines, and standards evolve for the medical, legal, and social sciences there is a need to disseminate this information worldwide through education, policy and training initiatives. If we are to significantly reduce the prevalence of child sexual abuse and sexual exploitation in its many manifestations, such efforts must be designed by and for the relevant individuals and systems in a state, country, or community. Any such training and education efforts shall remain open to the inclusion and adoption of culturally sensitive and culturally relevant alternatives.

Conclusion

That individual children are on occasions subjected to unwanted sexual activities has been acknowledged throughout recorded history. The formal identification of child sexual abuse as a significant and pervasive issue for children in all nations, from all cultural, linguistic and economic backgrounds is very recent.[15] The realization that child sexual abuse poses substantial risks to the physical and mental health and well-being of the individual child across his/her lifetime is more recent still.

Much has been done in the past fifty years in this field in all areas of the globe—to prevent, identify and treat the harm which arises from child sexual abuse—but much remain yet to be done. This paper (and the workshops which were instrumental in its development) is a small part of the ongoing iterative process of research, implementation and evaluation that is required to improve the lives of the world's children.

References

1. David Finkelhor, Richard K. Ormrod, Poly-victimization: A neglected component in child victimization, Child Abuse & Neglect, 2007; 31(1):7–26.

2. Convention on the Rights of the Child, http://www.unicef.org/crc/

3. Elizabeth D. Jones, Karen McCurdy, The links between types of maltreatment and demographic characteristics of children, Child Abuse & Neglect, 1992; 16(2):201–215, (http://www.sciencedirect.com/chiabuneg/article/pii/014521349290028P)

4. Runyan, Desmond K, Prevalence, Risk, Sensitivity, and Specificity: A Commentary on the Epidemiology of Child Sexual Abuse and the Development of a Research Agenda Original Research. Child Abuse & Neglect, 1998; 22(6):493–498.

5. ISPCAN Training Materials http://www.ispcan.org/?page=Training_Materials (accessed 25.7.12)

6. Organization of African Unity, African Charter on the Rights and Welfare of the Child, 11 July 1990, CAB/LEG/24.9/49 (1990), available at: http://www.unhcr.org/refworld/docid/3ae6b38c18.html (accessed 23 July 2012).

7. United Nations Millennium Development Goals (http://www.un.org/millenniumgoals/) accessed 25.7.2012

8. National Sexual Violence Resource Center http://www.nsvrc.org/publications/prevention/public-health

9. Finkelhor Gérard Niveau, Cyber-pedocriminality: Characteristics of a sample of internet child pornography offenders, Child Abuse & Neglect, 2010; 34(8):570–575.

10. Margaret M. Rudin, Christine Zalewski, Jeffrey Bodmer-Turner, Characteristics of child sexual abuse victims according to perpetrator gender, Child Abuse & Neglect, 1995; 19(8):963–973, (http://www.sciencedirect.com/chiabuneg/article/pii/014521349500058G)

11. David Finkelhor, Epidemiological factors in the clinical identification of child sexual abuse, Child Abuse Neglect, 1993; 17(1):67–70, (http://www.sciencedirect.com/chiabuneg/article/pii/014521349390009T)

12. Risk Factors for Child Sexual Abuse, DAVID FINKELHOR, University of New Hampshire, LARRY BARON J Interpers Violence March 1986; 1(1):43–71.

13. Trauma-Focused Cognitive-Behavioral Therapy tfcbt.musc.edu

14. Cohen and Manarino, Parent-Child Interaction Therapy J Interpers Violence November 2000; 15(11):1202–1223.

15. Acknowledgments The preparation of this paper was made possible by the generous contributions by numerous experts to the ISPCAN Denver 'Thinking-Space' 2011: Child Sexual Abuse and the APCCAN Conference in Delhi. A particular thanks is due to the Staff and Executive Council of ISPCAN for their support and input. The ISPCAN Denver 'Thinking-Space' 2011: Child Sexual Abuse was funded by by the Oak Foundation (Switzerland).

7

Child Sexual Abuse in India

Swati Y Bhave, Anjali Saxena

Introduction

Child Sexual Abuse is the most heinous of all sexual crimes that can be perpetrated against children. Most of them suffer silently and often bear the mental and emotional scars for their entire life. The few who build up courage to complain about the abuse are not taken seriously; they are often disbelieved and many times silenced especially if the perpetrator is a close family member or a well-known member of society.[1]

WHO defines an adolescent as being between 10–19 years old. In "The Protection of Children from Sexual Offences" Bill 0f India 2011, passed recently, a child is up to 18 years of age.[2]

Definition and understanding of (Child sexual abuse) (CSA)[3]

Sexual abuse broadly can be divided into four categories:

1. Child Sexual Abuse- Any sexual behavior or activity involving a child in the context of a relationship or responsibility, trust or authority.
2. Commercial sexual exploitation of children/child prostitution/Child sex tourism.
3. Sexual violence through Harmful and Traditional Practices—Child Marriage/Religious dedication, Devdasi, bacha baazi.
4. Sexual violence against children Facilitated by ICT's Information and communication Technology—Child sexual Abuse images (child pornography) and online sexual exploitation.

Child sexual abuse

Sexual abuse is inappropriate sexual behavior with a child. It includes fondling a child's genitals, making the child fondle the adult's genitals, intercourse, incest, rape, sodomy, exhibitionism and sexual exploitation. To be considered 'child abuse', these acts have to be committed by a person responsible for the care of a child (e.g. a baby-sitter, a parent, or a day care provider), or related to the child. If a stranger commits these acts, it would be considered sexual assault and handled solely by the police and criminal courts.[4] This was traditionally the understanding, and sexual abuse and sexual assault were so differentiated.

However, as per the newly passed landmark Bill 'The Protection of Children from Sexual Offences Bill, 2011', Bill No. XIV of 2011 of India.

According to the Bill the offences are grouped into following categories:[2]

Penetrative sexual assault

A person commits "penetrative sexual assault" if he penetrates his penis into the vagina, mouth, urethra or anus of a child or makes a child do the same or inserts any other object into the child's body or applies his mouth to a child's body parts. If however the child is between 16 and 18 years, it shall be considered whether consent for the Act was taken against his will or was taken by drugs, impersonation, fraud, undue influence and when the child was sleeping or unconscious. The penalty is imprisonment between 7 years and life and a fine.

Aggravated penetrative sexual assault

The Bill penalises "aggravated penetrative sexual assault." Such an offence is committed when a police officer, a member of the armed forces or a public servant commits penetrative sexual assault on a child. It also includes gang penetrative sexual assault and assault using deadly weapons, fire or corrosive substance. The Bill also covers assault by staff of private hospital and staff of an educational institution if the child is in that institution. Penetrative sexual assault shall be considered aggravated if it injures the sexual organs of the child or takes place during communal violence or the child becomes pregnant or gets any other threatening disease or is below 12 years. It also covers cases where the offender is a relative of the child through blood or adoption or marriage or foster care or is living in the same household. The penalty is imprisonment between 10 years and life and a fine.

Sexual assault

A person commits "sexual assault" if he touches the vagina, penis, anus or breast of a child with sexual intent without penetration, or makes the child do the same to him or any other person. If the child is between 16 and 18 years, it shall be considered whether the consent was taken against the child's will or by threat or deceit. The penalty is imprisonment between three to five years and a fine.

Aggravated sexual assault

The offence of "aggravated sexual assault" is committed under similar conditions as for "aggravated penfetrative sexual assault". The penalty for the offence is imprisonment between 5 to 7 years and a fine.

Sexual harassment

A person is said to commit sexual harassment upon a child when such a person with sexual intent uses words, gestures, pornographic material, or exhibiting of child's body parts.

A person shall be guilty of using a child for pornographic purposes if he uses a child in any form of media for the purpose of sexual gratification through representation of sexual organs of a child or using a child in sexual acts or other types of obscene representation. The penalty is rigorous imprisonment for up to 5 years and a fine. On subsequent convictions, the term of imprisonment is up to 7 years and fine.

- The Bill also includes penalties for storage of pornographic material and abetment of an offence.
- An offence committed under this Act shall be reported to either the local police or the Special Juvenile Police Unit who has to report the matter to the Special Court within 24 hours. The police also have to make special arrangement for the care of the child. In case a person fails to report a case, he shall be penalized. Also, the Bill includes penalties for making false complaints.
- Each district shall designate a Sessions Court to be a Special Court. It shall be established by the state government in consultation with the Chief Justice of the High Court. The state government shall appoint a Special Public Prosecutor for every Special Court. The Court shall, as far as possible, complete the trial within one year. The trial shall be held in camera and in the presence of the child's parents or any person trusted by the child.
- The guardian of the child has the right to take assistance from a legal counsel of his choice, subject to the provisions of Code of Criminal Procedure, 1973.
- If an offence has been committed by a child, it shall be dealt with under the Juvenile Justice (Care and Protection of Children) Act, 2000.

The WHO estimates that 150 million girls and 73 million boys under 18 years have experienced forced sexual intercourse or other forms of sexual violence involving physical contact, though this is certainly an underestimate. Much of this sexual violence is inflicted by family members or other people residing in or visiting a child's family home—people normally trusted by children and often responsible for their care. A review of epidemiological surveys from 21 countries, mainly high- and middle- income countries, found that at least 7% of females (ranging up to 36%) and 3% of males (ranging up to 29%) reported sexual victimization during their childhood. According to these studies, between 14% and 56% of the sexual abuse of girls, and up to 25% of the sexual abuse of boys, was perpetrated by relatives or step parents. In many places, adults were outspoken about the risk of sexual violence their children faced at school or at play in the community, but rarely did adults speak of children's risk of sexual abuse within the home and family context. The shame, secrecy and denial associated with familial sexual violence against children foster a pervasive culture of silence, where children cannot speak about sexual violence in the home, and where adults do not know what to do or say if they suspect someone they know is sexually abusing a child.[4]

Reporting of child sexual abuse

The parents and family very often do not want report sexual violence against their child some of the reason include.

a. They feel the child's future will be besmirched. In many of the countries arranged marriage are still the norm and virginity is a key issue
b. If the abuser is a family member—aunt, father, grandfather, etc. then to protect the abuser the abuse is not reported
c. Family honor—exposure would bring disgrace to the family
d. Fear of the offender who may be more powerful economically or socially
e. Media exposure
f. Lack of a reporting and response system to which all have access
g. Even where systems exist, lack of awareness or confidence in the system
h. Long process of investigation and justice in courts.

A study on Child Sexual Abuse carried out by Save the Children and Tulir in 2006[4] looked at the prevalence and dynamics of child sexual abuse among school going children in Chennai. The study was conducted with a view to add to the scarce indigenous body of knowledge on child sexual abuse and with the aim of breaking the silence around the issue, dispelling certain myths and providing research based information on child sexual abuse. The team followed major ethical standards of confidentiality, freedom to participate, informed consent and a multi-disciplinary team. The major findings of this study include:

1. Out of the total of 2211 respondents, 42% children faced at least one form of sexual abuse or the other

2. Among respondents, 48% of boys and 39% of the girls faced sexual abuse
3. The prevalence of sexual abuse in upper and middle class was found to be proportionately higher than in lower or in lower middle class
4. Sexual abuse was found to be prevalent in both joint and nuclear families
5. Majority of the abusers were people known to the child and strangers were a minority
6. Sexual harassment in public places and exhibitionism was higher by strangers
7. Sexual abuse of children was very often a pre-planned insidious abuse of a relationship by an abuser over the child.

Statistics of child sexual abuse in india based on ministry of women and child development report of 2007[4]

In order to examine the incidence of sexual abuse among child respondents in India, a questionnaire was administered to 12,447 children belonging to the five different categories including children in family environment, children in schools, children in institutions, children at work and street children. The study looked into four severe forms and five other forms of sexual abuse.

Out of the total child respondents, 53.22% reported having faced one or more forms of sexual

Abuse that included severe and other forms. Among them 52.94% were boys and 47.06% girls. The age wise distribution of children reporting sexual abuse in one or more forms showed that though the abuse started at the age of 5 years, it gained momentum 10 years onward, peaking at 12–15 years and then starting to decline. This means that children in the teenage years are most vulnerable.

The study looked at gender-wise break up of children who were subjected to one or more forms of sexual abuse in the sample states. The significant finding was that contrary to the general perception, the overall percentage of boys was much higher than that of girls. In fact 9 out of 13 States reported higher percentage of sexual abuse among boys as compared to girls, with states like Delhi reporting a figure of 65.64%.

Among different evidence groups, highest percentage of children who faced sexual abuse was those at work (61.61%).

Out of the total child respondents, 20.90% were subjected to severe forms of sexual abuse that included sexual assault, making the child fondle private parts, making the child exhibit private body parts and being photographed in the nude. Out of these 57.30% were boys and 42.70% were girls. Over one-fifth of these children faced more than three forms of sexual abuse. Amongst these sexually abused children 39.58% were in the age group of 5–12 years, 35.59% in the age group of 15–18 years and 24.83% in the age group of 13–14 years.

Missing children and adolescents[5]

Children and adolescents may run away from home due to domestic problems or lured by child traffickers. Trafficking in women and children is the most abominable violation of human rights. There has been a known association between missing children and trafficking.

The National Human Rights Commission in association with other organizations spearheaded action oriented research on the same. In 2003 they reported that an average of 44,476 children are reported missing in India every year. Most of these become victims of trafficking or are sexually exploited.

India by conservative estimates has three to five lakh prostitutes, being a major destination for trafficked children from within India and adjoining countries.

Rape on children and adolescents[6]

Every year the National Crime Records Bureau releases national data on crimes committed in the country. The incidence of rape has seen an increasing incidence over the years. In the report of 2011 Madhya Pradesh has reported the highest number of Rape cases (3,406), Molestation (6,665) and Importation of girls (45) accounting for 14.1%, 15.5% and 56.3% respectively of total such cases reported in the country, followed by Uttar Pradesh and Maharashtra.

Offenders were known to the victims in 92.9% of Rape cases. 10.6% were under 14 years of age, and 19% were in their teens. This data may be an underestimate, since it takes into account only the registered crimes.

Conceptual and behavioral definitions of child sexual abuse[1]

"Child sexual abuse occurs when a child is used for sexual gratification of an older adolescent or adult. *"Any sexual behavior directed at the dependent developmentally immature child and adolescent that they do not comprehend fully, to which they are unable to give informed consent. It involves the exposure of a child to sexual contact, activity or behavior and may include invitation to sexual touching intercourse or other forms of exploitation such as juvenile prostitution or pornography."*

Forms of abuse sexual behavior[7]

1 An adult exposing his/her genitals to or persuading a child or adolescent to do the same
2 An adult touching a child or adolescent's genitals or making a child or adolescent touch the adult's genitalia
3 An adult involving a child or adolescent in pornography, either by exposing a child or adolescent to pornographic material or using child or adolescent to create pornographic material
4 An adult having oral, vaginal, anal intercourse with a child or adolescent
5 Any verbal or other sexual suggestions made to a child or adolescent by an adult
6 An adult persuading a child or adolescent to engage in sexual activity.

If an older adolescent manifest such a behavior to a child it will also constitute child sexual abuse.

Age of consensual sex

The legislation to protect children below 18 years from sexual abuse became a reality on 23rd May 2012 'Protection of Children against Sexual offences Bill'.

The is a path breaking bill dealing exclusively with sexual offences against children providing for stringent punishment up to a life term imprisonment. The section seven of the bill provides for "no punishment" if the consent for sexual act has been obtained with a person aged between 16 and 18 years.[2,8] The bill provides for treating sexual assault as "aggravated offence" when it is committed by a person in position of trust or authority over a child including a member of the security forces, police officer, public servant, management or staff of a children's home, hospital or educational institution.

Children at risk of sexual abuse include the following

- Lack of sexuality education that makes children aware of sexual abuse and empower to protect them
- Poverty—high-risk of getting sexually abused or sexually exploited because of poor socio-economic conditions. Child prostitution is a social evil due to poverty
- Children who are isolated from others with few friends and little contact with siblings are at greater risk
- Children who are abandoned or who live on the streets (street children in general) with/without adult caregivers are the most vulnerable
- When children and adolescent do not get the love and care from their parents—can involve in sexual activities, which they feel is a form of emotional support
- Broken families or single parents: due to lack of adequate supervision
- Children with low self-esteem some children—due to failure in academic life. May fall prey to sexual activity considering it as an achievement
- Parental factors—loss of job, substance abuse like alcoholism, drug addiction
- Mentally and physically challenged children
- Children who feel they are unloved or uncared are more susceptible to become prey to child predators.

Adults need to take the following measures to prevent SCS (a)

- Teach children to trust their feelings and that it is okay to say "NO" when someone they know and care about does something they do not like.
- Set and respect family boundaries
- Speak up when inappropriate behavior is seen or reported
- Talk about sexual abuse and teach proper names of body parts to children
- Educate children about the differences between safe touch and unsafe touch and that secrets about touching are not okay
- Children also need to know that people they know are capable of hurting them
- Encourage, affirm, and acknowledge a child's opinions and feelings-giving them sense of self esteem and confidence
- Involve your child in setting up a safety plan that is easy to remember
- Make a list for yourself and the child- whom to call for advice, information and help.

Mental status of child/adolescent with sexual abuse[1]

- The basic feeling are loss of trust, feeling of fear, feeling of guilt and shame, helplessness, doubt about the own perception of reality, and speechlessness. Children and adolescents find it difficult to break the silence, especially in cases of incest.
- Enforced secrecy and a child's fear of destroying the privacy and security of the family are powerful obstacles to disclosure.[9] The main factors are obligation to maintain secrecy under multiple threats and the dependency in relation between victim and the perpetrator.
- Child sexual abuse can be characterized as a "Syndrome of Secrecy and Dependency", also known as the child Abuse Accommodation syndrome[10] There is a strong conflict of loyalty as the victim both fears and loves the perpetrator in most of the cases. Perpetrator almost always succeeds in convincing the child of his/her own responsibility and guilt for being abused.

Child and adolescent sexual abuse in observation homes on streets[11]

A study of physical and sexual abuse and behavior problems against boys in a child observation home in Delhi by Pagare et al. reported sexual abuse in 38.1% of children, amongst these sexually abused children, physical signs were seen in 23.8% and behavior signs were seen in 16.3%.

A multi-centric study of street children project also revealed that older boys pimp for foreigners and commercial sex workers.[12]

Some researchers have documented cases of sexually transmitted diseases among children below 14 years which may be considered as signs of sexual abuse.[13]

Juvenile sex offenders

On an average 10 rape cases against juveniles are registered every month as per a national newspaper report in 2005.[14] Police records state that in up to 30% of rape cases the offender is a juvenile.

"At a very young age, juveniles from poor classes get exposed to the world of poverty and hunger. But to believe that such acts are not prevalent in juveniles from middle or rich classes would be wrong. To a large extent their cases do not get reported.

Most of these accused themselves first become victims of sexual abuse and when they get an opportunity, they tend to do the same. Many of these juveniles make girl friends in school at age 12 or 13 years and go for consensual sex".

Juveniles commit such acts (as told by juveniles themselves): out of curiosity. The might be indulging in substance abuse.

- Provoked after watching pornographic films and magazines.

Pedophile[7]

Is defined as a person who has an identifiable sexual preference with regard to pre-pubertal children and will frequent locations that attract children

Profile of the adult sex offender[1, 4]

- A study of adult sexual offenders found that the sample of offenders studied claimed to have a special ability to identify vulnerable children, and to use that vulnerability to sexually abuse the child
- It was also found that offenders systematically desensitize children to touch
- Offenders described the use of adult authority, adult physical presence and efforts to isolate the victim from others, as a means of controlling the victim
- Offenders use a number of strategies to gain access to children and to enforce their victim's silence, including threats, force, bribery, acts of cruelty and other forms of physical and psychological coercion
- Contrary to popular belief, the abuser is not always sexually pervert in the park or, the mentally unstable man walking the street, etc
- Studies reveal that in 80% of the cases, the perpetrator is either related or known to the victim
- Children and adolescents living in parental homes are more likely to be abused by adults from within the family or known friends circle and the chances of a child being abused by a stranger are very less

- Sexual abuse was found to be significantly associated with domestic violence, solvent/inhalant use and working status. Children on streets or observation homes are more likely to be abused by strangers.

Pedophilia

It is very sad to know that Pedophiles justify their behavior. Organizations such as the North American Man Boy Love Association (NAMBLA) and the René Guyon Society challenge the assertion that sexual abuse is bad because of its effects on children.[15] They Question "what is wrong about sex between adults and children?"[1]

These organizations argue that what we label as harmful effects are not the effects of sexual abuse but the effects of societal condemnation of the behavior. Thus, children feel guilty about their involvement, suffer from "damaged goods syndrome,"[16] have low self-esteem, are depressed and suicidal, and experience helpless rage because society has stigmatized sex between adults and children. According to their argument if society would cease to condemn the behavior, then children could enjoy guilt-free sexual encounters with adults. Such organizations also argue that we, as adults, are interfering with children's rights, specifically their right to control their own bodies and their sexual freedom, by making sex between children and adults unacceptable and illegal.

How can we respond to this argument?

We need to see that this opinion does not percolate into more minds. It is true that many of the effects of sexual abuse at least indirectly derive from how society views the activity. However, the impact also reflects the experience itself. Because the adult has more power, he/she has the capacity to impose the sexual behavior, which may be painful, intrusive, or overwhelming because of its novelty and sexual nature. This power may also be manifest in manipulation of the child into compliance. The child has little knowledge about the societal and personal implications of being involved in sex with an adult; in contrast, the adult has sophisticated knowledge of the significance of the encounter. The child's lack of power and knowledge means the child cannot give informed consent. Finally, although in some cases the adult may perceive him/herself providing pleasure to the child, the main object is the gratification of the adult.[17]

Effects of sexual abuse on its victim

The Impact of Sexual Abuse: can be classified as short term and long-term effects.[18]

Finkelhor[19] whose conceptualization of the traumatogenic effect of sexual abuse is the most widely employed, divides sequele into four general categories, traumatic *sexualization*, *betrayal*, *stigmatization* and *powerlessness*. Each has varied psychological and behavioral effects.

Traumatic sexualization

This is an adverse psychological outcome of sexual abuse, which is aversive feelings about sex, overvaluing sex, and sexual identity problems. Behavioral manifestations of traumatic sexualization constitute a range of hypersexual behaviors as well as avoidance of or negative sexual encounters.

Feeling of betrayal

In family member abuse there is a great sense of betrayal. This is a person whom the child trusts and who is expected to care for and protect the child. The child feels betrayed and hurt by the actions of this person. If the parents show helplessness in this matter then the child feels betrayed by the parents, and the child experiences a loss of trust in and disillusionment in the parental ability to protect and care for the child. The child begins to search for a persons she/he can trust. The child develops dependency and shows clinging behavior

and the child may develop an impaired ability to judge people. They can also develop mistrust or misjudgment in relationships. As adults they may also have disastrous or abusive marriages.[7]

Stigmatization

Common psychological manifestations of stigmatization are what Sgroi calls "damaged goods syndrome"[16] and feelings of guilt and responsibility for the abuse or the consequences of disclosure. The child feels he is doing something wrong, feels she is dirty and carried a heavy burden all the time. These feelings are likely to be reflected in self-destructive behaviors such as substance abuse, risk-taking acts, self-mutilation, suicidal gestures and acts, and provocative behavior designed to elicit punishment. There is a sense of worthlessness and poor self-esteem.[7]

Powerlessness

The psychological impact of the trauma of powerlessness includes both a perception of vulnerability and victimization and a desire to control or prevail, often by identification with the aggressor. As with the trauma of betrayal, behavioral manifestations may involve aggression and exploitation of others. On the other hand, the vulnerability effect of powerlessness may be avoidant responses, such as dissociation and running away; behavioral manifestations of anxiety, including phobias, sleep problems, elimination problems, and eating problems, and revictimization.[7]

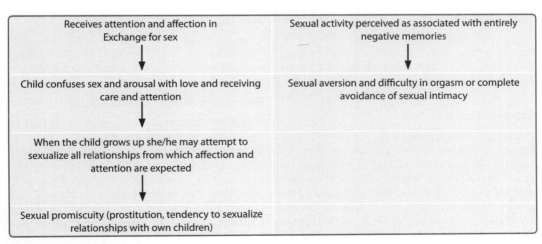

Source: (Graphics) FACSE[7]

Every child is vulnerable, dependent, innocent, and needy. Child is sexually abused: (physical, emotional, mental violation. A child is physically weaker and developmentally immature as compared to the older adolescent or adult abuser. Unable to stop the abuse a child feels powerless, anxious and unable to control his/her own life as the child grows she/he may feel anxious and unable to cope up. A tendency to run away from problems can be seen. Child can also feel despair and depression and the possibility of revictimisation. There is also potentiality for aggression and of becoming an abuser Source.[7]

The survivor's cycle[7]

Childhood

There is a negative sense of self

The child feels: "I'm a bad person; everyone is better than me. I don't deserve better. I'm a phony. If they really knew me they'd dislike and get disgusted by me. I deserve what I get; I don't know who I am".

Abuse causes of confusion

"What's he doing? I don't understand what's happening to me. I don't like this but how can I stop it? What is normal? Where can I be safe? I can't do anything right. I don't know what's real, what is right? I'm trapped: It's my fault. I must keep the secret to survive. I'm responsible. I didn't stop it or tell anyone. I'm responsible for what I've become. I can't change my life or myself or anything.

Self-estrangement

"I'm always wrong; I can't be like everyone else. I'm not normal. I'm not important. No one cares how I feel. My feelings don't count. What I want doesn't matter? I don't want to be me."

Survival skills

I have to hide inside myself, I have to protect myself. I can't let people see who/how I really am. How can I keep from exposing the real me. The consequences depend upon how quickly the adolescent confides with the parents or trusted adults and reveal the abuse? The initial effects of sexual abuse usually occur between two years of termination of abuse and depend upon the circumstances of abuse and child/adolescent's developmental status.

Adolescent will need family support, extra-familial support, sense of spirituality and high self-esteem. This will help in early recovery.

Reclaiming self[7]

Self-awareness

"I value and use my thoughts and feelings. I can make mistakes, everyone does. I can learn new things and be flexible. I appreciate myself."

Empowerment

"The abuse was not my fault. I can shed the guilt and shame: they're his, not mine. I did the best I could, as a child, living under those conditions. I'm remarkable for having endured abuse and its consequences".

Self-acceptance

I know myself. I like who I am. I respect myself for having lived through the abuse(s) of my childhood. I am strong and able to learn and change when I want or need to. I deserve to be loved and respected by others".

Clarity

I was sexually abused. I can separate out, who I am from what I've thought and felt about myself, because of being abused. I have personal right. I have the right to set and enforce boundaries and limits. I must respect my perceptions. I am much more than a sexual abuse survivor.

Survival skills

I can be myself to myself and others. These skills have helped me to survive. Now I can choose which ones to keep or change and which to put aside".

Recovery from sexual abuse

This depends upon the harm done to the victim, age of the child, duration, frequency, degree of the abuse. It also depends upon the relationship of the abuser to the child. It is important for professionals, particularly if they dedicate a substantial part of their careers to intervening in sexual abuse situations, to distance themselves from their visceral reactions of disgust and outrage and rationally consider why sex between children and adults is so objectionable.

Sexual abuse in boys

Many people seem to believe that rape happens only to women.[20] They are cautious about girls; mothers also talk to girls about sexuality. But since it is a belief that boys are safe, boys are not given important safety instructions. With the result boys are often subjected to sexual abuse, often by older friends or male relatives. Male rape is not understood by many and hence rarely reported. Male rape survivors think so too, and they may feel isolated and alone. If people in our community believe that, they may further this sense of isolation on the part of male rape survivors. Both homosexual and heterosexual males can get raped. Rapists who rape males are heterosexual in 93% of the cases.

Male rape victims share many of the feelings as female sexual assault survivors. They may feel guilty, powerless, concerned regarding their safety, denial, shock, anger.

Strong or weak, outgoing or withdrawn, homosexual or heterosexual, old or young, male or female, no one does anything that justifies sexual assault.

Role of care givers

- All adults who are involved in looking after children should be aware and educate themselves about the various aspects of child sexual abuse.
- Victims are often unable to speak due to different reasons—threat, fear, shame, and guilt.
- Therefore indirect, non-verbal clues, behavioral disturbances, psychosomatic, psychiatric and seldom physical symptoms are often the only way to recognize sexual abuse.
- There is no specific CSA symptom or syndrome.
- Age appropriate sexual behavior is an important but not totally specific clue.
- Most important element of the diagnosis is the disclosure and therefore depends heavily on our ability to speak with children.

Adverse behavioral

Have you ever seen someone playing with a child and felt uncomfortable about it? Maybe you thought "I'm just over-reacting", or "He really doesn't mean that" Don't ignore the behavior; learn how to ask questions about what you have seen. The checklist below offers some warning signs:

Do you know an adult or older child who:
- Shows undue attention toward a child

- Insists on hugging, touching, kissing, tickling, wrestling with or holding a child even when the child does not want this affection
- Is overly interested in the sexuality of a particular child (talks repeatedly about the child's developing body)
- Constantly maneuvers to get time alone or insists on time alone with a child
- Spends most of his/ her spare time with children and has little interest in spending time with someone their own age
- Buys children expensive gifts or gives them money for no apparent reason
- Frequently intrudes a child's privacy, for instance walks in on the child in the bathroom.
- Allows children to consistently get away with undisciplined behavior.

Helping a victim[1]

When a child discloses that she or he has been sexually abused, she or he is entrusting you with a part of her life that is painful, frightening and vulnerable. It is important to refer the child to a well-trained professional person who has been trained to handle such case. Timely medical examination, specially testing and treating sexually transmitted disease is as important as counseling and emotional rehabilitation.

Ideally the perpetrator should be reported and legal process set in motion. As per the Bill of 2011 it is mandatory to report, and this may be difficult because when sexual abuse is committed by a family member the parents will be reluctant to make it a police case. All efforts should be made to remove the child from a surrounding that is a risk for further abuse.

Role of parents, teachers and other caregivers in preventing child abuse sexual abuse

Based on informal studies by Tulir in India it is estimated that 30% of the children will experience some form of sexual abuse, assault, or exploitation before they reach the age of 18 years.[21]

Most cases of child abuse occur because adults are failing in their duty toward protection of children. It is every ones duty to give children age appropriate sex education and make children aware of what is good touch and bad touch, so that they are aware of important facts of sexual abuse and are able to protect themselves. Simple instructions like saying NO shout for help and inform trusted adults are important to be imbibed 'Children should be listened to when they report abuse even if it is from a well-known member of the community, teaching institution or an important member of the family. Most often children are not believed or silenced. It is also very difficult for them to report somebody whom they love or are in a position of authority. Adults who indulge in child sexual abuse use a lot of tricks to first trick the victim and then use threats to keep continuing the abuse. It is important to prevent sexual abuse as it often leaves a child scarred for life. But equally important is rehabilitation of child after a child is subjected to sexual abuse. They need to be freed from the guilt, shame and helped to start a new life leaving behind the trauma.[21]

Important messages for personal safety[1]

- Self–esteem should be built in every child. Children with good self-esteem better able to protect themselves against abuse
- They should become assertive and learn various methods to say NO
- They should learn to say NO to sexual advances made by anyone both known and unknown
- Adults should give children age appropriate information about sexuality and, skills, to prevent abuse
- They should learn to protect their body and explain to them that no one has a right to touch them in any inappropriate fashion. This rule applies to even near and dear ones
- They should not become friendly with strangers and get tempted by chocolates, toys and other things
- They should never keep secrets with other people apart from parents
- They should not feel guilty or ashamed of the acts done to them. the offender is to blame not them.

Adapted from *Tulir Centre for Prevention and Healing of Child Sexual Abuse, Chennai, India.*[21]

Role of NGOs[21-26]

- These play a very useful/effective role in coordinating with police, legal system, community health facilities

- May give shelter to these adolescent children and act as a bond between these victims and their relatives
- If parents refuse these adolescent children, these NGOs may have to give emotional support, medical support and rehabilitate them
- There is need for a No Objection Certificate taken from the concerned education authority in cases any external agency/volunteer seeking to conduct any programme in schools
- There is need to implement life skill education in all the educational institutions and personal safety teaching
- All education/residential institutions should have a counselor/child psychologist/social worker and a grievance box should be placed in all above institutions.

Summary

- Child sexual abuse (CSA) violates a child's fundamental human rights and has an adverse effect on their emotional and psychological development which can last throughout their life time
- Schools and teachers have an important role to play in prevention, detection and management for CSA victims and are crucial in breaking this cycle of violence and preventing further physical and emotional damage to the child
- Children should be given age appropriate sexuality education and empowered to understand and develop skills to protect themselves from CSA. Parents and schools have a major role in imparting this education
- All care takers should receive education and training to detect, prevent and deal with CSA.

Acknowledgement and permissions

Some material in this chapter has been reproduced with permission from the chapter on Sexual Abuse in children and adolescents by Agarwal Kiran and Bhave Swati Y., Bhave's Text book of Adolescent medicine—Chief editor Dr Swati Y Bhave 1st edition. Jaypee brothers medical publishers New Delhi.

References

1. Agarwal Kiran, Bhave Swati Y Sexual abuse in children & adolescents. In Bhave's Text book of Adolescent Medicine 1st Ed. New Delhi: Jaypee brothers Medical Publishers; 2006

2. 'The Protection of Children from Sexual Offences Bill, 2011', Bill No. XIV of 2011as introduced in the Rajya Sabha, Shrimati Krishna Tirath, Minister of state in the Ministry of Women and Child Development. http://www.prsindia.org/billtrack/the-protection-of-children-from-sexual-offences-billtext.pdf, accessed September 01, 2012.

3. Damodaran Andal (VP Indian Council for Child Welfare, Tamil Nadu, India). Overview of Asia Pacific Region-recognition of CSA as a societal problem, prevalence, and steps to develop systems of response-challenges and good initiatives. APCCAN-2011, New Delhi.

4. Ministry of Women and Child Development Government of India. Study on Child Abuse India 2007. A report prepared by Dr. Loveleen Kacker, IAS, Srinivas Varadan, Pravesh Kumar: 17: 71–102.

5. The National Human Rights Commission Report on Trafficking in women and children 2003. Available from UR htt://www.nhrc.in/documents/reportontraffickinginwomenandchildren2003.pdf. Accessed on September 01, 2012.

6. The National Crime Records Bureau Report 2011. Available from URL: http://ncrb.gov.in. Accessed on August 31st, 2012.

7. The Forum against Child Sexual Exploitation (FACSE). Available from URL: www.facse.com. Accessed on August 31st, 2012.

8. http://itannu.wordpress.com/2012/05/16/child-sexual-abuse-in-india/TNN May 23, 2012, 04.47AM IST.

9. Shonali Prakash: I love daddy, but I hate him. Health, The Week, August 26, 2012: 18–27.

10. Roland C Summit. The child abuse accommodation syndrome. Child Abuse and Neglect, 1983; 17:177–193.

11. D Pagare; "A study of physical & sexual abuse and behavioural problems amongst boys in a child observation home in Delhi". MD Thesis, University of Delhi 2004. Guides: Dr. G S Meena, Dr. Malti Mehra, Dr. R. C. Jiloha, Dr. M. M. Singh, Department of Community Medicine, Maulana Azad Medical College, New Delhi.

12. Reducing risk behavior related to HIV/AIDS, STDs and drug abuse. (1996) Jyoti Mehra (Ed).National report, NACO,UNDCP,UNICEF,WHO.

13. Pandhi RK, Khanna K, Sekhri R. STD in children. Indian Pediatr 1995; 32(1).

14. Hindustan Times, N.Delhi, Sept. 5, 2005- Juvenile rapists claim innocence wish they could turn clock back.

15. National Clearing House on Child Abuse and Neglect Information, U.S.A.

16. Sgroi, Handbook of Clinical Intervention in child sexual abuse. Lexington books, Lexington, MA,1982.

17. D. Finkelhor, "What's Wrong With Sex between Adults and Children," *American Journal of Orthopsychiatry* 49 (1979): 692–697. Forum against Child Sexual Exploitation (FACSE)

18. Brown A. and Finkelhor D. (1986) "Initial and long-term effects:" A review of the research in D. Finkelhor (Ed.). A source book on childhood sexual abuse. Beverly Hills, CA: Sage, pp: 143–179.

19. Finkelhor D, Sourcebook on Child Sexual Abuse.

20. National Campaign against Child Sexual Abuse (Human Rights Law Network).Available on URL:http://hrln.org. Accessed on August 31st, 2012.

21. Courtesy data available from Tulir Centre for the prevention and healing of child sexual abuse, Chennai, India.

22. Conte J. R. Wolf. S. and Smith T. What sexual offenders tell us about prevention strategies. Child Abuse and Neglect 1989; 13:293–301.

23. Hobbs J. C., Hanks H. G. and Wynne J. M. (1993) Child Abuse and Neglect: A Clinician's handbook. Edinburgh, Churchill Livingstone.

24. Adol Sexual Abuse – Course Manual for Adol Health Part II Indian Perspective (IAP-ITPAH).

25. Seshadri S., Ganesh A. and Kumar L. (1994) Childhood sexual abuse of girls, Bangalore, India. Report published by SAMVADA.

26. ISPCAN "World Perspective on Child Abuse 2004" – Defining child maltreatment in India (India report).

27. F. Porter, L. Blick, and S. Sgroi, "Treatment of the Sexually Abused Child," in S. Sgroi, ed., *Handbook of Clinical Intervention in Child Sexual Abuse* (Lexington, MA: Lexington Books, 1982), 109–146.

28. The Velvet Blouse. Sexual exploitation of children. National commission for Women, Government of India, 1997.

8

Medical Evaluation of Child Sexual Abuse

Martin A Finkel

Introduction

Few forms of child maltreatment are as challenging for the clinician than evaluating the child suspected of being sexually abused. As in all forms of child abuse understanding a child's experience requires the collective insights of the disciplines of medicine, child protection, law enforcement and mental health to fully appreciate what the child experienced and to be able to assess the impact of that experience. If one considers a suspicion or allegation of sexual abuse a puzzle than it is readily apparent that there are many pieces to the puzzle. Unlike physical maltreatment where the child presents with a physical injury, something that can be seen directly with the naked eye or through imaging sexually abused children infrequently present with physical signs of genital, anal or extra-genital trauma. Sexually transmitted infections are found in approximately 3% of cases and forensic evidence is rarely found after 24 hours if at all.[1,2] It is precisely the absence of physical findings and laboratory results that makes the diagnosis so challenging for the clinician.

The reality is that sexual victimization of children remains a significant societal issue and primary care clinicians are on the forefront when it comes to responding to a concern of sexual abuse. Child sexual abuse (CSA) cases represent approximately 9% of the case load of child protective services (CPS) in the United States and does not represent the universe of abuse but rather cases that come to the attention of CPS for a variety of reasons.[3] Population surveys of adults reflect that 1 in 4 girls and 1 and 7 boys have experienced some form of sexually inappropriate contact by the age of 18 years.[4] In the United States the national trends suggest that there is an deceasing prevalence of CSA. The reasons for such are not clear although may be related to public awareness of the legal implications of sexual abuse and prevention efforts which have dramatically increased over the last 20 years.[5] Although there has been this trend in the US, in those countries where the issue of CSA is just being addressed and little is known about actual prevalence it may be some time before public awareness and systems responses will be sufficient to reduce sexual victimization. Regardless CSA will continue to be a societal problem and all professionals need to develop the requisite skills to respond to the investigative, protection, medical and mental needs of child victims. Primary care clinicians, schools and the community at large have a responsibility to provide anticipatory guidance regarding children's rights to personal space and privacy as a step toward primary prevention.

Role of the health care professional

The health care professional should play an important role in the prevention and detection of child sexual abuse. It is incumbent on health care professionals to educate caretakers and patients in age appropriate ways about personal space and privacy, OK and not OK touching, teach the appropriate names for private parts so children have the language to communicate, encourage age appropriate independence in regard to bathing and anogenital care. All of these issues make up the cornerstones of primary prevention that should be integrated into our routine anticipatory guidance. As pediatricians we have all assumed the responsibility to provide anticipatory guidance regarding back to sleep safety, car safety, bicycle safety, water safety, environmental safety and it is now time to address the issue of personal space and privacy as soon as children are young enough to begin to take responsibility for their own genital/ perianal care and bath themselves. Children should be taught the appropriate names for their private parts rather than the silly names that are frequently used so they have the language to communicate clearly using the appropriate terms what they may have experienced if touched inappropriately. Pediatricians have an ideal opportunity to provide anticipatory guidance during a child's annual physical and just before conducting an anogenital examination. Prior to conducting the anogenital examination the doctor can determine the names they use for their private parts, talk about okay and not okay touching, instruct on what to do if touched or made to do something inappropriate. Once this has been discussed the doctor can then explain the need to proceed with the anogenital examination. By routinely incorporating the anogenital examination as a part of the annual physical the doctor increase their comfort level and experience in identify problems and variations of normal anatomy. The pediatrician also demonstrates to the parent and child the importance of an examination of the private parts and the examination becomes an expectation just as listening to a child's heart.

In United States less than 10% of suspected sexual abuse cases are reported to child protective services (CPS) by medical professionals.[3] The response of the medical professional to concerns of possible sexual abuse will be slightly different depending on whether they are a primary care provider, a child abuse specialist, an emergency room physician, school nurse or nurse practitioners where they practice independently. The primary care provider can best serve their patients needs by identifying specialists in their community that are experienced in diagnosing and treating sexual abuse. The decision as to whether a child undergoes an immediate examination following disclosure is best determined by simply asking when was the last time something happened.[6]

The traditional window regarding the potential to identify acute signs of injury and collect forensic evidence is 72 hours. Most children who disclose sexual abuse do so long after the last contact and infrequently present with acute signs of trauma. The response by the primary care doctor who receives a call from a caretaker expressing a concern for sexual abuse should not be one of simply sending the patient to an emergency room but rather asking some screening questions that help in triaging the case; When was the last contact with the alleged perpetrator?, Does the child have any anogenital complaints and is the child safe.

If there is no need for an immediate examination based on the screening questions and the child is safe the most appropriate step is to make a referral to CPS/LE and then make arrangements for follow-up comprehensive medical evaluation by a community specialist. In those case where the history suggests the contact was recent and there is the potential to identify "evidence" than an immediate referral is made for a medical examination.

Clinical presentation of suspected child sexual abuse

Medical professionals are in a position where they will need to respond to the concern of possible sexual abuse in the context of the following possible scenarios;

1 A disclosure in the context of providing anticipatory guidance regarding body safety,
2 A caretaker expresses concerns about possible sexual abuse because of their child's behaviors, anogenital complaints, direct observation or a response to direct questions,
3 Physical examinations findings (genital, anal, extragenital) reflective of acute or healed trauma, a sexually transmitted infection (STI) or pregnancy in an adolescent.

Conceptually disclosures of sexual abuse can be broadly categorized as occurring as the result of: (i) a purposeful disclosure, (ii) an accidental disclosure or (iii) an elicited disclosure.[7] Each of these disclosure scenarios occurs for different reasons which are important to understand. Purposeful disclosures occur because the child has made a conscious decision to tell because they want the abuse to stop, fearful that the activities will progress over time, that other individuals many times siblings or cousins are considered at risk if they don't tell, worries about their body, they no longer can keep their feelings inside or other permutations and combinations of these factors.

Purposeful disclosures in many ways are the optimal type of disclosure in great part because they allow for planned intervention. Once reported the focus shifts to understanding what the child experienced, assessing non-offending parental support to assure protection and scheduling of the medical examination in the right environment in a non emergent manner.

Accidental disclosures by definition imply that neither the child nor the perpetrator was prepared to share the "secret" and thus have the potential to precipitate a crisis. When an accidental disclosure occurs an appropriate response must be mobilized with a primary focus on making sure the alleged perpetrator has no contact with the child to avoid threats, intimidation or attempts to undermine the credibility of the child and assure safety. Elicited disclosures occur as a result of a variety of circumstances which might include a behavioral observation, a limited statement by child that raises a concern, a physical sign or symptom, discovery of a written statement in perhaps a diary, high-risk behaviors and/or caretakers intuition that results in someone asking a probative question that raises either further suspicion or confirms concern and that leads to a report.

Making a decision to report

Reporting is easiest when the presenting concerns are clear and unambiguous. In circumstances in which there is uncertainty as to whether to report it is advisable to call the CPS screening unit and presents the concerns and ask for advice.

Not uncommonly parents will raise concerns which are vague and will require some degree of probative questioning to clarify the basis of the concern and determine whether the threshold to report is met. The challenge for the clinician is that it is not typically one piece of information that will confirm a concern but rather a combination of history, behavioral changes, psychological and/or physical signs and symptoms that must be considered collectively.[6]

Once a decision to report is made than a decision regarding the place for and timing of a comprehensive medical evaluation must be made. It is particularly important to attempt to minimize

the number of physical examinations a child must undergo and every attempt should be made to assure that the initial examination will address the child's medical needs. Follow-up examinations will be necessary if a child experiences physical trauma to observe and document the healed residual and to assure effective treatment for a sexually transmitted infection.

Medical evaluation

All children who CPS and/or law enforcement are investigating for the concern of possible sexual abuse should have a comprehensive medical evaluation. Some CPS/LE professionals erroneously believe that children should only be referred for medical examinations if there is the potential to collect "evidence". The purpose of the medical examination from a health care providers perspective is that medical examination is justifiable for two primary purposes. (i) To diagnose and treat any effect from the sexual contact which can simply be said for "abnormality" and (ii) for the purpose of assuring physical intactness and well being best referred to as "normality". Whether the examination is conducted for either the purpose of diagnosing abnormality or normality the examination should be of great therapeutic value to the child and caretaker.[8]

It is important that CPS/LE are aware of how the medical examination will be conducted so they can explain to the caretakers the reasons for the examination and that it is not something that will be traumatic to their child but potentially of great value.

In the context of the medical history an important question for all children to be asked is whether they have any worries or concerns about their body because of what they experienced. When given an opportunity to respond to the question of worries about their body children frequently express idiosyncratic concerns about their body that add credibility to the history and reflect concerns that speak to the reality of the psychological impact of their experience.

Obtaining a medical history when sexual abuse is suspected

The most available form of "evidence" in cases of child sexual abuse is what the child has to say. This "verbal evidence" can best be obtained within the context of the doctor taking a medical history from the child. After all it is the child who knows what they experienced. It is incumbent on the doctor to know how to obtain a detailed medical history in a manner that is non-leading, not suggestive, empathetic, non-judgmental and facilitating. Ideally when the medical history is obtained from the child it should be done independent of any accompanying caretaker. Children may be reluctant to share specific details about the sexual interactions in front of their caretaker in great part because of embarrassment, shame, culpability or simply they don't want their parent to be upset. The information skillfully obtained during the medical history from the child will be quantitatively and qualitatively different than the information they are likely to share with CPS or law enforcement. There is a special relationship that children have with a doctor, a relationship of confidence and trust that doctors can help. As many a child has said; "I can tell you because you're a doctor."[9]

The ability to obtain a history of any "disease" entity begins with understanding how a given disease unfolds clinically. Sexual victimization of children is not a capricious activity but follows a well understood conceptual framework. The medical history should attempt to obtain details that reflect each of the components of the "disease." The work of Finkelhor & Browne and Summit have helped to articulate the nature of sexual victimization of children and the sometimes idiosyncratic and un-intuitive nature of this form of victimization.[10,11] The most difficult challenge for the doctor is not the anogenital examination but rather the ability to conduct a medical history in a developmentally appropriate manner that obtains information about events that are inherently embarrassing and for which children may express shame and fear of consequences of disclosure.

Preparing the child for the medical history

When meeting with the child for the first time attempt to engage the child in conversation that is introductory and explains who you are and what you do. Ask the child if they know why they are here to see you. If based on the preliminary history it is not anticipated that there will be a need for blood work or procedures which are physically intrusive let the child know. Children are particularly fearful of needles and telling them that there won't be any shots or needles will immediately decrease their anxiety. If the child states that they don't know why they came then a statement such as "My name is Dr. .... and I am a kids doctor. One of the things I do that is different than most kids doctors is every day. I have a chance to talk to and examine kids just like them when there is a worry that they may have had something happen to them that could be confusing or difficult to understand by someone they know and should trust. That happens to a lot of kids and I understand that happened to you. Is that true?"[8] This introductory statement is modified based on preliminary details available.

A response to the child's acknowledgement that something happened could be; "Most kids don't tell about those things why did you decide to tell?" Children who experience sexual abuse are not provided an opportunity to consent to the sexual activities yet many times responsible for their own victimization. Therefore, it is important to ask questions to find out who they think is responsible for what had happened to them and if they think it is their fault then this should be addressed. Because the medical evaluation should be therapeutic for the child always ask: "Do you have any worries or concerns about your body because of what happened or what you had to do?" This question frequently provides insight into alterations of body image or concerns about body intactness and/or sexually transmitted infections. If the child doesn't express any concerns one can state; "Some kids have expressed worries about... do you have any of those worries?"

The following represents areas of the medical history that should be addressed with the child and can result in a much more complete understanding of the child's experience.

1. Circumstances and reasons surrounding disclosure
2. Access and opportunity for the alleged perpetrator to have contact with the child
3. Details of the first inappropriate sexual interactions and the progression of the sexual contact over time. Specific questions regarding genital-urinary and gastrointestinal signs and symptoms temporally associated with the specific sexual contact
4. Statements made to the child regarding secrecy, threats and intimidation and/or child's perceived consequences

5. Worries or concerns about body image
6. Questions that elicit specific details surrounding sexual interactions with a focus on signs and symptoms that may have medical significance and provide insight into the potential for physical injury or contracting an STD
7. Questions that clarify child's perception of the interaction particularly around the issue of penetration
8. Exposure to pornography or having photographs taken of them
9. Recantation.

Documentation of the medical history

Just as it is important to ask questions in a manner that is appropriate it is equally important to preserve the medical history obtained from the child in a manner that is an accurate reflection of what the child said. It is unacceptable to simply ask questions, listen to the child's response and then record one's recollection of that history or to summarize the clinical history. Although time intensive it is best to record in writing the exact questions asked of the child and the child's verbatim response. All records, notations should be both available and legible in the medical record. It is these notes that are used to formulate a type written report for the medical record and/or consulting entity.[12,13]

Physical examination

All children who are suspected of experiencing inappropriate sexual contact deserve a comprehensive medical evaluation. Most examinations can be completed in a non-emergent fashion in a comfortable and appropriate setting as most kids do not disclose immediately following sexual contact. Children whenever possible should experience only one physical examination by a skilled individual who is familiar with the special needs of child victims and has the time and sensitivity to conduct the examination in a manner that can be not only medically complete but therapeutic for the child. With few exceptions children should be seen by clinicians who will conduct a head to toe examination and not just a genital examination. Head to toe examinations in addition to providing a message to the child that all parts of their body are important also allow for the identification of extra-genital trauma.

An emergent examination is justifiable under the following circumstances:

1. Complaints of genital and/or anal discomfort
2. History of genital/anal bleeding
3. Last contact within 72 hours and potential to identify and collect biological fluids that may have been transferred
4. Need for medical intervention such as pregnancy prophylaxis, treatment for STI's and repair of injuries
5. To meet the emotional needs of the child/caretaker and to assure safety

Positioning the child

The genital examination in the female prepubertal child is conducted in the supine frog leg position as well as the knee chest position which provides an alternative view of the hymenal membrane. The knee chest position is awkward for children but can be particularly helpful when the child's hymen is redundant. The knee chest examination should be routine to confirm any physical findings observed in the supine frog leg position that the clinicians interprets as a diagnostic finding. On occasion concerning physical findings in the frog leg position will appear normal or persist confirming the observed finding. In the prepubertal child positioning along with the use of the simple technique of labial separation and traction is all that is generally necessary to visualize all aspects of the hymenal membrane. The hymen in prepubertal children is exquisitely sensitive to the touch and the use of a Q-tip to probe the tissue is not indicated. Instilling warm water or saline into the vestibule can help to reduce the cohesive forces of the moist tissues and in effect unfold the adhered membrane resulting in more complete visualization of the membrane edge. Speculum examinations are not indicated in prepubertal children except under the infrequent circumstance where the child has significant genital trauma and is being examined under anesthesia to assess the extent of the intra vaginal trauma or remove a foreign body.

The perianal area of the male or female child can be examined by having the child flex their legs onto the abdomen followed by a simple separation of the buttocks. An acceptable alternative approach is to examine the perianal area is the lateral decubitus position.

In the pubertal child the knee chest position is not routinely utilized as the position of choice for the female genital examination is the supine lithotomy position. In the lithotomy position with the use of labial separation and labial traction it is possible to visualize all the structures of the vaginal vestibule including the edge of the hymenal membrane circumferentially. Because the hymenal membrane of the pubertal child is estrogenized the tissue becomes redundant and elastic. The redundant folds of the hymen may create the impression that there could be an interruption in the integrity of the hymenal membrane edge as the result of blunt force penetrating trauma. To fully visualize the edge and differentiate initial observations that could be interpreted as abnormal the edge must be visualized completely and the use of a saline moistened Q-tip to unfold the edge of the hymen that follows the edge circumferentially can be helpful. The decision to use a vaginal speculum to examine the cervix and the posterior portion of the vagina is determined on a case by case basis. If the clinical history suggests vaginal penetration in a pubertal child then with the adolescents' cooperation a speculum examination is warranted and provides for more complete assessment for sexually transmitted infections.

Most female examinations following genital to genital contact in the prepubertal child will not demonstrate any acute physical findings. Prepubertal children who experience genital to genital contact do so generally within the vaginal vestibule and do not experience penetration into the vagina per se. Prepubertal children who experience true vaginal penetration will likely demonstrate healed residual generally in the form of a hymenal transaction. Once a child is pubertal the hymen develops elasticity and distensibility that makes it very difficult to determine if the child has experienced vaginal penetration unless the exam is done acutely.[14,15]

Sexual activities may include anal penetration in either males or females with genitalia or a foreign body. Depending upon the degree of force, the use of lubrication and the "cooperativeness" of the victim there is a spectrum of residual from none to significant trauma. In addition to anal trauma there may also be frictional trauma to the tissues of the gluteal cleft when a penis is rubbed between the buttocks. The degree to which more than external visualization of the external sphincter is necessary will be determined by the child's history. Anoscopy or sigmoidoscopy is most likely to be needed in acute cases where there is concern for the assessment of internal trauma than extends beyond the external sphincter.

Residual to oral genital contact is not common but when present following fellatio may be observed as palatal petechiae and/or contusion with or without labial frenulum tears. The likelihood of positive findings in the oral cavity is directly related to the degree of force used. Bite, suction or pinch marks may be seen on the penis. Extragenital trauma in the form of ligature, hand marks, bite marks or concomitant residual to physical abuse may be observed on the skin.

Less than 5 % of all children will have physical findings that on their own are diagnostic.[16,17,18] Of all the factors to consider the single most important factor in most cases that can lead to substantiation is the child's medical history. The clinician can enhance the diagnostic certainty of inappropriate sexual contact in girls by focusing the medical history on eliciting historical details regarding signs and symptoms temporally related to the sexual contact for which the child would have no alternative way of knowing other than experiencing such. DeLago et al. found that in a 2008 study of 161 girls between 3 and 18 years that 60% of the girls experienced one or more symptoms/signs with 53% of the sample complaining of genital pain, 37% dysuria and 11% bleeding following sexual contact with no alternative explanation and the direct result of the genital contact. Forty eight percent of girls who reported genital to genital contact had dysuria compared to 25% not reporting genital–genital contact, 72% complained of genital pain/soreness compared to 32% not reporting genital to genital contact, and 16% had bleeding compared to 4% of those not reporting genital-genital contact.[19] This study emphasizes the importance of a detailed medical history from the child.

Enhanced visualization and visual documentation of physical findings

Increasingly the use of colposcopy has become standard practice when examining the genital and anal tissues of children evaluated for possible sexual abuse. Colposcopy as applied to the examination of children is the adaptation of this gynecologic instrument to provide a magnified view which can result in improved definition of acute or healed injuries that are otherwise difficult to fully appreciate with the naked eye. Colposcopes differ in their magnification capability but generally vary from 3.75 to 25X depending upon the manufacturer. The instrument is non-invasive and when equipped with a video feed allows the examiner and the patient to observe the examination on a video monitor. The child's ability to observe the examination can help demystify what is occurring and provide the child with a sense of participation and control throughout and facilitate cooperativeness of the patient. The colposcope is equipped with a "red free" filter which appears as a green light and enhances the visualization of acute mucosal injuries and healed injuries.

Digital photographs and/or HD video documentation should always be obtained in circumstances in which there is a physical finding that will be interpreted as diagnostic and be used to formulate an opinion. By doing this the child will not require a repeat examination should there be a challenge to the interpretation of a finding when an expert is asked to provide a second opinion. Instead the expert can review the image of the finding(s) initially observed. Alternatives to visual documentation with a colposcope include hand held digital still and/or video cameras. When children have physical examination findings that are non-diagnostic yet they remain at risk it is reasonable to either record the examination on video or obtain still images of the genitalia/anus for future reference if there is a concern. The visual documentation of examinations also allows for peer review or consultation.

Sexually transmitted infections

When children experience inappropriate sexual contact they are also at risk for acquiring a sexually transmitted infection (STI).[20] The spectrum of STI's includes *Neisseria gonorrhea, Chlamydia* trachomatis, *Trichomonas vaginalis*, herpes simplex virus, human papillomavirus (HPV), syphilis, hepatitis and human immunodeficiency virus (HIV). Beyond the perinatal period when children present with clinical findings of an STI the obvious implication is that the child came in contact with infected genital secretions. Young children who acquire a STI can be a challenge in understanding how they acquired the infection as they require genital/perianal care and may not be sufficiently verbal to provide a history that explains the mode of transmission. It is well documented that caretakers can transmit the common HPV responsible for the common hand wart to the perianal area in the process of caretaking. When HPV presents in children who do not require genital/anal care tracking the mode of transmission may be difficult because of the time interval between contact with the virus and the clinical appearance of warts which can be at a minimum of 3 months. A popular yet scientifically unsupported mode of transmission of STI's is through innocent contact with infected secretions from inanimate objects such as toilet seats or through co-bathing/shared wash cloth. Fomites remain a mode of transmission that requires further research. For the clinician sometimes it is difficult in spite of thorough investigations to understand how usually younger children acquire an STI.

When a child is being evaluated for possible sexual abuse the clinician must make a decision regarding screening and/or treating for STI's. In the prepubertal child STI's have a low prevalence rate and the decision to screen or treat is tailored to the presenting history. The clinician obtains and weighs information regarding the type of sexual contact and the risk for transmission of a STI, offender's history of STI when available, physical signs and symptoms and the time interval between last sexual contact when making a decision to screen and/or treat presumptively. As a general rule prepubertal children are not routinely screened nor presumptively treated but rather decisions to screen and/or treat are individually tailored. Adolescents are potentially at greater risk for acquiring a STI if their victimization has contributed to the child engaging in high-risk behaviors with other sexual partners. Just as in the prepubertal child decisions to screen and/or treat are individually tailored. When the offender is a stranger and the history suggests contact with potentially infected genital secretions screening and presumptive treatment including HIV prophylaxis is warranted. The American Academy of Pediatrics (AAP) Red Book and the Center for Disease Control (CDC) guidelines for screening, testing and treatment should be referenced for the most up-to-date clinical information.[21]

Formulation of a medical diagnosis of child sexual abuse

The medical diagnosis is the work product of a comprehensive medical assessment of the child alleged to have been sexually abused. As such, the diagnosis must be formulated in a manner that is clear, educative to those who utilize the opinion, balanced and defensible.[12,22] The clinician should prepare every report anticipating the potential that CPS and/or law enforcement will request an expert opinion which then leads to the potential for an appearance in court. When called to court the clinician plays an important role in explaining the basis of one's opinion and the science that supports such. When formulating the diagnostic assessment, the clinician must consider and incorporate salient aspects of each of the following:

- Historical details and behavioral indicators
- Symptoms and signs that result from the contact
- Acute genital/anal injuries and/or chronic residual
- Forensic evidence
- Sexually transmitted diseases.

The clinician's written report in addition to providing the diagnosis also allows for an opportunity to explain why discrepancies can exist between the child's perceptions of what he or she experienced and why physical examination findings might not be present, the healing of injuries and the significance of specific historical details provided by the child. Recommendations for further laboratory testing, treatment of STI's, follow-up examinations should be noted.

For every child who has experienced sexual abuse the primary impact is psychological and the clinician should provide recommendations for a complete psychological assessment of the impact of the child's experience which then serves as the basis for therapeutic intervention that follows. There is now a body of evidence based literature known as Trauma Focused Cognitive Behavioral Therapy (TF-CBT) which when used by mental health clinicians has been demonstrated to provide objective and measurable therapeutic outcomes for children who experience sexual abuse.[23,24]

Conclusion

The medical provider plays an important role in diagnosing and treating children suspected of sexual abuse. The medical literature which provides the science behind our understanding of the diagnosis of sexual abuse has mushroomed over the last 30 years and continues to evolve contributing to the refinement of our diagnostic acumen, our understanding of the therapeutic needs of children and our ability to provide recommendations to colleague in child protection to assure the safety and continued well-being of children. Sexual abuse continues to be a serious threat to the emotional health and development of children. We all have a responsibility to learn more about early recognition and double our efforts to provide anticipatory guidance to children regarding their right to personal space and privacy and the prevention of sexual abuse. This chapter serves as an introduction to understanding and addressing the medical diagnostic and therapeutic needs of children suspected to experience sexual abuse.

References

1. Christian CW, Lavelle JM, De Jong AR, Loiselle J, Brenner L, Joffe M. Forensic evidence findings in prepubertal victims of sexual assault. Pediatrics 2000; 106(1 Pt 1):100–4.

2. Siegel RM, Schubert CJ, Myers PA, Shapiro RA. The prevalence of sexually transmitted diseases in children and adolescents evaluated for sexual abuse in Cincinnati: rationale for limited STD testing in prepubertal girls. Pediatrics 1995; 96(6):1090–4.

3. US Department of Health and Human Services, Adminis-tration for Children, Youth and Families, Children's Bureau. Child Maltreatment 2010; 2011.

4. Finkelhor D, Hotaling G, Lewis IA, Smith C. Sexual abuse in a national survey of adult men and women: prevalence, characteristics, and risk factors. Child Abuse & Neglect 1990; 14(1):19–28.

5. Finkelhor,D., Jones, L. and Kopiec, K. Why is Sexual Abuse Declining? A Survey of State Child Protection Administration. Child Abuse & Neglect, 2001; 25(9):1139–1158.

6. Kellogg N, American Academy of Pediatrics Committee on Child Abuse and N. The evaluation of sexual abuse in children. Pediatrics 2005; 116(2):506–12.

7. Alaggia R. Many ways of telling: expanding conceptuali-zations of child sexual abuse disclosure. *Child Abuse & Neglect*. 2004; 28(11):1213–1227.

8. Finkel MA. The Evaluation. In: Finkel MA, Giardino AP, eds. *Medical Evaluation of Child Sexual Abuse: A practical guide*. 3rd ed. Elk Grove Village, IL: American Academy of Pediatrics; 2009: 19–52.

9. Finkel, MA. "I can tell you because you're a doctor" *Pediatrics*, 2008; 122(8):422.

10. Finkelhor D, Browne A. The traumatic impact of child sexual abuse: a conceptualization. American Journal of Orthopsychiatry 1985; 55(4):530–41.

11. Summit RC. The child sexual abuse accommodation syndrome. Child Abuse & Neglect 1983; 7(2): 177–93.

12. Myers JEB. Legal issues in the medical evaluation of child sexual abuse. In: Finkel MA, Giardino AP, eds. *Medical Evaluation of Child Sexual Abuse: A practical guide*. 3rd ed. Elk Grove Village, IL: American Academy of Pediatrics; 2009: 313–340.

13. Finkel MA, Ricci LR. Documentation and Preservation of Visual Evidence in Child Abuse. Child Maltreatment 1997; 2(4):322–330.

14. Finkel MA. Physical Examination. In: Finkel MA, Giardino AP, eds. *Medical Evaluation of Child Sexual Abuse: A practical guide*. 3rd ed. Elk Grove Village, IL: American Academy of Pediatrics; 2009: 53–105.

15. Kellogg, ND, Menard, SW, Santos A. Genital anatomy in pregnant adolescents: "Normal" does not mean "Nothing Happened". *Pediatrics*. 2004; 113(1):e67–69.

16. Heger A, Ticson L, Velasquez O, Bernier R. Children referred for possible sexual abuse: medical findings in 2384 children. *Child Abuse and Neglect* 2002; 26:645–659.

17. Adams JA, Harper K, Knudson S, and Revilla J. Examination findings in legally confirmed child sexual abuse: It's normal to be normal. *Pediatrics*. 1994; 94:148–50.

18. Adams JA, Kaplan RA, Starling SP, Mehta NH, Finkel MA, Botash AS, Kellogg ND, Shapiro RA. Guidelines for medical care of children who may have been sexually abused. *J Pediatr Adoles Gyn*. 2007; 20(3):163–172.

19. DeLago C, Deblinger E, Schroeder C, Finkel MA. Girls who disclose sexual abuse: urogenital symptoms and signs after genital contact. *Pediatrics*. 2008; 122(2):e281–286.

20. Siegel RM, Schubert CJ, Myers PA, Shapiro RA. The prevalence of sexually transmitted diseases in children and adolescents evaluated for sexual abuse in Cincinnati: rationale for limited STD testing in prepubertal girls. *Pediatrics*. 1995; 96(6):1090–1094.

21. Centers for Disease Control. Sexual Assault or Abuse of Children. Sexually Transmitted Diseases Treatment Guidelines, 2010.

22. Finkel MA. Documentation, Report Formulation and Conclusions. In: Finkel MA, Giardino AP, eds. *Medical Evaluation of Child Sexual Abuse: A practical guide*. 3rd ed. Elk Grove Village, IL: American Academy of Pediatrics; 2009: 357–370.

23. Deblinger E, Mannarino AP, Cohen JA, Steer RA. A follow-up study of a multisite, randomized, controlled trial for children with sexual abuse-related PTSD symptoms. *J Am Acad Child Adolesc Psych*. 2006; 45(12):1474–1484.

24. Deblinger E, Steer RA, Lippmann J. Two-year follow-up study of cognitive behavioral therapy for sexually abused children suffering post-traumatic stress symptoms. *Child Abuse Neglect*. 1999; 23(12):1371–1378.

9

Child Trafficking in Asia-Pacific Countries

PM Nair

Introduction

Nothing debases, disempowers and demolishes human lives and dignity more than human trafficking, especially Child Trafficking (CT). It is the most hope hensible form of human abuse, neglect, exploitation of the individual.

Human trafficking is demand-driven. There is so much demand for children, both boys and girls and, therefore, CT is indeed a major organized crime and a major human rights violation across the world. Children, being more vulnerable than adults, are easy targets of human predators. They can be made to work even in the most difficult, obnoxious and hazardous situations where adult do not venture. Children are not aware of their rights and, therefore, their exploitation remains unnoticed. As a consequence, they are the ones who are more violated and exploited.

The investment, costs and the overheads are much less in children, than in to adults. Therefore, there is a huge economic gain in exploiting children than exploiting adults. Human predators capitalizing on child trafficking generate huge amount of funds which are neither unfathomed nor estimated. Therefore, child trafficking is indeed the gravest form of exploitation that we see in today's context. It is indeed a concern for all human beings, if one is human-rights oriented. If one is not part of the problem, one has to be part of the solution.

Dimensions of child trafficking

Generally speaking, CT can be classified into three categories:

- CT for commercial sexual exploitation
- CT for exploitative labor
- CT for other types of exploitation.

Trafficking for **sexual exploitation** could be brothel based and non-brothel based. CT can be for several exploitations which take please under he façade or legal activities like massage parlours, bar tending, tourist circuit, false marriages, pornography, etc.

Exploitative labor includes agricultural labor, industrial labor, domestic labor, labor for other entertainment businesses, trafficking for beggary, trafficking for couriering of drugs, arms, explosives, etc., trafficking for militancy, extremism, naxalism, etc.

Other types of CT include trafficking for organ sale, illegal adoption, etc.

The NHRC research[1] shows the following facts:

- Trafficking in children surpasses trafficking in adults
- Trafficking in children is the worst form of child exploitation, as it involves a 'basket of crimes' and Human rights violations
- The demand for children in trafficking increases every year
- There is a high demand for children in sexual exploitation, exploitative labor and all other types of exploitations
- Many children who are trafficked into exploitation continue be remain in exploiter even when they became adults
- The profit generated by traffickers by trafficking children is much more than that of adult trafficking

- The factors which push valuable children into trafficking include lack of awareness, illiteracy, lack of parental care and attention, poor or distorted law enforcement, lack of redressal of grievances, economic disparities in society and the patriarchal mindset prevalent in several sections society.

Regional trends of human trafficking

No place or region can be said to be free from child exploitation as it could be a source, transit area or demand area.

Europe and Central Asia

Intraregional trafficking is the major pattern reported for human trafficking in Europe and Central Asia. UNODC found that almost all of the countries in this region are both origin and destination countries for intraregional trafficking, except Tajikistan and Turkmenistan which are exclusively countries of origin for trafficking victims. The Eastern Europe and Central Asia region is not a major transregional destination, but victims originating from this region are identified in Western and Central Europe as well as neighboring Asian countries.

The majority of trafficking victims in Europe and Central Asia are adult women, and sexual exploitation is the most common form human trafficking in this region. However, trafficking for forced labor accounts for over one-third of the total number of victims identified by state authorities in Western and Central Europe as well as in Central Asia. Women and men are also exploited in domestic servitude and forced labor in agriculture, construction, fishery, manufacturing, and textile industries. Children are trafficked for the purposes of sexual exploitation, forced marriage and forced begging.

South Asia

UNODC's global report indicates that intraregional trafficking affects Nepal and Bangladesh as origins of trafficking victims and India as a destination country. The United States Department of State reports that Bangladeshi men and women willingly migrate to Middle Eastern and South Asian countries for work through recruiting agencies, and the recruitment fees contribute to the placement of workers in debt bondage or forced labor once overseas. Bangladesh and India also experience domestic trafficking.

Victims of trafficking in South Asian are mainly adult women and children of both sexes. Trafficking for sexual exploitation is again the most common form of trafficking reported, yet trafficking for domestic servitude and forced labor are equally prominent in the region. A significant number of forced labor cases in brick kilns, rice mills, agriculture, and embroidery factories are reported in India. Children are often trafficked for the purposes of sexual exploitation, forced marriage, forced begging, and forced labor in brick kilns, carpet-making factories, and domestic service. According to the US TIP Report, Afghan boys are promised enrollment in Islamic schools in Pakistan, but instead are trafficked to paramilitary training camps by extremist groups. In Nepal and Pakistan, one of the major forms of human trafficking is bonded labor.

East Asia and the pacific

UNODC reports that East Asian countries exhibit the most complex human trafficking flows as this region has the widest range of transregional trafficking between countries of origin and the destination of victims. For example, Thai victims are found in Southern Africa, Europe and the Middle East while Chinese victims are identified in Europe, the Middle East, the Americas and Africa. Intraregional trafficking is also a major issue as victims from the East countries are largely trafficked to Australia, Japan and Malaysia. Many countries within the East Asia region are countries of origin for trafficking victims.

Women and girls are the primary victims of trafficking in this region, particularly for the purpose of sexual exploitation and forced marriage. Men are also victims of trafficking. They willingly migrate for work in the region and are subsequently subjected to conditions of forced labor in the agriculture in the agriculture, construction, finishing, manufacturing, plantation, and service (hotels, restaurants, and bars) sectors. Children in this region are often trafficked for the purpose of sexual exploitation, domestic servitude, and forced begging.

Profiling a victim of CT

It is not possible to wholly fathom the mind of the victim. The trauma varies from victim to victim, depending on the circumstance to which he/she was exposed during and after trafficking. However, a profile of the general features would present the following:

- Displaced (from the community)
- Alienated (from near and dear ones)
- Isolated (from one's own environment)
- Physically assaulted/injured/wounded
- Raped or sexually assaulted/abused/violated
- Starved of proper food/food that one is used to or likes to have
- Starved of sleep and rest
- Deprived of normal routine that one was used to
- Infected with several diseases
- Deprived of hygiene
- Subjected to miscarriage/abortion
- Deprived of medical care and attention leading to further complications
- Debt bonded
- Intimidated
- Enslaved
- Deprived of entertainment
- Subjected to forceful addictions of tobacco, smoke, drugs, alcohol, spurious addictives, etc.
- Psychologically/emotionally disturbed, with thoughts and feelings such as:
  - Helplessness and withdrawal
  - Dissociation
  - Coping mechanism of normalization and shaping (the experience as something 'that has to happen')
  - Self-blame and identification with aggressor
  - Distraction
  - Foreshortened view of time
  - Subjected to psychiatric disorders, including post traumatic stress disorder, depressive disorder, dissociative disorder, psychotic disorder and eating disorder.

Discussions with survivors show that virgin girls have been subjected to a 'break in' process where the victim is raped and subjugated to sexual intercourse by the brothel manager or anybody in command and control of the brothel, as and when she is brought to the brothel. The **'hardening process'** involves psychological abuse, threats and intimidation which range from severe beating, gang rape, denial of food, to burning with cigarettes, etc. The sense of rejection, betrayal and numbness that a women or girl goes through is beyond comprehension. The girls succumb to this and accept prostitution as the way of life, as thus have no other choice. The case of victims trafficked for labor or other types of exploitation are no different. Several children trafficked for camel racing has broken limbs. Children have are deliberately maimed for begging. There have been instances of organ trafficking.

Missing children

One of the important dimensions of child abuse and neglect is that of missing children countries. police stations and statutory agencies; many times it is never reported. Therefore, the available data may be only a tip of the iceberg. The NHRC study (*op cit*) shows that children go missing mostly due to violations and exploitation at home, including neglect, lack of care and attention, etc. The response systems are also shockingly lopsided. A study for UNICEF, undertaken by Bhamathi in 1994, has pointed to the unknown and possible linkages between trafficking and missing children. The NHRC study shows that during the beginning of the century, 44000 children were reported missing in India, out of which 11000 are never traced, therefore, there is an area backlog of 11000 children who continued to remain untraced and in wilderness. Case-studies developed from different parts of the country showed that many such children reported missing were indeed trafficked and many were rescued after several months or years from different places of exploitation. The NHRC research uncovers the vicious linkage between the missing children and CT.

A study conducted by an NGO, Bachpan Bachao Andolan (BBA), released in 2011 shows that the average annual reporting of missing children has gone up to 1,20,000 and that among them 40,000 remain untraced. A comparison of the data presented in the NHRC study (2004) and the data of BBA study (2010) shows that in six year's time, the number of children reported to be missing has gone up three times. It is indeed an alarming number. The study also shows that the percentage of untraced children has also increased from 25% in the NHRC study period to 33% in the BBA study period. This shows that the response systems of tracing children have become more inefficient or are less concerned.

The existing response systems

The response to child trafficking and related issues in the Asia-Pacific region is uneven. Even within the countries, the situation is quite uneven. In fact, the response can be classified into two: the '**good part**' and the '**bad part**'.

1. Unfavorable Across the region the positive indicators are as follows:
   - Increased awareness of the public to child trafficking
   - Qualitative improvement in the response systems, at least at certain places
   - Synergy between law enforcement agencies and NGOs in addressing child trafficking
   - Involvement of corporate and business houses in prevention and protection processes
   - Judicial intervention and outreach with several judgment and pronouncements from the child rights perspective
   - Media attention to the issues of child rights has improved in some places
   - Budgetary support in addressing child trafficking, abuse and neglect has generally improved
   - Several UN agencies, especially UNICEF and UNODC have made strident initiatives in flagging the issues in the international and national agenda and facilitating positive action in addressing the problem
   - Several new dimensions in trafficking has been exposed
   - Research, both macro and micro, has been undertaken thus facilitating understanding of the core issues
   - The findings of research have made an impact in the response system
   - Synergy among the stakeholders has been instituted at several places, which has lead to addressing the issues in a holistic manner
   - The need for integrated action on all the three fronts, viz. **P**revention, **P**rotection and **P**rosecution has been recognized and is being implemented at least in certain places.

2. Unfavorable aspect:

   Despite all the improvements which have been noticed across the regions of the world, the problem of child trafficking persist. Major challenges and issues are as follows:
   - Lack of priority among the response systems
   - Lack of synergy among the various departments of government and among government sector and NGO
   - Lack of coordination between rescue and rehabilitation measures
   - Response systems are violative and unrefined, and lead to victimization of victims and exacerbation of the harm to the victims
   - Insensitive handling of the issues by all responders and lack of their training and orientation
   - Lack of resource materials and facilities in addressing the issues
   - Poor linkage between source and destination points
   - Anonymity of the offender
   - Nexus among the various offenders and responders.

The available research studies have brought out several reasons for Continuations and child trafficking.

- There is no voice for children except in certain islands of excellence, which are disparate and are not institutionalized.
- As more awareness and more attention have been bestowed on the issues of CT, it was observed that the problem of CT is graver, deeper and wider. The response systems are found to be irresponsive, delayed, callous, inadequate, violative and retrogressive. Therefore, the gap between the problem and the response has widened.
- Accountability mechanisms are bureaucratic, often toothless, serving political agenda and not a human rights agenda. They are often ill-equipped and ineffective. The following facts:
  - Served need explanation and thousands of children below 16 years are HIV positive and they are languishing in Homes without care and attention?
  - As per the law, rape of a child under 16 years entails the gravest penalty like life imprisonment in India, but the offenders are not brought to book.
  - About 100,000 children are reported missing every year in India and more than 40,000 of them remain untraced. the percentage of untraced children (to the number of those reported missing) has gone up to 33% during 2011 from 25% in 2004?

- A large number of cases of child sexual abuse (CSA) go unreported and untraced? My own research, shows that the police officers themselves have stated that more than 50% of the crime remains unreported (Ref.)
- Several crimes of CSA and commercial sexual exploitation (CSE) do not make headway as the medical reports are either not available or unduly delayed or are not in tune with the prosecution evidence?
- Sex ratio among children has been acutely skewed against girls and children despite all laws to prevent feticide, female infanticide, prenatal diagnostic tests, etc.
- Many 'marriage bureaus' have become 'trafficking bureaus' and are indulging in selling and buying of brides, forcing them to submit to 'multiple husbands' and are being traded and sold several times.
- Culturally sanctioned practices of child abuse and trafficking continue to exist despite legal provisions?

These questions emanating from the victims of CSA are only illustrative and not exhaustive. There are many more such questions which the child victims have and yet there is no institutionalized platform where these issues can be raised or redressed. We need to ponder as to how the existing institutions can be make accountable so that all such issues are addressed with celerity and certainty, and gravity that they deserve. We need to put in place an accountability mechanism and bring them to public glare, public debate and public scrutiny of all forms must be prevented. These are the questions that any child would like to ask to all the adults, all of us, those child protection is governace and involved in care as either parents or medical professionals or teachers or law enforcers or government servants or human rights activists and so on.

The role of media

The role of media in this context is extremely important. Media healthy constituted to the anti corruption crusade in during August 2011, drawing the attention of the whole world. Media has made tremendous impact in polity, economy, administration, development, defense management, etc. changes and dramatic turnarounds have been brought about by the media in several spheres of public concern. Unfortunately the field of CSA, remains a territory unchartered by the media. When will the media wake up to the distress calls from the children who have no voice? When will the media address the cause of 40,000 plus children who remain untraced every year? Will media address the concern of trafficked and exploited children in ensuring redressal of grievances? Will media help to address the issues of vulnerability in the interiors of the country, especially the tribal heartland where anti-socials entice, coerce and force them to join their stream and to take up serious crimes like waging war against the State or indulging in organized crimes like drug trafficking, arms trafficking, etc. We need to develop media involvement and media participation if we need to address such burning issues. We need to make it mandatory for the media to look into these concerns. We also need to bring in protocols for rights based reporting.

A vacuum of sorts

The intervention by the author in the interiors of the country, in different States, in addressing issues of national security, has shown that anti nationals prosper where the writ of the government does not run. At such places there is a vacuum. It is a vacuum of several constituents, the important ones being:

- Security vacuum
- Developmental vacuum
- Political vacuum.

There is a catch-22 situation as to which one should be or can be addressed first. And, indeed there is no panacea either. The fact of the matter is that one vacuum contributes or exacerbates the other. As a corollary, the positive improvement in one aspect has its positive reverberations on the other two. Therefore, it is better to start with any one of the three with an assurance that the other two aspects will be dove-tailed. Such a holistic approach can make a difference. However, in practice, it does not happen this way. There is neither synchronization nor cohesion among the stakeholders. Therefore, things deteriorate. This is obvious from the fact that many places are said to be 'liberated' in the interior parts of Indian heartland. The political vacuum can be addressed in many ways. The regular political process characterizing the democracy is indeed the final goal. Empowering people to raise their voice against exploitation, by anybody, is an essential ingredient of the political process. The principle of 'zero tolerance' to violations/exploitations/deprivation is the crux of the political awakening. Vulnerable children need to be identified and empowered so that such a process commences.

In this context the recruitment of vulnerable adolescents from certain naxal affected villages in different States in India, empowering, training and building their capacity to work as Security Guards and other unskilled or semi skilled vocation mostly at their door-steps, a process started by the author during 2011, is a good model in vogue. These adolescents and children would have been trafficked into commercial sexual exploitation and into militancy. However, making use of the government funds in the right direction and by networking with NGOs and local public leaders, hundreds of such vulnerable male and female adolescents and children were identified trained and employed as Security Guards. They are now living a life of dignity and are not available for exploitation. They have empowered themselves, their family, their community and thereby the nation. A small step to start with, but with a great potential to grow into a giant stride in bringing about public safety and security. The vacuum, mentioned earlier, has been addressed at least at the lowest level. Of course, this and similar efforts need to be replicated. This momentum can generate into a revolution which would bridge the gap and fill the vacuum for all the time to come.

Role of medical professionals in anti human trafficking

Though the role of medical professionals in AHT seems to be secondary, often it borders on the boundary of, or treads into, the realm of a primary service provider. The victim who is physically or sexually wounded looks forward to medical redressal as the first need. However, the medical professionals are called upon to perform a vast array of functions including age verification, expert opinion regarding the injury on the person, etc. Therefore, the menu of services they provide is also multifaceted.

*Give **priority** of attention to a trafficked victim* as this person is a victim of multiple abusers, multiple exploitation and multiple harm by multiple abusers.

*Appreciate the victim's position and respond with **empathy**,* even when the victim may be violent, angry, abusive, etc. due to the high level of trauma.

*Respect **human rights**.* The victim is a person whose human rights have been deprived and denied. The initial responders need to validate the harm, make the victim feel that she is only a victim and that she has a right to redressal and that it will be done. Also ensure her that there will not be any further violation from your side. Tell her that it is her right and your duty. And she has a right to demand best care and attention.

*Respect **gender rights**.* If it is a female victim who is not comfortable with a male doctor attending to her, do take the services of a female doctor or, if a female doctor is not available, keep a female nurse or another person to be with the victim during the entire process of examination, treatment and related activities.

*Do **not delay**.* Response delayed causes more trauma and harm. If there are several steps involved in medical attention, e.g., check-up by specialized doctors like gynecologist, pediatrician, etc. line up the appointments so that all activities move in a chain without break. Do not delay in giving reports of medical examination to the police/others concerned, as such delays defeat justice delivery process.

Age verification is an important task the medical professionals are required to attend to. Age of the victim has a lot of bearing on deciding about the nature of offence and the gravity of punishment to the offender. Further, it has several legal implications. If it can be proved that the victim was trafficked at an age when she was less than 16 years and that she was sexually assaulted, the offender becomes liable for rape even if the victim had consented. Moreover, if the offence was done in a hotel, the license of the hotel can be cancelled u/s 7A ITPA. Therefore, the age of the victim may be ascertained carefully. Benefit of doubt should go to the victim. If he/she is in trauma or if he/she is illiterate, the child may give a wrong age. The exploiters may coerce her to say she is an adult. Doctors have to go for scientific evidence, both direct and circumstantial. The Ossification test may not give a complete result, hence it may be seen along with other scientific parameters.

*Be a **good human being** also.* Doctors are healers before being treatment providers. More than medicine their words, demeanor and feelings towards the victim make all the difference.

In brief, medical professionals have specific role to play in **Protection, Prosecution** and **Prevention**. The post-rescue care needs to be professionally handled so that the victim is not victimized further. It calls for human rights oriented care and attention. As regards prosecution, the age determination and injury determination are important from the forensic point of view. The medical professionals will be called upon to testify in the court of law as experts. Their reports and findings facilitate investigation and help the investigators to take appropriate steps in investigating the crime on all aspects. As regards prevention, the role of medical professionals is generally not known, but it is a fact that well-counselled and rehabilitated person would not be re-trafficked. As a corollary, chances of re-trafficking are high if the post-rescue care and attention is poor or improper. Medical professionals, therefore, help in prevention.

Legal provisions

Several UN regional and national legislations and conventions are relevant in the context of CT. The list below explains the position.

- UN Convention on Transnational Organized Crime
- The Convention on the Rights of the Child, 1989
- The Optional Protocol to the Convention on the Rights of the Child on the Sale of Children, Child Prostitution and Child Pornography, 2000
- The Convention on the Elimination of All forms of Discrimination against Women, (CEDAW) 1979
- The Protocol to Prevent, Suppress and Punish Trafficking in Persons, Especially Women and Children
- Declaration on Social and legal principles relating to the Protection and Welfare of Children, with special reference to Foster placement and adoption, Nationally and Internationally, 3 December, 1986
- SAARC Convention on Regional Arrangement for the Promotion of Child Welfare, 2002
- The Constitution of India, Articles 23 and 24
- Substantive legislation, i.e. The Indian Penal Code
- Special Legislations like:
  - Immoral Trafficking Prevention Act (ITPA)- 1956
  - Child Labor (Prohibition and Regulation) Act, 1986
  - Information Technology Act, 2000
  - Juvenile Justice (Care and Protection of Children) Act, 2000
- State-specific legislations like:
  - Karnataka Devadasi (Prohibition of Dedication) Act, 1982
  - Andhra Pradesh Devadasi (Prohibiting Dedication) Act, 1989
  - Goa Children's Act, 2003.

Moving ahead

Considering the dismal picture that emerges from the existing response systems, it is obvious that we have miles to go. A lot needs to be done to address the issue of child abuse, neglect and child trafficking. Synergy of the stakeholders, committed participation by all stakeholders and concerted action by all of us is the essential *mantra*. The responses have to be human rights oriented and rights based. The following issues need to be taken forward:

- **Sharing good practices** with all practitioners in the region
- Developing **regional/national protocols for minimum standards of care and attention** for trafficked children. This should be rights based and victim centric
- **Sharing quality resource materials across the region** with all stakeholders
- **Empowerment/capacity building/training of trainers** in the region, with a view to build a BANK OF MASTER TRAINERS/EXPERTS, who are professionals and committed persons in the relevant field. The empowerment process can and should be done by facilitating the visit of such experienced and competent resource persons to the countries in the Region, which requires attention. A list of such resource persons in the region can be brought out in the conference and circulated to all participants so that their services could be utilized by them
- **Instituting rewards and recognition for the institutions and individuals** who make outstanding contributions in preventing and combating child trafficking. This should include Researchers, Academics, Medical professionals, Media, Law Enforcement officials and Activists who have contributed in strengthening the

system, empowering the responders, for undertaking innovative experiments in the field of child trafficking, etc.

Studies, research and reference materials

In the context of addressing CT, the following resource materials are of much relevance:

1. By UNODC (Dr P M Nair was the Project Coordinator of the UN Project on Anti Human Trafficking, run by UNODC in partnership with the Government of India, with funds from the US Government.)
   i. SOP on the Investigation of Trafficking crimes for sexual exploitation
   ii. SOP on the Investigation of Trafficking crimes for exploitative labor
   iii. Protocol for interstate transfer of trafficked victims
   iv. Manual for Psychosocial intervention
   v. Manual for Training Police on Anti Human Trafficking
   vi. Manual for Training Prosecutors on Anti Human Trafficking
   vii. Compendium of Best Practices by NGOs on Anti Human Trafficking
   viii. Compendium of Best Practices by Law Enforcement agencies on Anti human trafficking
   ix. Hand Book for Indian Police to address human trafficking crimes
   x. Protocol on setting up Integrated Anti Human Trafficking Units in India
   xi. Compendium on the Legal Framework
   xii. SOP on Prosecution of human trafficking Crimes
   xiii. Posters (8 numbers) on eight themes on trafficking
   xiv. Film on Anti Human Trafficking, titled "One Life, No Price", a Abraham. (Dr PM Nair is the Concept advisor for the Film produced by Touchriver Films, Hyderabad in 2007 for UNODC)

[All these materials are available on the website unodc.org/India.]

2. **Dr PM Nair**, "**HAND BOOK** for law enforcement agencies in addressing trafficking for sexual exploitation", published by UNODC and UNIFEM, 2005

3. **Action Research on 'Trafficking in Women and Children in India'** was a project of the **National Human Rights Commission (NHRC),** India during the period 2002–2004

4. *"Victims, Witnesses care and Protection", page- 42 of the **Hand Book for Law Enforcement Agencies in India on Trafficking in Women and Children for Sexual Exploitation, by P M Nair**, published by UNIFEM and UNODC, 2007)*

5. **Dr P M Nair**, "**Human Trafficking: Dimensions, Challenges and Responses**", published by Konark Publishers, 2010

6. **Protocol** on **Minimum Standards of Care and Attention** by **SARIQ**-2006

7. **UNICEF** Protocol for media in addressing child sexual exploitation and trafficking

8. **Dr Achal Bhagat**, *Mind of the Survivor",* SAARTHAK, 2004

9. **Dr Achal Bhagat** – *"Ensure", "Enable", "Outgrowing the Pain",* (UNIFEM, 2006)

10. **UNODC, New York, 2010,** Antitrafficking Manual for Criminal Justice Practitioners

11. Rulings of the Supreme Court of India, especially the following:
   - Sakshi Vs Union of India (which mandates in-camera trials of all cases of child sexual exploitation, use of screen in the court to protect the child victim from being exposed to the court scenes, provision of child mentor, etc.)
   - Praful Desai Vs Union of India—where teleconferencing has been allowed. This would facilitate victims not appearing in the court and also would avoid unwarranted travels.

10

Child Labor

Rajeev Seth

Introduction

Child labor constitues a serious violation of fundamental rights of children. From rights based perspective, there can be no excuse for existence of child labor. It deprives children of their childhood, their potential and their dignity, and that is harmful to their physical and mental development. Child labor is a global phenomenon; around 215 million children work, many full-time worldwide. It is essentially a socio-economic problem, inextricably linked to poverty and illiteracy. There is a consensus emerging that when a child is not in school, the child would perforce be part of the labor pool. In linking child labor to education, the tasks of eliminating child labor and of universalizing education have become synonymous.

There is an essential need to develop a comprehensive plan to withdraw children from work and mainstream them into schools, in order to provide them basic right to education. Considering the extent and magnitude of the problem, it is indeed a challenging task, but can be attained with concerted efforts at all levels of the Government, elected representatives, policy makers, international agencies, NGO's, educationist, child professionals, teachers, counsellors, *panchayats*, municipal councillors, child rights activists, parents and juvenile justice and child protection systems. Finally, we urgently need a movement against child labor rendering justice for all children and towards equity and democracy.

Definition

The International Labor Organization (ILO) has defined child labor as work that deprives children of their childhood, their potential and their dignity, and that is harmful to physical and mental development.[1] It refers to work that is mentally, physically, socially or morally dangerous and harmful to children; interferes with their schooling or requires them to attempt to combine school attendance with excessively long and heavy work.

Not all work done by children should be classified as child labor that is to be targeted for elimination. Children's or adolescents' participation in work that does not affect their health and personal development or interfere with their schooling is generally regarded as being something positive. This includes activities such as helping their parents around the home, assisting in a family business or earning pocket money outside school hours and during school holidays. These kinds of activities contribute to children's development and to the welfare of their families; they provide them with skills and experience, and help to prepare them to be productive members of society during their adult life.[2]

Magnitude of problem

Child labor is global phenomenon. Throughout the world, around 215 million children work, many full-time. They do not go to school and have little or no time to play. Many do not receive proper nutrition or care. They are denied the chance to be children. More than half of them are exposed to the worst forms of child labor such as work in hazardous environments, slavery, or other forms of forced labor, illicit activities including drugs, trafficking and prostitution, as well as involvement in armed conflict.[2]

India has the dubious distinction of holding the largest number of child laborers in the world today. As per the Census of India 2001, there are 13 million child laborers in the age group of 5–14 years. There is a consensus emerging that when a child is not in school, the child would perforce be part of the labor pool. It is estimated that out of school children constitute nearly 18 percent of children. In absolute numbers, the potential child labor pool remains very high at above 40 million.[3] Child labor is found in all the sectors of Indian economy such as

a. *Manufacturing sector:* Children are engaged in various manufacturing process of different home-based industries such as brassware, lock, match, firework, diamond cutting, gem polishing, glassware, carpet making, etc.

b. *Agrarian sector:* In rural areas, children are engaged in agricultural and allied occupations as a part of family or individual

c. *Service sector:* Self-employed invisible or wage-based employment.[4-6]

Categories of child labor

Child labor is a term that covers a range and variety of circumstances in which children work.[7] Children may be working as:

Street children

Children live on and off the streets, such as shoeshine boys, rag pickers, newspaper-vendors, beggars, etc. Most children have some sort of home to go back to in the evenings or nights (children on the street), while other set of street children are completely alone without home (children off the streets) and are at the mercy of their employers. They live on the pavements, in the bus stations and railway stations. They are at the mercy of urban predators, as also the police.

Migrant child labor

Millions of families are being forced to leave their homes and villages for several months every year in search of livelihoods. These migrations mean that families are forced to drop out of schools. All evidence indicates that migrations are large and growing. Children migrate from rural to the urban area or from smaller to larger towns/cities either with or without families.

Bonded child labor

Children who have either been pledged by their parents for paltry sums of money or those working to pay off the inherited debts of their fathers. Bonded children are in many ways the most difficult to assist, because they are inaccessible. If the carpet owner has bought them, they cannot escape. If the landlord in the village owns them, they will spend their life in servitude till they get married and can, in turn, sell their children.

Children used for sexual exploitation

Many thousands of young girls and boys serve the sexual appetites of men from all social and economic backgrounds. Factories, workshops, street corners, railway stations, bus stops and homes where children work are common sites of sexual exploitation. Almost all such children are betrayed by those they trust and end up getting abused! The physical health, danger of HIV/AIDS, sexually transmitted diseases and psycho-social damage inflicted by commercial sexual exploitation makes it one of the most hazardous forms of child labor.

Female working children, engaged in household activities

There are a large number of children, especially girls who are working in their own houses, engaged in what is not normally seen as "economic activity". These children are engaged in taking care of younger siblings, cooking, cleaning and other such household activities. The girl child begins her work by helping her mother with household chores from the age of four or five.[8] The problem of child labor situation is worse for girls than it for boys. A closer examination of the data reveals that more than 85% of female child workers are engaged in agricultural child labor.[9] The girl working children are usually low paid and work for longer hours.[10-11] Further, if such children are not sent to school, they will eventually join the labor force as one of the above categories of child labor.

Agricultural child labor

India is predominantly an agrarian country. Agriculture is one of the hazardous occupations from the standpoint of child health and safety. In general, higher susceptibility to ill health arises, because children are deputed to undertake adult jobs with their immature bodies and minds.[6] Between the age group of 8–14 years, majority of child workers are engaged in transplantation, crop watering, harvesting, irrigation, weeding, threshing and sowing. Children are employed in spreading fertilizers, insecticides and pesticides without any protection. They are also employed to operate modern powered agricultural machineries, making them more vulnerable to physical injuries.[10]

The UN Convention on the Rights of the Child (UN CRC), 1989; the National Commission for Protection of Child Rights (NCPCR) 2007 & Right to Education Act (2009).

The UN Convention on the Rights of the Child (UN CRC) is the first legally binding international instrument to incorporate the full range of human rights—civil, cultural, economic, political and social rights to a child.[12] By agreeing to undertake the obligations of the Convention (by ratifying or acceding to it), national governments have committed themselves to protecting and ensuring children's rights and they have agreed to hold themselves accountable for this commitment before the international community. States parties to the Convention are obliged to develop and undertake all actions and policies in the light of the best interests of the child.

The National Commission for Protection of Child Rights (NCPCR) was set up in March 2007, under an Act of Parliament of India.[13] The Commission's mandate is to ensure that all laws, policies, programs and administrative mechanisms are in consonance with the Child Rights perspective, as enshrined in the Constitution of India and also the UN CRC.[13]

Education is a crucial child right.[12] In linking child labor to education, the tasks of eliminating child labor and of universalizing education have become synonymous. One cannot be achieved without the other. In other words, the task of withdrawing a child from work becomes the same as inducting the child into school. A full time formal day school is the only form of school which guarantees the child the right to education.

The Right of Children to Free and Compulsory Education Act (RTE) 2009, passed by the Parliament of India, makes education a fundamental right for all children between the ages of 6 and 14.[14] The RTE Act makes elementary education free and compulsory. It sets quality norms for all school, working norms for teachers and mandates curriculum in all schools to be in consonance with constitutional values. It also mandates participation of civil society in the management of schools and reservation for children (25%) from the weaker section of the society. The RTE Act is implemented by the Government education department, while it is monitored by the NCPCR.

There is an urgent and essential need to develop a comprehensive plan to withdraw children from work and mainstream them into schools, in order to provide them basic right to education. This is indeed a challenging task, but can be attained with a united effort with a clear perspectives at all levels of the Government, elected representatives, policy makers, NGO's, education professionals, teachers, counsellors, *panchayats*, municipal councillors, child rights activists, parents and juvenile justice and child protection systems.

Constitutional provisions

Child labor is essentially a socio-economic problem, inextricably linked to poverty and illiteracy. All respective Government's have taken various proactive measures to tackle this problem. However, considering the extent and magnitude of the problem in developing countries, it requires concerted efforts from all sections of the society.

The Government of India formed the first committee called Gurupadswamy Committee to study the issue of child labor and to suggest measures to tackle it, way back in 1979. The Committee examined the problem in detail and made some far-reaching recommendations. It observed that as long as poverty continued, it would be difficult to totally eliminate child labor and hence, any attempt to abolish it through legal recourse would not be a practical proposition. The Committee felt that in the circumstances, the only alternative left was to ban child labor in hazardous areas and to regulate and ameliorate the conditions of work in other areas. It recommended that a multiple policy approach was required in dealing with the problems of working children.[15] Based on the recommendations of this committee, the Child Labor (Prohibition & Regulation) Act India was enacted in 1986.

The Child Labor (Prohibition & Regulation) Act 1986

The Child Labor (Prohibition & Regulation) Act 1986 outlines where and how children can work and where they can not. It defines a child as any person who has not completed his fourteenth year of age. Part II of the act prohibits children from working in any occupation listed in Part A of the Schedule; for example: catering at railway establishments, construction work on the railway or anywhere near the tracks, plastics factories, automobile garages, etc. The act also prohibits children from working in places where certain processes are being undertaken, as listed in Part B of the Schedule; for example: beedi making, tanning, soap manufacture, brick kilns and roof tiles units, etc. These provisions do not apply to a workshop where the occupier is working with the help of his family or in a government recognised or aided school.[16] The act calls for the establishment of a 'Child Labor Technical Advisory Committee (CLTAC)' which is responsible for advising the government about additions to the Schedule lists.

Part III of the act outlines the conditions in which children may work in occupations/processes not listed in the schedule. The number of hours of a particular kind of establishment of class of establishments is to be set and no child can work for more than those many hours in that particular establishment. Children are not permitted to work for more than three hour stretches and must receive an hour break after the three-hours. Children are not permitted to work for more than six-hour stretches including their break interval and can not work between the hours of 7 p.m. and 8 a.m. No child is allowed to work overtime or work in more than one place in a given day. A child must receive a holiday from work every week. The employer of the child is required to send a notification to an inspector about a child working in their establishment and keep a register of all children being employed for inspection.

Section IV of the act outlines various remaining aspects such as penalties. The penalty of allowing a child to work in occupations/ processes outlined in the schedule which are prohibited is a minimum of 3 months prison time and/or a minimum of Rs. 10,000 in fines. Second time offenders are subject to jail time of minimum six months. Failure to notify an inspector, keep a register, post a sign or any other requirement is punishable by simple imprisonment and/or a fine up to Rs. 10,000. Offenders can only be tried in courts higher than a magistrate or metropolitan magistrate of the first class. Courts also have the authority to appoint people to be inspectors under this act.

The technical advisory committee on the Child Labor (Prohibition & Regulation) Act 1986 child labor recommended domestic work and work in hospitality center as 'hazardous for children'. Effective October10, 2006, the Ministry of labor, Government of India baned on employing children below 14 years, as domestic help in these occupations. The ban was aimed at " ameliorating the condition of hapless working children from psychological trauma and even sexual abuse" The penalty for flouting this law is jail term ranging from 3 months to 2 years and fines that could range up to Rs 20, 000.[16]

Rehabilitation of child laborers and intervention strategies

All Government has taken proactive steps to tackle the problem of child labor through strict enforcement of legislative provisions along with simultaneous rehabilitative measures. State Government officials have conducted regular inspections and raids to detect cases of violations. Since poverty is the root cause of the problem of child labor, enforcement alone cannot help solve it. Recently, Government has been laying a lot of emphasis on the rehabilitation of these children and on improving the economic conditions of their families.[15]

The National Policy on Child Labor 1987

The National Policy on Child Labor 1987 seeks to adopt a gradual and sequential approach with a focus on rehabilitation of children working in hazardous occupations and processes in the first instance. The Action Plan outlined in the Policy for tackling this problem is as follows:

a. Legislative Action Plan for strict enforcement of Child Labor Act and other labor laws to ensure that children are not employed in hazardous employments, and that the working conditions of children working in non-hazardous areas are regulated in accordance with the provisions of the Child Labor Act.

b. The National Child Labor Project (NCLP) (1988) Envisages starting of projects in areas of high concentration of child labor. The scheme envisages running of special schools for child labor withdrawn from work. In the special schools, these children are provided formal/ non-formal education along with vocational training, a stipend of Rs.150 per month, supplementary nutrition and regular health checkups so as to prepare them to join regular mainstream schools.

National Resource Centre on Child Labor

The Child Labor Cell at V.V. Giri National Labor Institute NOIDA, UP India was upgraded as National resource centre on Child Labor in March 1993 (http://www.vvgnli.org/).[17] In addition of conducting research projects, the Centre also organizes various training programs to develop capabilities of individuals, groups and organizations working toward the elimination of child labor.

Indian Child Abuse Neglect & Labor group (ICANCL Group)

The Indian Child Abuse Neglect and Labor group (ICANCL group) (www.icancl.com) is a nationally registered society, started in 1996, under the framework of Indian Academy of Pediatrics (IAP) (www.iapindia.org). The Group realizes that the problems must be tackled at various fronts, jointly with other agencies and organizations interested in child welfare. Advocacy, information and sensitization are the crucial issues.

The main aims and objectives of the society are:

a. To advocate on children's behalf, inform and sensitize the community, formulate recommendations for welfare and protection of children, and demand rights of children;

b. To provide health care to the neglected, deprived, abused and exploited children and help in their protection and rehabilitation in cooperation and collaboration with various organizations and national and international agencies; and

c. To work with news media and information agencies toward bringing about social awareness and attitudinal changes, and seek community participation in child welfare activities.[18]

Membership is multidisciplinary professional and community members who are interested to prevent and manage Child Abuse, Neglect and Child labor. A National workshop was organized by Indian CANCL group, on the subject of Child Labor (1997) and a conference on 'Every Child in School' (2004)[19-20]. The following was the summary of the recommendations:

1. The definition of a 'child' has to include all children up to 18 years of age.

2. The Government should draw up a definitive health care policy for child labor—to be followed by the employers in the so-called non-hazardous jobs. This can include a provision of health cards for such children, regular check-ups and treatment, provision of relevant immunizations, mid-day meals and reproductive health. Such children should be included in the ESI program till child labor can be completely abolished.

3. Education is a fundamental right and is the responsibility of the State. It is the only answer to take children away from child labor and provide them right direction to their overall development.

4. In rural area, the responsibility for primary education should be with the village *panchayats*, block and districts officials. The panchayat must be given funds and empowered. The difficulties of child laborers in urban areas can be tackled with active participation of NGO's and welfare officers, whose job should be to ensure that every child is in school.

5. Once a child is in school, the health and nutrition problems must be addressed.

6. Adequate and effective legal provisions must be in place to ensure relief, compensation, reparation and restitution for forms of abuse, torture and exploitation.

The Way Forward and World Day Against Child Labor (June 12)

From rights based perspective, the National Commission for Protection of Child Rights (NCPCR), India considers that there can be no excuse for existence of child labor and violation of child rights.[13] There can be no discrimination between child labor and child work, or hazardous labor and non-hazardous labor. The definition of 'child labor' must include children working for the families in their own homes, children in agriculture work, work rendered by girls and all other forms of work that deprive children of their right to education in a full time formal school. In other words, the definition of child labor must be inclusive and recognize all forms of child labor as prohibited.

Each country's national policy on abolishing child labor must resonate with heroic accounts of young children who repeatedly risk their lives in their struggle to escape insults and humiliation in their work place. The policy must recognize their voices against loss of childhood, suffering and exploitation, hunger, lack of education, and the damage we cause them by not meeting their basic child rights.

The fundamental principles of any nation's child labor policy should be founded on the following truths: (a) that among other factors, child labor causes and perpetuates poverty; (b) non-economic factors play a significant causal role in sustain child labor; (c) lack of educational attainment is the most important non economic factor, which continues to entrench child labor generationally with in a vicious cycle of poverty; (d) child labor can significantly impede educational attainment for both out of school and in school children; (e) and poor families can and do send and support their children in school.

June 12 is the World Day Against Child Labor. This day brings the spotlight on the rights of children to be protected from child labor and other violations of children's fundamental rights. The urgent realization and effective implementation of the rights of the child are crucial for social justice and democracy. Children are not only adults of tomorrow, but are citizens of today and they need protection now.

On June 12, 2012, the National Commission for Protection of Child Rights (NCPCR), International labor Organization (ILO) and United Nations Children's Fund (UNICEF) reiterated and renewed their commitment toward justice for ALL children by enabling them to celebrate their right to grow, free from child labor, and receiving an education of quality in a formal school. At a public meeting, the above agencies called for: (a) Ratification of international instruments against child labor in an equivocal manner; Review of existing anti-child labor legislations and policies and adapting them to the Right of the Children to free and compulsory Education Act, 2009 and the Juvenile Justice (Care and protection of children) Act, 2000; universalization of secondary education for all children in the age of 14–18 years and further provision of opportunities to all such children who are out of school or educational institutions to get them back to the mainstream schools; and finally a movement against child labor rendering justice for all children and toward equity and democracy.

References

1. International Labor organisation: http://www.ilo.org/ipec/facts/lang--en/index.htm, accessed December 2, 2012.

2. The International Labor organisation: http://www.ilo.org/global/topics/child-labor/lang--en/index.htm, accessed Dec2, 2012.

3. Abolition of Child labor & Making Education a Reality for Every Child as a Right. NCPCR 2008, 1–40.

4. International labor Office, A bureau of statistics and special studies, Geneva :I L O, 1980.

5. Singh S,Verma RBS. Child Labor in Agriculture, Lucknow; Print House, 1987: 1–23.

6. Banerjee S R.Agricultural Child Labor in West Bengal. Indian Pediatr, 1993 ; 30:1425–28.

7. Abolition of child labor in India, strategies for the eleventh five year plan. Submitted by NCPCR to Government of India (2011). www.ncpcr.gov.in

8. Ghosh S.Discrimination begins at birth. Indian Pediatr 1986; 23:5–7

9. Rama Rao R. Child Labor –A demographic perspective. Social Welfare, 1986; 33:4–9.

10. Banerjee S R. Child Labor, Indian Pediatr. 1990; 27:3–6

11. Banerjee S R. Female Working Children, Indian Pediatr. 1990; 27:1153–1155.

12. UNICEF. Convention of the Rights of childhttp://www.unicef.org/crc/. Assessed Dec3, 2012.

13. The National Commission for Protection of Child Rights (NCPCR). http://ncpcr.gov.in/

14. The Right of Children to Free And Compulsory Education Act..http://ssa.nic.in/quality-of-education/right-of-children-to-free-and-compulsory-education-act-2009. Accessed Dec3, 2012.

15. Ministry of Labor, Government of India. http://www.labor.nic.in/ accessed Dec 3, 2012.

16. Child-Labor-Prohibition-and-Regulation-Act-1986. Accessed Dec 2, 2012. http://www.childlineindia.org.in/

17. V.V.Giri National Labor Institute. Towards Combating Child labor. Sekar Helen R. 2003 (http://www.vvgnli.org/)

18. The Indian Child Abuse, Neglect & Child Labor group, Indian Academy of Pediatrics www.icancl.com.

19. Proceedings from National workshop on Child Labor-Health Statistics, Indian CANCL, IAP & ILO (IPEC), New Delhi, India 1997.

20. Proceedings from National Conference on 'Every Child in School'. Indian CANCL group, New Delhi, India, 2004.(www.icancl.com).

11

Violations of Child Rights During Disasters

Naeem Zafar, Mehek Naeem

'Disaster is a crisis situation that far exceeds the capabilities' Quarentelly

Introduction

Pakistan has received more a number of Aerious disasters over the last decade. The mass influx of almost 5 million Afghan refugees after American attack on Afghanistan after 9/11 along with Pakistan's fight against terrorism almost collapsed the country economically and politically. War in Afghanistan (2001–present)). The massive earthquake that struck northern areas of Pakistan and Kashmir on October 8th 2005, took as many as 73,000 lives and rendered more than 2.5 million homeless Child Protection in Disaster Management in South Asia: A Case Study of Pakistan). In 2009 more than 3 million population of Swat District and adjacent areas in Khyber Pakhtunkhwa had to migrate overnight because of military action against terrorists by the Pakistan Army. Most of the displaced were women and children with an estimated 60% of this internally displaced population being children under the age of 18 years. In the following year the worst floods in the history of Pakistan submerged almost one-fifth of its land and affected more than 20 million population, again the worst affected were children and women. There have been many more natural disasters including earthquakes and floods during this decade but their toll has been much less than the above-mentioned calamities. The nation is also fighting terrorism as a front line state for the last 11 years. This has led to hundreds of suicide and remote bomb explosions all over the country. The economy is also virtually collapsed and social fiber is disrupted due to continuous war against terrorists from adjacent Afghanistan and militants from within Pakistan.

In this chapter, we discuss the rights of child that can be violated, their probable causes, the role of stakeholders and recommendations to minimize these violations.

United Nation's Convention on the Rights of the Child

United Nation's Convention on the Rights of the Child is a very comprehensive document, which has listed various rights of the child. It groups these rights into Survival, Development, Protection and Participation Rights, and explains each of these emphasizing the role of the state and society in providing all the rights to the child. Unfortunately even after more than two decades of signing and ratifying of this UN Convention by almost all countries of the world children are yet to receive these rights. Especially those living in the developing countries are still struggling for their governments to take action as the 20-year report of UNICEF (Ref The State of The World's Children) paints a dismal picture about its implementation.

Table 1 Survival Rights

Survival Right	Compromise in Emergency Situation
The Right to Life	Perinatal care, trauma, killing, use as soldiers, etc.
Health	Basic health infrastructure, Maternal and child Health, immunizations
Nutrition	Breastfeeding, scarce food supply, micronutrients
Shelter	Destruction, dangerous and open places
Registration at Birth	Documentation lack
Preservation of Identity	Illegal adoptions, trafficking, religious rights

As children are physically, psychologically, financially and socially dependent on their parents or caregivers for protection and support, they are the most vulnerable to abuse and neglect whenever any situation compromises the financial and social stability of the family and the community. This vulnerability increases dramatically during emergency situations when there is an unexpected turn of events resulting in an abrupt change in the child's physical environment and hence we see a steep increase in the violation of their Survival, Development, Protection and Participation Rights.

Every child has a right to life, adequate health and nutrition, a safe shelter and preserved identity. These Survival rights are fundamental for a child to stay alive, healthy and safe. However, during the early phase of an emergency situation, access to food, water and shelter become limited and there is inadequate sanitation within the area of destruction and displacement.

During an emergency, the already existing health services break down. Deliveries are conducted by untrained birth attendants in unhygienic environment with unsterile equipment. This causes a steep rise in perinatal mortality and morbidity. The infants are not vaccinated in time, the incidence of diarrhea and pneumonia rise exponentially due to overcrowding and bad sanitary conditions. Infant and children's mortality and morbidity is usually the highest at the onset of an emergency during the most threatening conditions (WHO Report on feeding children, 2004).

Infants and child nutrition also suffers due to food scarcity and a lot of cases of protein energy malnutrition and micronutrient deficiencies are seen after the disasters.

Children not only falter in growth but also become more vulnerable to infections due to relative immune deficiencies. Breast fed infants, although considered relatively safe are also at a high-risk of infections, as the mother struggles with challenges including threat to personal safety.

When the earthquake struck northern areas of Pakistan, children were in schools and the collapsing buildings injured and killed thousands of these children. Many more succumbed later due to non-availability of timely aid as the road structures were totally destroyed. Army helicopters and volunteers rescued many children but injuries required amputation of limbs in many survivors, in ill equipped make shift operating theatres by surgeons, who were not trained to manage trauma in emergencies. A surgeon admitted that if he did not have to perform so many surgeries in such taxing circumstances, he would have been able to avoid many unnecessary amputations.

Children are not a priority while feeding in a food scarce situation. There is insufficient food to fulfill the need of families, and thus children do not get enough food to sustain normal development. Children are more prone to ill effects of any physical injury or diseases and may become marasmic or fall prey to infections. During emergencies, due to limited resources and medical assistance, immediate medial attention to all is not always possible. In developing countries these injuries and illnesses could be especially problematic, in view of the already deficients facilities. For example, during Haiti earthquake, a high number of crush injuries were exacerbated by the pre-existing weak health system (Iezzoni and Ronan, 2010). Similarly in Pakistan earthquake majority of deaths occurred among children.

Epidemics usually follow emergency situations. Bad sanitation and limited access to clean potable water along with overcrowding, and limited health services and lack of vaccination against communicable diseases (measles and typhoid) may lead to rapid spread of diseases. During the Pakistan super floods, it was estimated that around 8 million people did not have access to clean water of which 3.5 million children were at a risk of potentially fatal water borne diseases (Solberg, 2010).

Preserving identity is vital for a child's wellbeing and existence. However during an emergency situation, when the parent/caregiver of the child is killed, injured or is missing, the child's identity becomes jeopardized. Illegal adoptions and trafficking takes place and the child is forced to change his/her identity. Children who are born during emergency situation, have no documentation records of their birth may face increased challenges during the coming months and years.

After the great Indian Ocean Tsunami of 2004, many children were abducted in the garb of adoptions. It led Pakistan Paediatric Association to convince the Khyber Pakhtunkhwa government to put a ban on all kinds of adoptions within two days of the earthquake in 2005. Thus a lot of children whose parents had perished in the disaster were saved from possible abduction. A very closely-knit extended joint family system came to the help of these children and these were taken care by the extended family till proper adoption mechanisms were set in by their own tribal system. This adoption ban was still valid in Khyber Pakhtunkhwa during the IDP crisis of 2009 and super floods of 2010 and hence the problem of abduction was automatically saved.

Children are frail, defenseless, and therefore, every child has the right to be protected. During an emergency, the child becomes more vulnerable to neglect, abuse and exploitation. Depending on the child's age, dependency, level of mastery and ability this may have a huge impact on his or her physical safety and psychological sense of security.

Psychological and behavior problems

In any disaster situation the psyche of children is totally neglected. They are usually taken as bystanders in the whole process of relief and are expected to stay out of way, and are never talked to, or taken into confidence. They are not provided any play activity and the essential need of education is also ignored. These children may suffer from serious psychological problems including anxiety, depression and 'post traumatic stress disorder'. However, the camp authorities seldom take any notice of the children's emotional needs. Caretakers often neglect children physically and emotionally when they are themselves stressed. Not enough

Table 2 Protection Rights	
Protection Right	**Compromise in Emergency Situation**
Neglect	Child Needs totally neglected
Emotional Trauma	No Psychological Services, PTSD care
Physical & Sexual Abuse	Increased incidence as child becomes more vulnerable
Trafficking and Abduction	Illegal Adoptions, Marriages, Sale of children
Lost and Missing Children	No mechanism to track missing children
Disabled Children	No support for mentally, or physically handicapped
Involvement in Conflict	Child Soldier, suicide bomber,
Refugee	Vulnerability in camps or outside
Child labour	Usually accepted in crisis situations
Juvenile Justice	No provision of Justice to Child victim or offender

attention is paid to their appearance, nourishment, and emotional well-being. For example, during the Internal displacement of people in Pakistan, there was absolutely no psychological counseling for children in the camps and host communities. Young girls showed clear signs of internalizing behavior and boys symptoms of exhibited externalizing behaviors. In Pakistan there are very few child psychologists in main cities, let alone present in remote rural areas where the major disasters hit. Hence psychologists are rarely seen playing their part either as volunteers or employees in any emergency situation.

Behaviors that may be otherwise objectionable during normal circumstances may become acceptable in disasters and crisis situation. As the caretaker goes through extreme emotions and distresses, domestic violence and punishment increases. There is an increased incidence of spouse abuse in the camps and consequently the mother then beats up the child. Any financial help may matter a lot to sustain the family so child labor also becomes tolerable in emergency situations. Trash picking and is one of the commonest modes whereby Afghan refugee children, both boys and girls, earn for their families. At the leaky Torkham border between Pakistan and Afghanistan, these children carry loads from one side of the border to the other. The adults are apprehended for smuggling, but these children often go 'un-noticed' by the border authorities.

Refugee children face additional challenges. The environment within camps is usually very harsh depending on the climate, number of people, resources and other factors. The security within these camps is low and the child becomes more vulnerable. Adolescents and youth in remote rural or urban areas may face reproductive health risks (Austin et al, 2008) and increased exposure to sexual coercion and violence (Lane 2008).

Table 3 Development Rights	
Development Right	Compromise in Emergency Situation
Education	Schools destroyed, No schooling, No priority to start school
Social Security	Pre emergency lack, total shut down as government fails
Leisure and Recreation	No Child play areas or time, No Psychological relief
Access to Information	Torn infra structure, Communication last priority
Conciense and Religion	No effort by relief agencies at its preservation

Missing children

There is no mechanism to track missing and lost children. Illegal adoptions take place and risks of sexual abuse, trafficking and abduction increase. A study conducted in Sierra Leone in 1999 found that 37 per cent of prostitutes were under the age of 15, and 80 per cent had been displaced by war (Red Cross World Disaster Report 2012).

In Pakistan after the earthquake many underage girls were married off to people coming from all over Pakistan to 'support' the poor families. There is no mechanism to track the future of these marriages.

Children are also killed as a part of civilian deaths during an armed conflict, and many times, young people are brain washed and used as soldiers by the different warring factions including religious organizations. Children of 16 years and below are also being trained by the militants to be used as suicide bombers.

In times of war and disaster, implementation of the law is at its lowest ebb. There are no provisions and no system for justice to the child victims and offenders. As the threshold for acceptance of crimes is very high, only the most heinous crimes are apprehended, all others are more or less accepted by the society.

While under the duress of an emergency, the normal child is deprived of his or her protection rights, the mentally or physically handicapped child fares even worse. There are no systems to ensure any special care for the disabled, and even the civil societies supporting the children forget the plight of these children and no provisions are made for their rehabilitation.

Development rights are fundamental for the child's mental growth and psychological well-being. Every child has the right to education, leisure and recreation, assess to information and choice of religion. Following a disaster or a crisis, giving children these development rights is an important step for their psychosocial rehabilitation.

The schools may be destroyed by a disaster, as we witnessed during earthquake, or they may have to be used as camps as happened in super floods. The education of the children is totally compromised due to school closure. Unfortunately in Pakistan schools are immediately closed in case of any small or big emergency (even after security alert), and remain closed for as long as any sign of emergency persists. On the on hand school closure or conversion may be essential in an economically compromised emergency situation, but on the other hand children suffer a lot. During the World War II, the rural schools remained open during the whole war in the UK and children from urban areas were moved to the rural areas for this purpose through "operation pied piper" and education was given its due recognition, and we can see the result of rebuilding of the nation immediately after the war (Children and World War Two) (Spartacus Educational). Whereas in Pakistan most of the school destroyed during the earthquake are still awaiting rebuilding after a lapse of many years.

In Pakistan, literacy rate among tribal areas of Baluchistan and Khyber Pakhtunkhwa is as

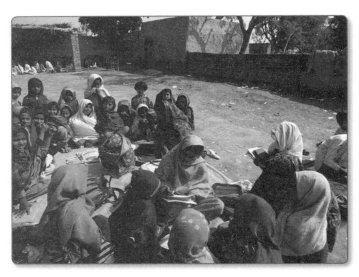

Figure 1 Makeshift class for girls

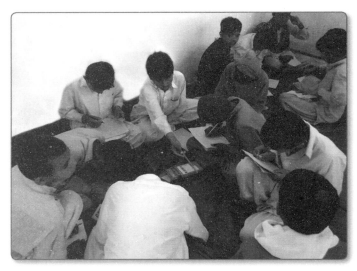

Figure 2 Boys studying

low as 7% in girls. During the conflicts in the past years, many girls' schools have been blown up by terrorists and the government has been very reluctant at rebuilding these schools. While interviewing internally displaced children, girls showed reluctance to join schools again. In the Swabi camps, no effort was made by the government to promote and provide education and very little effort was made by Non Government Organizations to advocate for this right of the child.

There is no element of social security in the predisaster times in most of the rural districts of Pakistan. Social Welfare department is one of the least active government departments and hence it comes as no surprise, when after a disaster is struck, there is no response on social welfare from the government. After the floods, when we were working in one of the less privileged districts of Dera Ghazi Khan, on a UNICEF project for psychosocial rehabilitation of children in 10 rural union councils, we involved the government

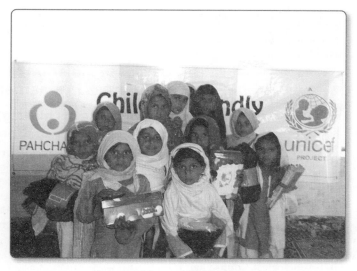

Figure 3 Girls at a child friendly space

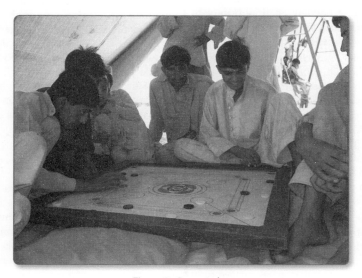

Figure 3 Boys at play

department of social welfare in that district. The department had the mandate of formation of child protection units in the area even before the floods, and we tried to create an opportunity to technically support the department to make such unit in the district, but except for a few meetings called in for that purpose, no concrete work could be done.

Little effort is made by the state for leisure and recreation during any disaster. Children had to play in the open amongst themselves. There was no adult supervision; they played a self-invented game in which children took sides of Taliban's or the militants, fighting each other. This game reflected their psychological state, but no efforts were made to promote other less destructive forms of play.

A child–right organization PAHCHHAN (Protection and Help of Children Against Abuse and Neglect) created Child Friendly Spaces during the IDP crisis of 2009 and floods in 2010 to provide not

Table 4 Participation Rights

Participation Right	Compromise in Emergency Situation
Right to express opinion	Children's opinion never sought
Freedom of thought	Only one-sided propaganda, No chance to get knowledge
Freedom of association	No children groups, no assemblies
Freedom of privacy	Child a property of adults, No private corners for children

only a space for the children to pass their time, but also to provide them an opportunity for leisure and recreation along with an effort to bring smile back to their life through psychological counseling. The children were extremely happy to come to these spaces and involved themselves in all the activities. They only needed an opportunity to forget the trauma at least for the time they were in the Child Friendly Space.

The child's belief system is also under a lot of threat in emergency situations. His existing beliefs are broken down and reconstructed again. The child's trust in his caretakers, religion or authority is broken. The child may also start to blame himself/herself. Virtually no attempts are made to restore this trust. This is quite evident in the case of Malalah Yousafzai, where a young girl lost trust in her own religious figures and spoke openly against them. She had to pay for it through an attempt on her life by one of the fundamentalists.

In most of the third world countries the only right to participation in governance to the general public is their right to vote once every 4 or 5 years. Children unfortunately do not have that right as well, hence any talk of participation right in our society is more academic and tokenistic than real. Child's right to access information, express opinion, freedom of thought, freedom of association, freedom of privacy are given the least priority under any circumstances. These are important for a child's sense of empowerment and are important to restore the child's trust after the disaster or a crisis. During an emergency situation no one is willing to speak to children, even in their own matters, or listen to their feelings. Formation of a child group is a luxury that the caregivers do not afford. When the children in Child Friendly Spaces formed groups, they were able to speak

for their own rights and actually support the authorities I providing support to their families.

Causes of violation of child rights in emergencies

Compromise of child rights before the emergency situation

One of the most important determinants in child protection issues is the situation of the children prior to the onset of emergency. This not only predicts the outcome of children after the disaster, but also reflects on the government's commitment and capacity to deal with children's issues.

Most developing countries are struggling to provide a child his/ her basic rights. These include the right to health, education, nutrition and social welfare. The infrastructure and resources are minimal to cater for the needs of general population, during normal circumstances. This situation is aggravated after an emergency situation. During the 2009 internal displacement of people in Pakistan, an extra load of 2.5 million people were added to the districts of Buner, Swabi and Mardan. The pre-existing issues in health services along with the addition of an influx of people led to a severe problems of maternal and child health services.

Post disaster, lack of resources and further aggravation of the compromised infrastructure may be especially problematic for developing countries. During the earthquake of 2005, almost all these facilities were severely damaged in the vast valleys of Khyber Pakhtunkhwa and Kashmir. Relief agencies immediately managed to install temporary hospitals but schools were given the least priority. Today, 7 years after the devastation most of the Government Schools are still not rebuilt.

Lack of disaster planning or policy

In most of the developing countries, disaster management starts after the disaster has struck, and there is virtually no planning on Disaster mitigation or anticipation. There are no policies on managing any emergency situation as a whole let alone specifically geared toward children.

According to the World Disaster Report, 2012, due to limited resources and capacity, most low-middle income countries are unable to allocate sufficient resources to disaster preparedness in their national plans. Alternately, some countries have started moving toward formulating such policies but their implementation is under question. The Government of Pakistan has formed a National Disaster Management Authority as an independent body to manage the disasters and it is working towards formulating such policies. They have not yet been able to formulate specific policies for children during disasters.

Children are not given priority in an emergency

During any natural or man-made calamity the initial focus is always diverted toward loss of lives and injuries. After securing these, the next effort is toward rebuilding and livelihood. All the relief effort is geared toward the provision of food, shelter and health. As the family is taken as one unit, the specific problems related to women and children are least acknowledged.

During the mass exodus of 2009 in Pakistan, on the second night, we received a frantic call from Mardan, explaining how thousands of women are in need of basic sanitary napkins overnight. Since they had to leave their homes in an hours notice, organizations, government, and people were ill prepared to deal with issues that may not seem as important at that moment in time. There were an estimated 40,000 pregnant women ready to deliver over the next couple of months, however there were no midwifery services available in any of these districts for them. Perinatal care was at its lowest and most of these deliveries were conducted by local untrained birth attendants with virtually no asepsis.

Psychosocial rehabilitation is another challenge faced by most developing countries. There is a lack of trained psychologists and related expertise. From our experience, working with psychologists during 2010 floods none of them was willing to stay for more than a week in the far flung district of Dera Ghazi Khan. This meant by the time the child opened up, they were ready to leave. Even the volunteer students training to be psychologists would not stay for a longer period of time. Any tangible counseling to the child was next to impossible. Moreover, the number of children requiring these services is always far greater than a psychologist can handle. The psychologists try to accommodate maximum number of children but end up providing quality services to very few.

As seen from the previous disasters in Pakistan and other developing countries, inside the camps and settlements children are usually expected to help mothers look for and collect food items from the donors and the authorities. They queue up in the ration lines, go out and help fetch water from distances. Alternatively, the girl child looks after the younger siblings while the mother is away. While doing these chores these children are vulnerable to all kinds of abuses. The child is already going through emotional distress and trauma due to change in environment. Furthermore, he/she is subjected to extreme emotional abuse. During disasters, the father, who under normal circumstances is the bread winner, is extremely frustrated at not being able to fend for the family He becomes outraged at minor issues and vents this anger on women in the house. These women having no other escape direct their frustrations to the children who ultimately take the brunt of all the anger of the family.

Children in camps are also vulnerable to physical and sexual abuse. Child labor becomes acceptable and they are expected to add to the family income.

Schools are the first institutions to be closed in any emergency, be it a large natural calamity or even a law and order situation in the city. They are the last to open when every thing else has settled down. Schools are used as camps, and even as sheds for the animals. In Pakistan, during elections, schools are even used as polling stations, and are closed for weeks.

Furthermore, children in camps do not have constructive activities and they feel useless. One of the most common activity is sitting on roadside watching buses go from one direction to the other and hoping some one in the bus would wave to them. Provision of recreation and leisure to children is a luxury that the authorities cannot afford during a crisis situation or later. The task is ultimately left to the NGOs working on children, who have limited resources and experience. Over the last three massive emergencies that Pakistan has faced the concept of Child Friendly Spaces has been increasingly practiced by the NGOs with the help of INGOs. PAHCHAAN was able to provide psychosocial support to about 5000 children in Swabi and Buner during IDP crisis and more than 20,000 children in rural areas of Dera Ghazi Khan

District which not only helped the children to cope better, but to handle the day to day conflicts in a much better way.

Lack of training of relief and rehabilitation workers

As there is no disaster anticipation or mitigation planning, the humanitarian workers only come out when a calamity hits hard. These workers have never received any formal or informal training in managing disaster situations. They are clueless to issues related to child protection during these challenging situations.

The organizations working on different development projects during normal time, take a disaster as an opportunity to expand their scope of work. They jump into different aspects of relief and rehabilitation. The existing staff then takes the lead and starts supervising the newly inducted personnel. As they themselves have no experience of working with the children, they do not plan any child-centered intervention for their staff.

Another problem arises when the donors require that local people be employed to run these projects. The concept is very pertinent to provide jobs to local people, empower them to work in their own areas and to involve local community for sustainable development beyond the project cycle. However, as the disasters tend to be most severe in the remotest places, it is usually difficult to find suitable human resource. As many different organizations start working simultaneously, the available resource demands extremely high salaries. Compromising the expected outcomes.

Moreover, training of the newly inducted human resource is also very problematic. Usually the relief and rehabilitation projects are very short in duration and do not contain any budgets for training. Even if training budgets are kept, suitable trainers are either not available or unwilling to travel distances. They are reluctant to train in far flung areas where they will not find comfortable and decent living conditions for themselves. Hence the staff either learns from his/her own experience or get more frustrated. In both cases, the ultimate beneficiary suffers as the resources are wasted and very little impacts generated.

Very limited quality research in disasters affecting developing countries

In an emergency situation, attention is paid on providing relief to the effected population. Documentation of these efforts is greatly neglected. Projects are usually awarded on concept notes and minimal documentation, budgets are calculated as ballpark figures and neither governments nor relief agencies provide any grant for quantitative and qualitative research. Some reports are generated by better organizations but are unable to find a place in peer review journals as they are classed as gray research.

Due to lack of evidence-based data, the current belief is not challenged and so the cycle of ignorance continues. Even though Pakistan has faced many large scale emergency situations over the past decade, we have very limited data on child protection issues we rely on the experiences from other countries of our region and around the world keeping cultural-religious differences in mind.

Reports compiled by child rights based organizations have been mostly conducted on a small sample/from anecdotal evidence, yielding less validity. These cannot be used to force any change in policy or planning of disaster management or mitigation.

Child rights based organizations are too few and small

There are many large National and International organizations working on different aspects of community development. These have some very small child rights cells or child related projects. Most of the dedicated child rights based organizations are small as they are mission oriented organizations. Most of their work is not related to children in emergencies. However, during emergencies, they find the need to support children, working beyond their capacities and capabilities. Hence, these organizations find it extremely difficult to cope with the challenges ultimately exhausting their resources and losing their focus of child rights.

Provision of relief is the mandate of large relief organizations. However, when smaller organizations start replicating the same efforts, they do not remain economically or programmatically feasible. Moreover, there is a lot of duplication of efforts between the small and large organizations, resulting in wastage of extremely scarce resources and neglect of other areas. During the 2005 Kashmir earthquake almost every individual philanthropist, every small and large Community Based Organizations (CBO), and every small and large NGO packed relief material, and headed to the north. Consequently, the roads were blocked, a lot of time was wasted and relief was provided to only those affected who could reach the roads. Due to unequal distribution of relief goods, those near the accessible roads got more than their requirements and wasted the relief goods, while those in the deep valleys were deprived of food and shelter. The Pakistan Army played an important role in proving services to people in these remote areas.

Role of NGOs/CBOs in optimizing disaster management

Strengthen the government initiatives

The governments are cognizant of the disaster management issues and are working toward solving it, each according to their own capacities and priorities. A National Disaster Management Authority (NDMA) has been formed at the highest level in Pakistan and is working independently on mitigating and managing disasters. It has a very close collaboration with the Pakistan Armed Forces and they have been pivotal in providing immediate relief and evacuation to the flood affected populations since the 2010 floods. The NDMA has also provided a lot of support in rebuilding after the earthquake and is providing the necessary training to personnel. It is also in the process of making policy and plans, although these are time consuming efforts, hopefully if the government will continues, Pakistan will be able to manage the disasters better in future. International Non-Government Organizations (INGOs), National level NGOs and locally Community Based Organizations (CBOs) should all contribute to the efforts of the governments, by supporting and assisting its initiatives but also by acting as a watchdog.

The International NGOs having vast experience of working in disasters are providing technical support to the government initiatives through policy dialogue and capacity building of government, besides providing funds. They are also providing relief and rehabilitation directly to the disaster affected. They need to continue and scale up this support even during the time of relative calm for disaster preparation, as they are the ones who have the capacity and the vision of disaster preparedness and mitigation. They should also dedicate some funds for research, as this is one of the most neglected areas in disaster preparedness. The INGOs and the government can take the help of NGOs and CBOs to conduct the research and make necessary policy changes according to its results.

INGOs should also be able to build the capacity of NGOs and CBOs to create a pool of volunteers ready to work at the time of disaster. This pool of volunteers can be trained at a minimum level during preparedness phase and can immediately go into action after a short training in case of an Emergency situation. NGOs and CBOs can become local partners for these trainings.

Collaborate with other NGOs to support their strengths

In social sector, as opposed to the corporate culture, benefit to the society is the primary driving force and services to the beneficiary is much more important than the growth of the organization. The organizations usually are not in competition with each other, rather they complement each other's work through mutual collaboration and formation of networks and partnerships. Different organizations have strengths in some different sector or approach. PAHCHAAN's strength is its Hospital Based Child Protection Program and its psychological support to the most vulnerable children. While working for psychosocial rehabilitation of children in Dera Ghazi Khan after the floods, PAHCHAAN collaborated with Pakistan Pediatric Association to formulate a Hospital based Child Protection Committee in the District Headquarter Hospital, and also trained not only the health professionals of the area but also teachers, and other duty bearers on child protection. On the other hand UNICEF had other partners in the same district working on education of children and on other different community uplift projects. Despite its efforts, and a mandate from UNICEF to steer a Child Protection Unit at the Social Welfare Department, PAHCHAAN could not bring them on one platform of child

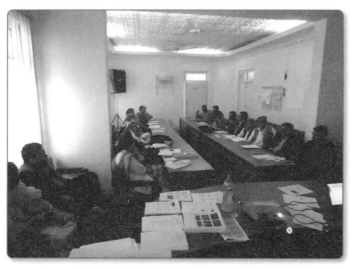

Figure 5   Meeting of the Disaster management cell of Pakistan Pediatric Association

rights and create a child protection net. Hence the close collaboration that was possible through local CBOs could not be done, the projects continued for their life cycle but no sustainable work could be done. An opportunity of rebuilding the society was therefore lost. It is imperative to think beyond the project, look beyond one's own domain and work collectively for the welfare of the community.

Stop riding the bandwagon

One of the most difficult things to do is to resist the urge of doing what every one else is doing and what every one else is expecting you to do. After a disaster strikes, survival of populations is the most urgent need of the communities. After the earthquake each and every individual of Pakistan was eager to contribute, each and every organization, small or large was willing to provide relief goods to the affected people. Trucks loaded with food and clothing were queued up on the highway to Balakot as far as the broken road would allow. Every doctor was willing to serve the needy, and the whole nation rose up to save the situation. However, donor fatigue set in very soon and after two months the survivors we left to brave the harsh winter on their own. PAHCHAAN, though in its infancy (being registered less than two months before earthquake) was able to mount a response of about 25 truck loads worth about Rs. 3 million including surgical, medical goods, food, clothing, bedding and tents and temporary

shelters, When later we needed support for child health, education and psychosocial rehabilitation, there was no support from the public. Similarly during the IDP crisis PAHCHAAN was forced by its members and volunteers to provide relief goods. However this time we did plan a psychosocial rehabilitation project and created child friendly spaces a month after the evacuation. During the super floods PAHCHAAN leadership was again pressed by its members and volunteers to provide relief to far flung areas of KP, and then Punjab and Sind provinces. This time, however, we decided against the immediate relief as by now NDMA was rather well established and the armed forces were doing a very good job at relief and any other relief effort from a small organization would not be cost effective or efficient. We focused instead on psychosocial relief of children and training of caregivers, of which PAHCHAAN already had the experience and could do much better than many. It was very difficult to say no to millions of rupees worth of donation, which would have brought PAHCHAAN into lime light and had satisfied the philanthropic desire of our volunteers and well wishers. PAHCHAAN, however, being a specialized child rights organization decided to do what it was good at not ride the bandwagon.

Do what you can do best

If you are an educationist, set up school systems, if you are good at marketing, collect funds, if you are a researcher, conduct studies, and if you are an IT professional, set up information systems. Do what you are best at, give your best in an emergency setting. It is not the time to learn new trades, these can be done during a long project, but it is bound to fail during a disaster. Even if seemingly you are doing well at some other field behold; the professional could have done much better. Pakistan Pediatric Association would never, e.g. set out to build homes or latrines. It has tried to set up water purification plants in Sind after floods, but after spending lacs of rupees, these plants have gone out of order for want of maintenance and local community involvement. Pure water is essential for child health but pediatrician is not the best person to set up installations. This decision has been criticized in the pediatric circles, and therefore PPA has now diverted its funds to the job it can do best.

Pakistan Pediatric Association has now established a disaster management cell, which has taken an initiative of formulating a curriculum on disaster management and creating provincial disaster management teams of pediatricians. Whatever little funds it has on its disposal will be used to train provincial trainers though a volunteer core team, meanwhile it will look for INGO funding to build a team of up to 300 pediatricians and doctors as local disaster managers for the health care of children. This is what PPA is best at, this is what it should do.

Be innovative, experiment! but document

PAHCHAAN bas been innovative and has tried to do certain things differently. During the internal displacement in 2009, PAHCHAAN involved a group of volunteers, who would sponsor and organize stitching of clothes for the displaced families. PAHCHAAN camp team would list the persons in the camp and take their body measurements, to be sent to a group of volunteers in different villages of Punjab through its main office in Lahore. In a few days the stitched clothes would reach the camp and the displaced children, women, and men would receive a gift of new clothes from their Punjabi brethren. This would not affect the self-esteem of the recipient and would inculcate a sense of brotherhood between the two provinces. PAHCHAAN even managed to arrange dowry clothes for many girls whose marriage was arranged by the camp authorities through the same channel.

Nestle was marketing a nutritious biscuit for infants and it donated a truck load of these biscuits during the IDP crisis. These biscuits were an ideal food for the infants and toddlers as these provided all the essential nutrients and energy, but were not to the taste of adults and hence were only consumed by the children. PAHCHAAN distributed these biscuits within the child friendly spaces. On the one hand these provided nutrition to the children, and on the other these were not

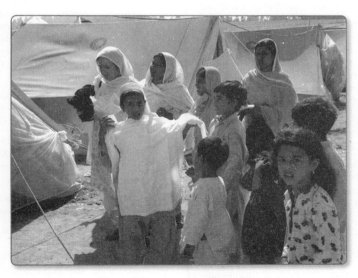

Figure 6 Inmates with fresh clothes

wasted or pilfered, as these were not a popular 'take away souvenir' for other camp management workers.

The only purpose of bringing up these two examples is to show that one should be innovative. The initiative should be properly documented, preferably as a case study or a through a small action research, so that its results can be validated. Unfortunately PAHCHAAN did not document these or other innovations, and the learning could not benefit other populations in other settings.

Disasters are best managed during a period of calm

Initiating a disaster response during a disaster is bound to bring disastrous results. All the learning from disaster management emphasizes the need to work before disaster at disaster preparedness and disaster mitigation.

The number of natural disasters has increased up to 4 times during the last two decades, and the world is expected to experience up to 500 natural disasters every year. It is better to be prepared now than to be caught by surprise (Natural Disasters Up More Than 400 Percent in Two Decades).

Conclusions

Children become increasingly venerable during emergency situations. Their Survival, Protection, Development and Participation rights are violated. The preexisting issues and vulnerabilities multiply the challenges that children face post-emergency situation.

Prior to emergency situation the government needs to develop and implement policies to minimize the damage. Basic training needs to be provided to experts as well as locals.

In our opinion, organizations need to evaluate its resources, capacities and capabilities. Child rights based organizations should restrict themselves to research, providing rehabilitation for children and capacity building advocacy around the issues of rights during emergency They should not try to compete with the more experienced and resourceful institutions like army, government, or large relief organizations but try to form collaborations with them.

Bibliography

1. Adirim, T. (2009). Protecting Children During Disasters:

2. Austin, J. et al. 'Reproductive health: a right for refugees and internally displaced persons' in Reproductive Health Matters, 2008; 16(31):10–21. Gaffney, D. A. 2006.

3. Halvorson, S. and Hamilton, J.P. 'Vulnerability and the Erosion of Seismic Culture in Mountainous Central Asia, Special Issue on Coping with Human Vulnerability in Mountain Environments' in Mountain Research and Development, 2007; 27(4):322–331.

4. Iezzoni, L.I. and Ronan, L.J. 'Disability legacy of the Haitian earthquake' in Annals of Internal Medicine, 2010; 152(12):812–814.

5. Javaid, Z., & Arshad, M. Child Protection in Disaster Management in South Asia : A Case Study of Pakistan. *Research Journal of South Asian Studies*, 2011; 26(1):191–202.

6. Lane, C. Adolescent Refugees and Migrants: A Reproductive Health Emergency. Pathfinder International, 2008.

7. Penrose, A., & Takaki, M. Children's rights in emergencies and disasters. *Lancet*, 2006; 367(9511): 698–9. doi:10.1016/S0140-6736(06)68272-X

8. Singapore Red Cross (2010), Pakistan Floods:The Deluge of Disaster - Facts & FiguresReport, 15 Sept 2010 Retrieved from https://mail-attachments.googleusercontent.com/attachem ent/?=2&ik=b82aa745ff&view=att&th=13b71e acf194da4&attid=0.10&disp=inline&relattid=f haec8t169&safe=1&zw&saduie=AG9B P-ri-vizDsL 9qljmRWDpf7j&sadet=1354962426362&sads=D0L WRGmFyY3pkkJFx2bYP96SEj8

9. Solberg, K. Worst floods in living memory leave Pakistan in paralysis. *The Lancet*, 2010; 376(9746): 1039–1040. doi:10.1016/S0140-6736(10)61469-9

10. The Aftermath of Disaster : Children in Crisis. *Journal of clinical psychology:in session*, 2004; 62(8):1001–1016. doi:10.1002/jclp Guiding principles for feeding infants and young children. *World Health Organization*.

11. The Federal View. *Clinical Pediatric Emergency Medicine*, 10(3):164–172. doi:10.1016/j.cpem.2009.06.005

12. Ul Haq, N. (2005). P AKISTAN E ARTHQUAKE 2005, Rescue, Relief, Rehabilitation and Construction. Retrieved from http://ipripak.org/factfiles/ff79.pdf

13. World Bank. Analyzing Urban Poverty: A Summary of Methods and Approaches. World Bank Policy

Count

1
2
3 ———————— 1306
4 —

chapls   8   —   210

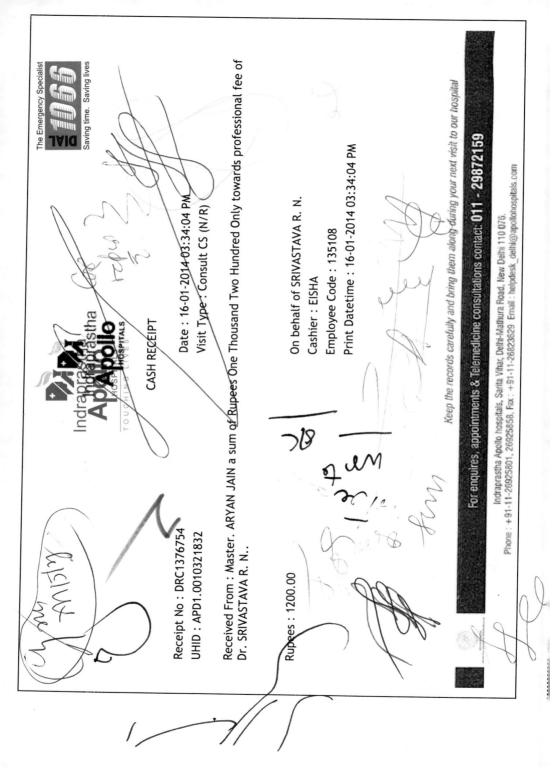

Indraprastha Apollo
Apollo
HOSPITALS
TOUCHING LIVES

The Emergency Specialist
DIAL **1066**
Saving time. Saving lives

CASH RECEIPT

Receipt No : DRC1376754
UHID : APD1.0010321832

Date : 16-01-2014 03:34:04 PM
Visit Type : Consult CS (N/R)

Received From : Master. ARYAN JAIN a sum of Rupees One Thousand Two Hundred Only towards professional fee of Dr. SRIVASTAVA R. N..

On behalf of SRIVASTAVA R. N.
Cashier : EISHA
Employee Code : 135108
Print Datetime : 16-01-2014 03:34:04 PM

Rupees : 1200.00

Keep the records carefully and bring them along during your next visit to our hospital

For enquires, appointments & Telemedicine consultations contact: 011 - 29872159

Indraprastha Apollo hospitals, Sarita Vihar, Delhi-Mathura Road, New Delhi 110 076,
Phone : +91-11-26925801, 26925858, Fax : +91-11-26823629 Email : helpdesk_delhi@apollohospitals.com

Research Working Paper 3399, written by J. Baker and N. Schuler. Washington DC: World Bank, 2004.

14. World Bank. Natural Hazards, UnNatural Disasters: Te Economics of Effective Prevention. Washington DC: World Bank, 2010.

15. World Bank. 'Conflict, security and development' in World Development Report 2011. Washington DC: World Bank, 2011.

16. *World Disaster Report 2012- Focus on forced migration and displacement.* (2012). Retrieved from http://www.ifrc.org/PageFiles/99703/1216800-WDR 2012-EN-LR.pdf

17. World Food Programme (WFP). Emergency Food Security Assessment Handbook. Rome: WFP, 2009, 2nd edition.

12

Child Neglect: Wider Dimensions

Aisha Mehnaz

Introduction

Child Abuse and Neglect (CAN) are of global prevalence not affected by ethnicity, religion, socioeconomic class or geographical areas. It remains an under reported issues every where. The overall picture of health, sanitation and education in children in South East Asian countries presents a very dismal picture (Table 1). The basic rights of children are violated; there is considerable morbidity and mortality arising from neglect in children belonging to underdeveloped and developing countries.

Even in developed countries like USA there are more than 3 million reported cases of CAN more than 2,000 death and 18,000 permanent disabilities occur every year because of CAN. Neglect is the commonest type of abuse identified in over 64.1% of cases, followed by physical abuse (16%) sexual abuse (8.8%) and emotional neglect (6.6%). Almost 80% perpetrators were parents.[1]

The situation is equally gloomy in Sout East Asia. In New Dehli Child abuse rate is over 83% with more boys (72%) than girls (65%) reported to be abuse, the perpetrators are again identified as family members.[2] Sri Lanka has 40,000 child prostitutes[3] in the country; their emotional, nutritional and physical neglect is not quantified.

In Pakistan no official data exist on various types of Child Abuse. Neglect is the commonest type of abuse reported in various studies. Among all types of child neglect, nutritional neglect is the commonest; nearly 40% of children in Pakistan less than 5 years of age suffer from undernutrition[4,5,6]. Nearly half are affected by stunting and about 9% by wasting, 36% or Urban and 44% of Rural Children are stunted, 79% deaths in children less than 5 years of age are associated with malnutrition. Those surviving the effect of undernutrtion in early childhood ends up as emotionaly depressed, stunted adolscents. Early marriage of such adolescent girl lead to the birth of another under weight, under nourished child and thus the vicous cycle goes on.

Before we discuss what are the factors affecting neglect, let us first look at the definition of neglect.

Definition of neglect

Child neglect is difficult to define. There is no consensus on its definition. Definition varies across discipline; it has to be considered in a societal context. More commonly neglect is defined as parental or caregivers acts of omission, such as inadequate supervison of a child.[7]

Although lack of parental or caretaker supervison and care is considered the prime factor behind neglect. The societal and environmental factors need to be taken into account in defining neglect and its causation.

According to WHO (1999) Neglect is the inattention or omission on the part of caregiver to provide for the development of the child in all spheres; health, education, nutrition, emotional developmental shelter and safe conditions in the context of resources reasonably available to the family or caretakers and causes or has a high probability of causing harm to the child health or physical, mental, social, spiritual, moral or social

Table 1 Profile of South Asia	Pakistan	India	Bangladesh	Afghanistan	Sri Lanka	Nepal
Population under 18 (thousands)	73,227	447,309	55,938	16,781	6,154	12,874
Population under 5 (thousands)	21,418	127,979	14,707	5,546	1,893	3,506
Infant mortality rate (per 1,000 live births) 2010	70	48	38	103	14	41
Under-Five mortality rate (per 1,000 live births) 2010	87	63	48	149	17	50
Maternal mortality rate 2008 (Adjusted)	260	230	340	1,400	39	380
Total % of population using improved drinking water sources (2008)	90	88	80	48	90	88
Total % of population with access to sanitation (2008)	45	31	53	37	91	31
Total adult literacy rate (%) 2005–2010*	56	63	56	–	91	59
Primary school enrollment ratio (net) male/female (2007-2010)*	72/60	97/94	86/93	–	95/96	-
Percentage of population below $1.25 per day 2000–2009	23	42	50	–	7	55
GNI per capital (US $) 2010	1,050	1,340	640	330x	2,290	490
Percentage of government expenditure allocated to:	Health	1	2	6	–	6	7
	Education	2	3	14	–	10	18
	Defense	13	13	8	–	18	9

Source: UNICEF. The State of the World's Children 2012 – Children in an Urban World. 2012.

X: Data refer to years or periods other than those specified in the column heading. Such data are not included in the calculation of regional and global averages.

*Data refer to the most recent year available during the period specified in the column heading.

development. This includes the failure to properly supervise and protect children from harm as much as is feasible.

Other defines neglect as when "Parents fail to meet the needs of an infant through lack of care and nurture which results in developmental consequences".[8]

While defining neglect one has to consider what constitutes "adequate care" of children, and what actions or acts of omission on parts of parents or caretakers constitute neglect, must these action or inaction be intentional or unintentional resulting from ignorance of child's development. The ultimate effect of these inaction affects the child's health resulting in actual or potential damage to their prospect of developing into a healthy adult.

Polansky's[9] conceptual definition of child neglect has taken these points into consideration and is well accepted he defined child neglect as "A condition in which a caretaker responsible for

the child, either deliberately or by extraordinary inattentiveness, permits the child to experience avoidable suffering and or fails to provide one or more of the ingredients generally deemed essential for developing a person's physical, intellectual and emotional capacities" this definition though include parental action which result in untoward consequences for the child but fail to specify the extent of harm to the child.

Neglect is often the most ignored and underrated of all types of child abuse. Many do not consider neglect a kind of abuse especially in a condition where the parents are involved as it is often considered unintentional and arise from lack of knowledge or awareness. This may be true in certain circumstances and often it results in insurmountable problem being faced by the parents.

There thus exist an ambiguity and vagueness regarding the definition of neglect.

In short any act or failure to act which presents an imminent risk of serious harm constitute neglect.

Child abuse happens with "regular" people. There is no easy way to identify someone who will abuse or neglect children. Some children are at higher risk by having special needs. Neglect can happen to any child, any age, including teenagers.

Types of neglect

Not only is it difficult to define neglect it is even more difficult to describe the many forms in which child neglect exist. Often more than one types of neglect co-exist greatly affecting the child physical and mental development, if not intervened and managed at early stage it inevitably leads to worse form of child abuse and exploitation.

Different types of neglect: This include

Physical neglect

It is the failure to supply the physical needs of a child such as maintaining proper hygiene, cleanliness, clothing, food, shelter and other physical needs of the child by parents or caretakers. Physical and emotional negelct is most prevalent in institutionlised children or children living in shelter homes, however it is as common at homes but the latter is less likely to become apparent easily.

Disciplining a child without causing physical injury may not be called physical neglect but often parents who are strict disciplinarian unintentionly cause their children to suffer emotionaly which may affect their apetite and dietary intake. On the other hand not teaching the children the basic ethics involve in human relationship may interfere with their prospect of adopting a humane attitude in their adulthood. Thus, there exists a very delicate balance in adopting the right attitude of disciplining the child and neglect.

Physical neglect also includes refusal or failure to provide or allow needed care in accordance with the recommendations of competent health care professionals for a physical injury, illness, medical condition or impairment. It also include failure to seek timely and appropriate medical care for a serious health problem which any reasonable lay man would have recognised as needing professional medical attention. Abondonement, expulsion, lack of supervision and custody issues are also considered as form of physical neglect.

Emotional neglect

It is the failure to provide, love, affection and emotional bonding to the child. Lack of positive attention, Ignoring or isolating the child, rejecting his demand, not comforting them when upset, absence of positive reinforcement and physical affection results in emotional abuse and/or neglect. There is an assault on child's self-esteem, mental health or social development. The offender most often is a parent or caretaker-someone whose approval is important to the child. It is sometimes coupled with physical abuse or neglect, but not always.

Emotional neglect has far more devastating and long lasting effect than physical neglect. It is essentialy the failure to provide a developmentally appropriate, supportive environment including the availability of a primary attachment figure, so child can develop a stable, emotional and social competencies commensurate with her or his personal potential, and in the context of the society in which the child dwells.

Nutritional neglect

It is the failure to supply the essential nutrients to the child necessary for his growth and development. Children whose growth fall below the third centile in height and or weight for no known medical reason have been designated "non-orgainic failure to thrive". All children whose development is significanlty affected by inadequate nutrional intake is classified as "acutely malnourished".

In the third world countries under nutrition is the most widely prevalent type of nutritional neglect, the perpetrators often love parents. Nutritional neglect commonly present as macronutrient deficiency disorders (protein energy malnutrition, marasmus and kwarshiorkor) or manifest as micronutrient deficiency disorders like ricket, iron deficiency anemia, etc.

The high mortality in the third world countries is primarily due to nutritional negligence by the parents, caretakers and health care providers. Epidemiological data from 53 developing countries indicate that 56% of child deaths were attritbutable to malnutrition.[10] It is the major determinant of outcome in children suffering from infectious diseases, another major problem affecting children in developing countries. The potential affect of malnutrition in infectious diseases is more apparent in mild to moderate malnutrtion than severe nutrition.[11]

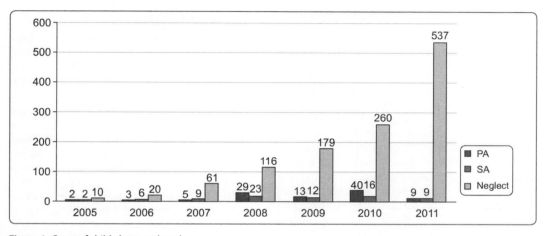

Figure 1 Cases of child abuse and neglect
Child Abuse Prvention Society /Hospital Child Protection committee, Civil Hospital Karachi.

In Pakistan the state of malnutrtion (undernutrtion) has worsened after the flood of 2010. The emergency threshold of malnutrtion established by WHO to trigger an emergency response is 15%.[22,23] After the flood the global acute malnutrtion rate in children between 6 and 59 months in Pakistan has risen to more than 21%. The data by Konpal, an NGO supporting the Hospital Child Protection Committee in Sindh (HCPC) has also shown a steady rise of nutritional neglect among all types of Child Abuse and Neglect (Fig. 1).

Overnutrition manifesting as obesity is also a fast emerging threat in developing countries. This is often due to failure of the parents to realize the optimum nutritive needs of the growing child. Rapidly improving economy of the developing nations and increase indulgence of the children in non-nutritive high caloric diet coupled with sedentry life style are often blamed for the rising incidence of obesity in the developing countries.

In most of the epidemiological studies only the socioeconomic status and its relationship with obesity has been studied. Little data is available on the relationship of maltreatment and/or neglect of children in childhood and obesity in later life. One potential mechanism is stress reulting from maltreatment causing children to react by increasing food intake and or decreasing activity.[11,12] Maltreatment in childhood has a close association with depression and anxiety and development of obesity in later life. Neuroendocrine responses to stress may alter the metabolism, activity levels or apetite, whatever

the mechanism is there is no denying the fact that there is dramatic rise in obesity in children in the developing countries. In developed countries obesity is considered a severe type of medical neglect requiring notification to child protection services. Unfortunately, the child protection services is in a state of infancy in most of the developing countries and has a long way to go. The rising epidemic of obesity should be recognized before it is too late.

Dental neglect

It is the consequence of nutritional neglect or the oral health of children. It is defined by the American Academy of Paediatric dentistry as "the willful failure of parents/guardian to seek and follow through with the treatment necessary to ensure a level of health essential for adequate function and freedom from pain and infection". Dental problems if left untreated lead to pain, infection and loss of function. These will ultimately adversely effects learning, communication, nutrition and other activities necessary for growth and development of a child.

Educational neglect

It includes failure to educate the child. Failure to enroll the child of a manadatoy scholl age group or causing the child to stay at home for non-legitimate reason like to work (within home or outside) or takecare of younger siblings, a practice commonly observed in South East

Asian Countries are the most common form of educational neglect.

The essential role of education in the intellectual and cognitive development of the child cannot be over emphasised. Education is the fundamental rights of every child. A number of developing countries have endorse the MDG 2 which obligates compulsory primary education for all children especially girls. Unfortunately in most countries including Pakistan the progress is slow. Recent humanatarian crises like flood of 2010-2011 during which 9,800 schools were washed away, security issues in armd conflict areas, destruction of school, high drop out because of economic reason are to name just the few obstacles toward achieving the goal. Neverthless denying this basic right of every child is the worst form of neglect the children of the south East Asian countries are subjected to and which is going to have serious long-term repurcussion.

Inattention to the special educational need of a handicapped child or a child with learning disorder or a mentally challenged child is also educational neglect. Habitual trauancy in situation where parents and guardian have been informed of the problem and had not attempted to intervene is also considered as a form of educational neglect.

Medical neglect

It includes failure to realise the medical problems in child. The neglect could be on part of health care providers, or by the parents or person incharge of the child. Witholding of a medically indicated treament in a sick child including appropriate nutrition, hydration and medication which will endanger the life of the child consititue medical neglect.

Child negelct in armed conflict or war affected zone

Children living in armed conflict areas are the most neglected population. Their health and education is severly compromised. Death of the parents or caretakers results in their physical, nutritional and emotional neglect. Many of these children are recruited as child soldiers or even as suicide bombers. Those survived suffer from worst psychological trauma. According to UNESCO 40% of primary school aged children.

Are living in conflict affected areas with 28 million living in conflict affected poor countries.[24]

Deprivation abuse

Neglect can be some time intentional. Deliberate withholding of basic needs of the child with intent to harm the child is called deprivation abuse. This act of omission merit immediate punitive action against the perpetrators.

However neglect in most part is unintentional on part of caretakers of the child, and is simply due to ignorance but is clearly an act of omission thus depriving the child of an environment conducive for his growth and developmnt. Neglect seems minor but has serious effects, stunting, Failure-to-thrive, developmental delay and behavioral disturbances all interfere with the development of a child into a mature and responsible adult.

Predictors of neglect

A number of predictors of child maltreatment has been identified in various setup.The four best predictors of child maltreatment includes family revenue below the poverty line, single working mother, young age mothers (first pregnancy occuring before the age of 21 years) and four or more children in the family. In developing countries there exist in addition other factors as well.

Poverty or poor socioeconomic status

It is a common belief that poor socioeconomic status is the much detrimental factor behind neglect especially malnutrition, the belief is not without justification. A substantive number of researchers have suggested that family income is strongly related to the incidence of abuse and neglect.[12]

As often it perpetuates conflicts with resultant violence. This lead to insecurity, emotional instability, depression and rejection in the mother, the primary caretaker of children which ultimately reflects in neglect of their children. This was observed also in our study[21] in which large family size >5 members (83%), poverty (90%), domestic violence (>75%) illiteracy (77%), addiction (43%), domestic violence (75%) and depression/anxiety disorders in mothers (80%)emerged as the most obvious risk factors affecting child care.

In USA it was found that children with families with annual income below $15,000 per year are more then 25 times more likely than children from families with annual income above $30,000 to suffer from abuse and neglect. However, there are other who argues that neglect is seen across all socioeconomic classes but affluent families are often given the benefit of doubt and cases from rich families are seldom brought to light as they are least suspected as they have better access to legal counsel. This may not be far from truth.

Female sex

There is plenty of evidence that female child is more likely to suffer from abuse and neglect especially nutritional neglect. In a patriachal society like ours male child is given preference over female child. The foods are preferentially served to male members including male off springs. Culturally male child is seen as superior to a female child as he is considered the future bread earners. He also shoulder the responsibility of carrying the family name forward. This is particularly true in the South East Asian countries. In most studies from the East female out numbered boys in all types of abuse and neglect. In the west although according to published statistics of child abuse and neglect 52% victims were female and 48% male, however most studies have shown no significant sex prediliction.

In Pakistan and Afghanistan (and perhaps in other Southeast Asian countries) a female faces discrimination, exploitation and abuse at many levels; girls are prevented from exercising their basic right to education—either because of traditional family practices, economic necessity or as a consequence of the destruction of schools by militants. Girls and young women continue to suffer from what the United Nations Committee on the Rights of the Child calls "inhumane customs and rituals", including forced marriage and so-called "honor" killings. Women are also subjected to local customs and cultural practices which all too frequently restrict their mobility, bar them from working, and see them victimized by violence and abuse.

Inadequate parenting skills

Poor nurturing qualities of mother, lack of knowledge concerning child developmeent, and deficient problem solving skills have been found to be closely related to mothers whose children are negelcted. Bouscha and Twenty[13] found that mothers of neglected children interacted least with their children compared with mothers of non-maltreated children. Several studies have indicated least or negative interaction between neglected children and their parents.

Maternal problem

Maternal problems like mental and psychiatric illnesses, e.g depression, substance abuse, domestic violence has been found to be closely linked with child neglect.[14-16] Mother's inadequacy in child care is often found to be related with neglect especially nutritional and medical neglect like delay in seeking health care. Very young mothers or overaged mothers, multiparous mothers, overworked and socially isolated mothers are more likely to suffer from depression Intellectual impairment and lack of education are also found to be closely associated with neglect

Maternal drug or substance abuse

A high rate of substance or drug addiction among the family members including mothers have been identified in number of reported cases of child neglect. In one study an incidence as high as 28% of drug abuse was found in the families of children who are neglected. Substance abuse is also a major problem in the South East Asia and the problem is escalating. Another disturbing aspect is the high consumption of non-nutritive substances like beetle nuts, gutka (mixture of tobacco and beetle nuts) niswar (a form of snuff used particularly by people of Afghan and Pathan origin). The practice is particularly rife in subcontinent. On an average it costs 100–150 Rupees per household which poses a great economic constraint on the families with poor resources. More often these substances are purchased by compromising the purchase of food items particularly those essential for children. A number of studies have a direct correlation of child nutritional neglect with the substance abuse and addiction. This has been our observation; the misplaced priorities in resource constraint communities are affecting the children nutritional status badly.

Environmental factors

This plays an important role in the causation of negelct especially in the presence of other factors like poverty, unemployement or large family size, etc. Environmental factors like pollution, war, mass exodus or immigration due to war, exposure to guns and violence (domestic and street violence) injuries to family members threatens child protection. Most parents are not able to cope with the strains resulting from environmental hazard and the changes that occur because of it, as a result they experience difficulty in providing care to their children.[17]

Disasters and emergency situation

Children are the worst affected population in all natural and man created disasters. Medical and nutritional neglect is extremely common. Pakistan has been hit by the disaster of unprecedented nature during the last decade. During the earhthquake of 2005 more than 10,8000 people were affected (50% were children and women, 19,000 < 5 years of age). During Flood 2010 and 2011 more than 3.5 million and 1.7 million children were affected (UNICEF 2011). malnutrition has worsened during last 5 years. Malnutrition has increased from 40% in 2007[18] to >50% in 2010.[19]

Psychological problems and emotional trauma are immense during emergency situation. Depression, fear, anger, frustration, helpless ness, psychosomatic symptoms like headache. Sleep disturbances, bowel disturbances are identified in these children with increasing frequency. Long-term psychological disturbances like PTSD, psychosomatic problems. Substance abuse were the other observed phenomena.

Factors present in children leading to neglect

Children need adult assistance to remain safe.

Elements that make children more vulnerable include young age, physical or mental disability, Illnesses, provocative behavior, non-assertive behavior, traumatic and, stressful situation. Even older children (preadolescents, teenagers) can be vulnerable.

Premature infant, children with terminal or intractable disease, children suffering from psychological trauma or grossly abused children are more likely to be nutritionaly negelcted. One imporatnt characteristic common to all these children are their failure to communicate their need

to their caretakers. As in most circumstances these children remain passive, they do not cry or complain to indicate their need, often the caretakers consider that child need is being met. The child therefore is left alone and slowly become isolated and neglectd.

Several studies have identified LBW and prematurity as risk factors for neglect especially the nutritional neglect[20] and medical neglect, the latter partly due to increase demand for frequent hospital visit which poses economic as well as emotional stress to the mother and the family, and the former simply as mother do not realize the nutritional need of the child. This again is due to the interplay of several factors like large family size, too closely spaced pregnancies, birth of girl child and rapidly changing socioeconomic and geopolitical situation.

Children with disabilities are more likely to be neglected. Families with disable children are often depressed and are not physically or psychologically prepared to provide extra care and support to the extra need of their special child. The medical and nutritional need is mostly neglected in such children.

Children placed in institutional care are more likely to suffer from emotional and nutritional neglect. UNICEF estimates that the total number of children placed in insittutional care in the world is 2.2 million which they admit are the gross under estimate. Children are placed in these insititution for a number of reason mainly poverty, death of one or both the parents, seperation, divorce, domestic violence, family feud or family breakup.Children seperated from their families during disasters or living in war affected or conflict zone are also sent for institutional care. The paid staff in these institution are often not trained to take care of the emotional, medical and nutritional need of these children. Many poverty stricken parents believe that putting their children into institution is the best way of providing good nutrition, education and health but they do not realise the harmful impact it leaves on child emotional and physical development.

These institutions are both state owned and private, the latter are established by NGO, Individual or faith based organizations. A number of such organizations have sprouted in South East Asia; mostly they are unsupervised and unchecked. The best interest of child is not considered, rather to achieve their objectives emotional abuse or nutritional deprivation is practiced.

Intervention and management

There is substantive evidence that child neglect particularly nutritional neglect is multi-factorial in nature therfore requires a multi-disciplinary approach. There is need for the development of programmes that integrate child development, health and nutrition. The intervention are needed at multiple levels as isolated intervention will not produce the desired results.

The families were neglect is present require not only immediate but long-term intervention as there is likelihood of rcurrence of neglect of children in such families. In all intervention program directed toward CAN, neglect is often given least priority. The emphasis is mainly laid on child sexual and physical abuse. However, it has to be considered while panning an intervention program for CAN that if neglect not detected and intervened earlier invariably and in most instances it ends up in physical and other type of abuse. Principles of effective prevention and intervention of neglect should consider the following while planning the strategies for prevention of CAN.

Identification of high-risk families

A number of studies have identified that children coming from families with low income group, unemployement, addiction in family members, domestic violence, and low literacy level are more likely to neglect their children. Intervention should be directed at multiple levels depending upon the family need.

a. Providing job opportunities or giving loans for setting up of small business.

b. Providing free education to their children and setting up of adult literacy centres in areas where high-risk families reside.

c. Setting up of detoxification centre where addicted memebers in the high-risk families are provided free treatment and counselling.

d. Low income housing scheme to provide safe and affordable shelters.

e. Capacity building of parents specially mothers in providing care and protection to their children. Konpal child abuse prevention society has an ongoing training program for mothers admitted in hospitals with neglected children. Theses mothers while in hospital are given training in basic hygiene, nutrition, breaset feeding, immunization, conflict management and child protection. Multiple modalitis of teaching like discussion, multimedia presentations, role play and hands on training are mployed to impart information and education to the mothers. Significant change in the mothers knowledge and attitude was found in these mothers.

f. Effective use of print and electronic media. The impact of media in raising awareness about various forms of neglect cannot be overstated. Unfortunately, the electronic media in the developing countries are not playing their role in educating the massess about the neglect. Simple messages on prevention of abuse and neglect if aired through media can have a more lasting impact. This combined with one to one consultancy to the affected families by the professionals will produce a convincing results.

g. Involvement of socialy isolated families in social activities like group discussions, recreation activities, etc. is essential, unless the affected families are part of the social network of the society any efforts to bring about the reformative and corrective changes will be ineffective.

Outreach programs

Most of the affected families have limited resources and are isoltaed. Out reach should be designed to take information, education and intervention (dietary, medicinal and social) at theire door step. In a limited scale UNICEF and WHO has initiated therapeutic feeding program at the country level by some countries including Pakistan which particularly proved affective during the flood of 2010. There is need to have more sustainable and concrete steps. Involving CBO and local country leaders and decision makers who can understand the family and their environment will prove more benficial in the long run compared to short-term project. This has been observed during the flood of Pakistan, RTUF (ready to use food) for the children was distributed to the flood affectes families free of cost, but once the supply was exhausted the families were left with the same problem of malnutrition. Every effort should be geared toward the capacity building of the families and providing opportunities for income generation to the affected families.

Empowerment of the families

Empowerment of the families in general and high-risk families particularly to solve their own problems will be the most essential and crucial step and will go a long way in alleviation of neglect.

Setting up of help line and home visiting programs

This may prove an effective intervntion for families who like to sek help of the professionals. One of the problem health care providers faced in sustaining intervention program with the families of neglected children is lack or loss of communication once the families leave the health care setup.A help line and home visiting program will help in forming good communication with the families and sustaing intervention program. This will also decrease the drop outs. Appointment of Medical social officers' and involvement of volunteers may produce good results.

Improving the competencies of service providers

It is most essential that service providers, program managers, medical social officers, and health care professionals involved in the management of negelct are culturally competelt and should have diverse knowledge and skills about the high-risk families and their problems leading to neglect of their children. Such persons involved in intervention program should also consider the religion and socio-cultural background of the targetted family's involved in nglect of their children before embarking on any intervention program.

Inclusion in education program and curriculum

Including the priniciples of essential child care practices and dangers of child abuse and neglect in education curricula is an important and early intervention measures. The undergraduate curri-culam of medical students should also incorporate the dvelopmental needs of the child. The physical and emotional needs of the child should be included in the training of adolscent male and female from their early formative years. This will be an asset to them when they become adult and assume the responsibilties of parents.

"Much of the next millennium can be seen in how we care for our children today. Tomorrow's world may be influenced by science and technology, but more than anything, it is already taking shape in the bodies and minds of our children."

Kofi Annan,
Secretary-General of the United Nations

References

1. http://www.childwelfare.gov/systemwide/statistics/can.cfm visited 18 august 2010.
2. http://www.mahendraap.wordpress.com/2007/05/04. visited 12 sept 2010.
3. Zero tolerance for child sex tourism in Sri Lanka. www.unicef.org/media, 2006.
4. State of World's Children.2009UNICEF, Basic Indicators, 176–7.
5. Black RE, Morris SS, Bryce J.Where and Why 10 million children dying everywhere. Lancet; 361:22, 2003.
6. Presentation by Joint scretary (2007) Ministry of social welfare.National consultation organised by SC-UK.august 2009: 26–3(4.5.6.678 editoria)
7. Office of human dvelopment services, CFR S1340.2 definitions.Washington DC: US.Department of Human Health Services 1987.
8. Maria scannapieco, Kelli Connel – Carick, Understanding child maltreatment: an ecological and developmental perspective. Oxford University Press, 10 fb, 2005.
9. N.E Polansky et al.Damaged parents, an anatomy of child neglect.Chicago IL.University of Chicago press 1987.
10. Bulletin of WHO, 1995: 73(4).
11. Pelletier DL, Frongillo EA Jr, Schroeder DG, Habicht JR. The effects of malnutrition on child mortality in developing countries. Bull World Health Organisation. 1995; 73(4):4438.
12. Cappelleri, J; Eckenrode, J., Powers, J. The epidemiolgy of Child Abuse: Findings from the second National incidence and prevalence study of child abuse and neglect. American Public health, 1993; 83:1622–1624.
13. Bouscha DM and Twentyman CT.Mother-child interaction style in abuse, neglect and control

groups: naturalistic observations in the home.J Abnormal Psychol. 1984:93–106.

14. A Rahman, H Lovel, J Bunn. Mother's mental health and Infant growth: a case–control study from rawalpindi, pakistan, Blackwell Publishing Ltd, childcare, health and development, 2004; 30:21–27.

15. Vikram Patel et al.Gender, poverty and postnatal depression: A study of Mothers in Goa, India. Is J Psychiatry 159:1, January 2002?

16. R.Taj, K S Sikander. Effcts of maternal depression on Breast Feeding.JPMA, 53(1) Jan 2003.

17. Wolfe, D.A 1991, Preventing Physical and emotional abuse of children, The Guilford Press, New York. 18. Pakistan Demorphic health Survey, MOH 2008.www.healthsysytemspak.com http://www.

18. Pakistan flood, uncover dire nutrtion situation, 2010, UNICEF.www.unicef.org/infobycountrypakistan

19. Benedict MI, White RB, Wulff LM. Selectedperinatal factors and child abuse.Am J Public health 1985; 75:780.

20. A Mehnaz, A mala, N shah, Uzma ET al. Psychosocial determinants of malnutrition. 2009, konpal/chk, (under publication)

21. www.sparcpk.org

22. Save the children USA, acute malnutrition survey sheet.save the children.org.292

23. UN educational scientific and cultural organisation (UNESCO). The hidden crises: armed conflict and education.2011 unesdoc.unesco.org

13

Abuse and Neglect of Children with Disabilities: Under a Veil of Secrecy

Renu Singh

Introduction

Child abuse continues globally under a veil of secrecy, with perpetrators going scot free, since there is an entrenched belief and misconception in majority societies that child abuse is non-existent. Children living in poverty and belonging to marginalized communities are those who are most 'at risk' of being subjected to abuse and neglect. Amongst these, children with disabilities form an acutely vulnerable group and their voices and abuse remains 'silent' and 'hidden'. According to WHO child abuse or maltreatment "constitutes all forms of physical and/or emotional ill-treatment, sexual abuse, neglect or negligent treatment or commercial or other exploitation, resulting in actual or potential harm to the child's health, survival, development or dignity in the context of a relationship of responsibility, trust or power". This paper embraces this definition and neglect is subsumed as a sub-set of abuse and covers all kinds of deprivation that children will encounter, including failure by caregiver to provide need-based care (if financially and emotionally able to do so). It is critical that issues related to children with disabilities are addressed as part of the wider mainstream activities to stop abuse against children, else we will continue to live with the problem for decades to come.

Children with disabilities

Right at the outset, it is pertinent to note that children with disabilities are 'children first' and respond and react to neglect and abuse in a similar manner to the *normal* (sic) child. While the magnitude and numbers of children with disabilities vary across nations, depending on the specific definition of disability, the World Health Organization's estimates that 10% of the world's young people—are born with a disability or become disabled before age 19 years. A recent report by UNICEF's Innocent Research Center (2007), estimates that there are approximately 160 million children with disabilities in the developing world. Various researches have revealed that children with disabilities have increased vulnerability to neglect and abuse (Sullivan and Knutson, 2000; Children's Bureau 2006).[1] Children who live with sensory impairments such as visual, hearing and speech impairments as well as intellectual disabilities would undoubtedly be especially vulnerable. While the amount of research available on this population is extremely limited, particularly for disabled children in the developing world, current research indicates that violence against disabled children occurs at annual rates at least 1.7 times greater than their non-disabled peers UNICEF, 2005. A quick review if existing literature amplifies that most of prevailing studies have been undertaken in Northern countries and research on the subject in developing countries like India, remain oblivious to the situation of children with disabilities. The only major study on child abuse in India (MWCD, 2007), does not have any evidence related to children with disabilities. This is despite the fact that India has a newly amended Juvenile Justice (Care and Protection of Children) Act, the Integrated Child Protection Scheme (ICPS), drafted the Protection of Children from Sexual

Offences Bill 2011, signed the United Nations Convention on the Rights of the Child (UNCRC) and ratified the UN Convention on the Rights of the Disabled (UNCRPD). Under Article 19 of the UNCRC children with disabilities have a right to be protected from all forms of physical or mental violence, injury or abuse, neglect or negligent treatment, maltreatment or exploitation, including sexual abuse. Children with disabilities are often the victims of neglect from family members, victims of abuse at the hands of strangers or those who are meant to be their protectors as well as neglected by well-meaning policy makers and bureaucrats, who fail to deliver a safe, nurturing environment. Abuse and neglect has immense long-term ramifications—the worst being the end and crushing of childhood and associated dreams the young child with disability may hold dear.

Emerging models of disability

There has been a number of developments during the past decade, questioning the 'medical model' of disability which although well intentioned, concentrated on "care" and "cure", thereby imposing a paternalistic approach to working with people with disabilities and assuming that the impairment was largely responsible for the perceived disability. Today increasingly the new paradigm of disability called the '*social model*', maintains that disability is a product of an interaction between characteristics (e.g. social and personal qualities) of the individual and characteristics of the natural, built, cultural and social environments. The problem with disability is not the disability or the person with disability, but rather the way that 'normalcy' is constructed to create the 'problem' of disability. Personal characteristics, as well as environmental ones, may be enabling or disabling. This argument of this model from a sociopolitical viewpoint emerges that disability stems from the failure of society to adjust to meet the needs and aspirations of a disabled minority and its strength lies in placing the onus upon society and not the individual. This also allows 'people with disability not to be homogenized into a group or groups according to impairments, and provides space for individuals not to be recognized as 'spastic' but as an individual with a number of strengths and an impairment such as cerebral palsy.

The World Health Assembly approved the International Classification of Functioning, Disability and Health (ICF, 2001), which makes a distinction from the International Classification of Impairment, Disability and Handicap (ICIDH) (1996) which used the terms impairment, disability and handicap. The ICF is extremely appropriate for heterogeneous populations of different cultures, age groups and gender. In ICF, all the three dimensions, functioning disability and health condition of the individual are viewed as interactive and dynamic. The personal as well as contextual factors of environment is also to be given due consideration. Not withstanding all the above, disability continues to be viewed in many societies as a 'curse' and labels such as 'cripple', and 'handicapped' continue to be used by society and policy documents.

Research evidence

The marginalization of children with disabilities is evident from the limited evidence that exists in the research domain, with scant scientific exploration of child abuse related to children with disability. This is clearly not a priority on the research agenda. In 2008, there were 758, 289 substantiated cases of child abuse and neglect in the United States (Children's Bureau, 2009), while a study in USA (Charlton, Kliethermes and Taverne, 2004) showed that sixty-four percent of children that experienced maltreatment had a disability. The research also stated that children with disability were up to 10 times as likely to be victims of sexual abuse as compared to typically developing children. According to research performed by the Boys Town National Research Hospital, children with disabilities were found to be at greater risk of becoming victims of abuse and neglect than were children without disabilities. The study showed that children with disabilities are 1.8 times more likely to be neglected, 1.6 times more likely to be physically abused, and 2.2 times more likely to be sexually abused than children without disabilities (Sullivan and Knutson, 2000). A recent scoping study that reviewed research about child abuse, child protection and disabled children published in academic journals between 1996 and 2009 revealed a strong association between disability and child maltreatment, indicating that disabled children are significantly more likely to experience abuse than their non-disabled peers. It is evident that children with disabilities tend to be maltreated and subject to neglect and abuse in multiple ways and this seems to vary with the disability type. For example, children with behavioral disorders were assessed to be at highest risk for all types of abuse and neglect (Hibbard, Desch, Committee on Child Abuse and Neglect, and Council on Children with Disabilities, 2007)[2] and children with chronic illnesses or multiple disabilities with higher dependency on caretakers place them at higher risk. An exploratory investigation conducted in East African countries of Kenya, Uganda and Tanzania (DCCD, 2007) found that majority of children with disabilities were likely to experience debilitating forms of criminal neglect and cases of near starvation, extreme deprivation and total abandonment were recorded. In particular girls with mental disabilities were found to be prone to be sexually violated (DCCD, 2007 p.7).

Situational analysis India

The data collected by the Census (2001) and National Sample Survey (NSSO, 2002) for persons with disabilities in India was broadly categorized into persons with visual, hearing, speech, locomotor and mental disabilities are show in (Table 1). The discrepancy in the figures from the Census, 2001 and NSSO, 2002 are an indicator of the lacunae in statistics available regarding children with disabilities.

Of the 21 million disabled population of the country (Census, 2001), children with disability comprise 1.67% of the population in the age group 0–19 years (Table 2) and 35.29% of the total population with disability. The categories of disability as framed in the Census still continue to follow the 'medical model' using unacceptable labels such as 'mental disability'.

This data needs to be analysed within the larger context of children in India, who continue to be one of the most neglected in the world. This is evident from the fact that out of the 26 million children born annually, nearly two million die before completing 5 years of age, half of these deaths occurring within the first month after birth. Nutritional conditions continue to be poor; 48 percent of children under 5 years of age were stunted, 20 percent wasted, 43 percent underweight, and 43 percent were moderately or severely anaemic according to the NFHS-3. All these are causal factors leading to children acquiring disabilities one of the main factors causing this is the lack of neonatal care and absence of medical facilities to address complication during birth like asphyxia. Many disabilities, e.g. intellectual, physical, multiple and speech impairments have the highest onset during childhood and early childhood care particularly health services are critical for children with disabilities and their long-term prognosis. Another critical area of the health system that

Table 1 Comparative Figures on Persons with Disabilities (In lakhs)

Disability	NSSO, 2002	Census, 2001
Locomotor	106.34	61.06
Visual	28.26	106.35
Hearing	30.62	12.62
Speech	21.55	16.41
Mental	20.96	22.64

Source: NSSO 2002 & Census, 2001

Table 2 Child Population with Disability, Census 2001

Total Population with Disability	21906769	Type of Disability				
		In Seeing	In Speech	In Hearing	In Movement	Mental
Population with Disability 0–19 years	7732196	3605553	775561	90452	2263941	796689
Children with Disability share of total population 0–19 years	1.67%	0.78%	0.17%	0.01%	0.48%	0.17%
Children with Disability share of total disabled population	35.29%	33.9%	47.26%	23.02%	37.08%	35.19%

Source: Census of India, 2001

has major impacts on the prevalence of disability is reproductive, maternal and child health. There is a large body of literature that underscores the importance of maternal factors such as education, nutrition and health care for child health outcomes. Unfortunately, access to care during pregnancy and delivery is poor in India and continues to adversely affect numbers impacted by disability.

Causes of abuse and neglect of children with disabilities

Poverty remains a significant confounding factor in defining child neglect. To understand the multiplicity of causal factors leading to abuse of children with disabilities it is critical to examine the various contexts in which the child exists from an ecological systems perspective. The Ecological Theory (Bronfrenbrenner, 1979) is an appropriate model since it visualizes children's development as being influenced by the interplay between 'nested systems' such as the *Micro* system (which is the immediate setting for the young child—mostly home and center based ECD services); the *Meso* system (which constitutes the interactions and inter-relations between different settings such as home, day care center, immediate community, school, Early Intervention Centre, Hospital, etc.); the *Exo* system (which shows how the *micro-* and *meso-* systems are related to broader societal organizations and their worldviews, policies), and the *Macro* system (which is at a higher level of generality, and which gives continuity to the form and content of all the other three systems).

Abuse at micro level

The child with disability is definitely at a much higher degree of vulnerability and the unfortunate but bitter truth is, that children with disabilities often become the recipients of abuse from birth itself. In some societies, the practice of 'infanticide' (also known as 'mercy killing') still occurs, where disabled children may be killed either immediately at birth or at some point after birth; and sometimes years after birth. Disabled girl infants and girl children are much more likely to die through 'mercy killings' than are boy children of the same age with comparable disabling conditions (UNICEF, 2005). Even if the

child with disability is allowed the 'right to life', the birth of a child with disability is interpreted as a 'curse from God' and the mother faces maximum 'blame' and taunts for having the child. Since there is complete absence of sensitivity amongst service providers and lack of 'role models' for families, the future looms dark and heavy for the young child with disability. Families, particularly parents, go through grief and shame on the birth of a child with disability, and often they are provided aninsensitive and 'hopeless' prognosis by medical practitioners, often resulting in rejection, and/or even abandonment of the young child. Societal pressure, prejudices and complete absence of counseling services lead parents to despair, often foreseeing social isolation for their child and themselves. Belief in 'karma' and myths such as 'sins of the last birth having caused disability', and societal prejudices against children with disabilities adds further barriers to, the nurturing care, the child with disability desperately needs. Girls with disability carry the double burden of both disability and prejudices based on gender discrimination and people with disability continue to be trapped in poverty. Parents with limited social and community support may be at especially high-risk for maltreating children with disabilities, because they may feel more overwhelmed and unable to cope with the care and supervision responsibilities that are required. Thus not only the child, but also his/her family faces maltreatment and neglect in the form of lack of access to guidance, support systems and provision of basic health and phychosocial needs for holistic development of children with disabilities.

In India as well as other developing countries, children with mild intellectual impairments and sensory impairments often remain undiagnosed, till a very long period of time. Parents remain ignorant about the child's impairment and may respond to a child's behavioural characteristic, e.g. communication difficulty or non-compliance with physical abuse. This is even more pronounced for behaviorally challenging behavior. Lack of respite or family support mechanism, to provide the immediate caregivers with respite can lead to an increased risk of abuse and neglect. As the child with disability grows, he can become an easy target for abuse—emotional, physical and sexual because their intellectual limitations may prevent them from being able to discern the experience as abuse and impaired communication abilities may prevent them from disclosing abuse. It is often familiar people in the child's environment who are the perpetrators. A Ministry of Women and Child Development study in 2007 on child abuse found 53% children reported one or more forms of sexual abuse and 50% of the abusers were known to the child or were in a position of trust and responsibility. Even though no empirical data for abuse of children with disabilities exists in India, it is certain that given the dependency of children with disability on caretakers, they are definitely in a more vulnerable position. Societal prejudice and negative attitude toward recognizing the rights of children with disability further compounds this situation. Guilt and fear of 'ruining the family name' (sic), does not allow children with disabilities, to even mention their torment and the perpetrators go scot free. In many a case, non-verbal and intellectually impaired children may not be able to even understand and comprehend the abuse they are undergoing and the incident goes unreported. Lack of acknowledgement of the scale of the incidence of neglect and abuse, further leads to families not addressing this rather sensitive issue and children with disabilities can go through life without any training and information about abuse, neglect, and exploitation as well as personal safety strategies. Continuous devaluation at the hands of family members, peers and society at large, often results in the child with disability resigning himself/herself to the situation and attributing the event as 'fate', ending up with low self-esteem, resentment and frustration. Since the perpetrators may be family members and associated closely to the child and are often the caretakers of the child in different situations, reporting becomes even more difficult. Thus, children with disability are at risk of emotional, physical, sexual abuse and are often subjected to social ostracisation and isolation when they do have the courage to report abuse. A qualitative study (West, Gandhi and Palermo, 2007) which explored children with disabilities perceptions on abuse, had a participant lament "people find it easier to ignore, neglect somebody who's blind or can't move, or you know, it's easy because people do not listen, you know". Thus, children with disabilities remain one of the most vulnerable and marginalized groups of children, at a high-risk of being abused physically, sexually and emotionally.

Challenges and gaps in the mesosystem

Despite the Persons with Disability Act, 1995 (PWD Act) having early intervention as a key focus, fifteen years has seen no efforts made in this direction. The Integrated Child Development Services (ICDS) and the National Rural Health Mission (NRHM) has had no convergence with the Ministry of Social Justice and Empowerment (responsible for implementation of the PWD Act) and personnel like ASHA workers and Anganwadi workers who are the first contact with families at the village level, have absolutely no idea about screening, making referral of 'at risk children' or providing parents and the child home-based training and stimulation. Due to absence of accessible rehabilitation services, the child with disability born in a remote village in a poor family has limited chances of getting early intervention services she/he deserves and becomes a victim of gross neglect.

Research and literature abound with examples of how development in the first five years of a child life, constitute the most important years of her life, with proof of how later intervention does not have the same impact. The role of preschool education in the age group three to six then takes on tremendous importance, particularly in light of the criticality of intervention in the early years for children with disabilities. According to the NSSO Survey, 58th Round (GoI, 2003), the proportion of disabled persons of age 5–18 years who attended the preschool intervention programme is only about 13 per cent of the disabled persons. This is because services are not ready to respond effectively and provide accessible equitable services to children with disabilities. The proportion of population with disabilities accessing early childhood services in urban areas is 20 per cent, while rural areas are estimated only at 11 per cent. *Surprisingly, a higher proportion of disabled girls attended the preschool intervention programme in urban areas, although the proportion was higher for boys in rural areas.* This data is exceedingly important, since the poor levels of attendance in preschool demonstrate the abysmally poor early intervention services available for young children with disabilities.

Census 2001, revealed that only 7% of disabled persons in rural areas and 17% of disabled persons in urban areas were educated up to the secondary level or above. Though the Sarva Shiksha Abhiyan has witnessed a large increase in enrolment rates, children with disabilities form the largest percentage of out of school population (SRI IMRB 2009) with 34.12% of children with disabilities in the age group 6–14 years out of-school. Furthermore the fact that many of these children are unable to access the curriculum and face taunts at the hands of peers and abuse from teachers who remain unable to address diverse needs in the classroom, adds to the unfortunate situation that children with disabilities face.

The XI Plan Sub Group Report on Child Protection mentions 'lack of lateral services linkages with essential services for children, e.g. education, health, police, judiciary, services for the disabled' (p.17) as a gap. It also mentions the risk of neglect, child labor, rape, abuse, trafficking, etc. for children with disability. In 2005, the National Human Rights Commission (Sen 2005) estimated that almost half of the children trafficked within India are between the ages of 11 and 14 years; they are subjected to physical and sexual abuse and kept in conditions similar to slavery and bondage. According to International Labor Organization (ILO) estimates, 15 per cent of India's estimated 2.3 million commercial sex workers are children. Though we have no data on the number of children with disability who are trafficked, it is no surprise that there numbers will be very large. Children with disabilities are seen as a huge source of income by traffickers, especially in the begging industry or in brothels. Their lack of participation or perceived value to the family, or even in some cultures a sense of shame or embarrassment to have a disability in the family, means that families may even seek out traffickers to relieve themselves of responsibility. Traffickers can capitalise on this by deliberately sourcing children born with disfigurements and sending them onto the streets to beg. Many hearing and speech impaired girls are seen in red light areas and subjected to economic and sexual exploitation. Despite all the efforts state governments have not been able to address and provide adequate services to stop exploitation of children with disabilities and the rehabilitation package needs immediate rethinking. Children with disabilities in institutional care are at immense risk as well, since there are no safeguards and mechanisms to assure children's safety and the ICPS has still to see the light of day.

Once again the fact that neglect and abuse is pervasive and needs to be acknowledged as a societal problem is not accepted. There is no sensitisation and training of service providers such as teachers, rehabilitation professionals, police personnel, etc. to provide information and counselling to children with disabilities on self-protection/risk reduction skills. Extensive research in this area reveals a clear correlation between the provision of such education and decreased vulnerability to abuse, neglect, and exploitation. However, even rehabilitation professionals are 'burying their heads in the sand' and do not wish to believe that abuse and neglect of children in general and children with disabilities has reached endemic proportions.

Challenges at the exo- and macrosystem

India does not allocate sufficient funds for child protection and this remains a major challenge. It is unfortunate that the share of resources for child protection in the National budget remained an abysmally low 0.034% in 2005–2006, with no increase in 2006–2007. What is worse is the fact that much of the funds allocated for implementation on Integrated Child Protection Scheme in the XI Plan remain unspent. It is no surprise that in light of the absence of an adequate mechanism for capturing and protecting children–there is a complete vacuum of empirical data regarding abuse and neglect of children with disabilities in India. This unfortunately, remains true for a large number of nations. One of the major reasons is that there is no Internationally agreed upon definition for "disabilities" and nation states vary even in their approach to collecting census data on persons with disabilities. Institutions for disabled children are often at the bottom of government priority lists and lack adequate funding, consistent support or oversight from government or civil society. Institutions are often overcrowded, unsanitary and suffer from lack of both staff and resources and many incidents of unreported abuse occur in homes for children and orphanages. Hibbard et al. report that, "schools, programs and institutions may have a disincentive to recognize or report child maltreatment because of fear of negative publicity or loss of funding or licensure".

Conclusions and recommendations

Children with disabilities are immensely vulnerable to abuse and neglect and unless child protection systems are strengthened for all children including children with disabilities, this situation will continue unabated. To curb violation of children with disabilities particularly gender based violence, it is essential that we first and foremost recognize their rights to a safe childhood. The lack of research and data collection on abuse of children with disabilities must find a priority in the XII Plan. Policy makers and advocates of children with disabilities must know the magnitude of population with disability as well as numbers of children subjected to abuse and neglect. Through research, the nature and pattern of existing abuse and neglect of children with disabilities must be captured and adequate financial and human resources made available to address this menace. To address the social exclusion and neglect that children with disabilities face right from birth, professionals and personnel must be trained to provide families and children with disabilities access to inclusive services that are adapted to meet their individual needs, particularly health, early intervention, education and appropriate counseling services. Abuse occurs in various settings such as homes, community, schools, institutional settings, etc. and dependence on others puts them at great risk. Many of these environments are not governed by any prescribed 'Standards of Care'. The latter need to be developed and implemented through a robust monitoring mechanism set up at District and sub-District level across the country. Not only do children with disability need to be empowered to seek help and support against neglect and abuse, but current myths and misconceptions associated with abuse and neglect of children with disabilities need to be addressed at all levels through a large scale campaign. Civil society can play a particularly important role in addressing community attitudes and behaviors through media, advocacy as well as community participation. A robust child tracking system must capture data regarding children with disabilities and ensure protection from trafficking, begging, physical and sexual abuse through provision of quality inclusive services. A Disability Council for Protection must be constituted at state level within the Disability Commissioners Office and mechanism to provide justice to abused children provided. Disability Training for parents as well as personnel working in various departments and settings such as schools, child protection centers, police stations, ICDS Centers, hospitals and medical centers, homes and special education institutions, not forgetting bureaucrats and the legal fraternity must be undertaken with firm resolve. The only solution to address the silent suffering of children with disabilities and realize their rights is to mainstream disability and strengthen the judicial, legal and service systems to provide protection, support, treatment and education to children at large and those with disability in particular. There is an urgent need for enhancing social participation of children with disabilities to decrease their vulnerability. As a first step we must recognise, acknowledge and address the lack of acceptance and response to abuse and neglect of children with disability, that has remained shrouded under a veil of secrecy for generations. We have to address the issue at all levels—micro, meso- and exosystems. All children, including children with disabilities have the right to grow in a safe and protective environment and all of us have to ensure we create a safety net for them across—we owe it to them!

Bibliography

1. American RT, Baladerian NJ. (1993) Maltreatment of Children with Disabilities. Chicago, IL: National Committee to Prevent Child Abuse.

2. Bronfenbrenner, U. (1979). The ecology of human development. Cambridge, MA: Harvard University Press.

3. Census of India (2001). Government of India. Accessed from: http://www.censuindia.net.

4. Charlton, M, Kliethermes, M. & Taverne, A. National Child Traumatic stress Network, (2004). Facts on traumatic stress and children with developmental disabilities Los Angeles, CA, Accessed from: http://www.nctsnet.org/nctsn assets/pdfs/reports/traumatic stress developmental disabilities final.pdf.

5. Children's Bureau (2009) U.S. Departments of Health and Human Services, Administration for children and Families, Washington, DC Accessed from http://www.acf.hhs.gov/programs/cb/pubs/cm08/index.htm.

6. Dutch Coalition on Disability and Development (2007) Hidden Shame: Violence Against Children in East Africa, Terres de Hommes, Nederland.

7. Government of India (1996) The Person with Disabilities (Equal Opportunities, Protection of Rights and Full Participation) Act, 1995, New Delhi, Ministry of Social Justice & Empowerment.

8. Government of India (2003) Disable person in India: NSSO 58th Round (July-December, 2002) Report No. 485. New Delhi: National Sample Survey Organisation, Ministry of statistics and Programme Implementation.

9. Hibbard, Desch, & American Academy of Paediatrics Committee on Child Abuse and Neglect and Council on Children with Disabilities Paediatrics, 2007: 119(5).

10. Hibbard, Desch, & American Academy of Paediatrics Committee on Child Abuse and Neglect and Council on Children with Disabilities Paediatrics, 2007:119(5).

11. Ministry of Human Resource Development (2009) Survey on Out of School Children in the age group 6-4 years, New Delhi: SRI-MRB.

12. Ministry of Women & Child Development (2007) Study on Child Abuse: India 2007, Government of India.

13. National Family Health Survey (2007), Ministry of Health & Family Welfare, Indian Institute of Population Sciences, Mumbai.

14. National Human Right Commission, UNIFEM (2005). A Report on the Trafficking of Women & children in India, New Delhi.

15. NSSO (2002). Disabled Persons in India. Website of the Office of Chief Commissioner of Persons with Disabilities in India. Accessed from: htpp://www.ccdisabilities.nic,in/disability%20india.htm.

16. Stalker, K. And McArthur, K (2011), child abuse, child protection and disabled children: a review of recent research. Child Abuse Review.

17. Sullivan, P.M., & Knutson, J.F. Maltreatment and disabilities: a population-based epidemiological study. Child Abuse & Neglect, 2000; 24(10):1257–1273.

18. UNICEF (2007) innocent Research Centre: Promoting the Rights of Children with Disabilities, Innocenti Digest No. 13, October 2007.

19. United Nation Children's Funds (UNICEF) (2005) Violence against Disabled children: Summary Report. UN Secretary General Report on Violence against Children: Thematic Group on Violence against Disabled Children, Finding and Recommendations.

20. West B, Gandhi S, & Palermo D.G. (2007) Defining Abuse: A Study of Perceptions of People with Disabilities Regarding Abuse Directed at People with Disabilities Studies Quarterly, Fall 2007, Vol 27,4.

21. World Health Organisation (1999): Report of the Consultation on Child Abuse Prevention; Geneva. Accessed from: http://www.who.int/violence injury prevention/violence/neglect/en.

22. World Health Organisation (2001) International Classification of Functioning, Disability and Health (ICF). Accessed from www.who.int/icidh.

Section 3

Protection and Prevention

14

General Comment 13 on Article 19 of the Convention on the Rights of the Child – Essential Elements of Child Protection Systems

Joan van Niekerk

Introduction

The United Nations Convention on the Rights of the Child was developed and adopted by the General Assembly of the United Nations in 1989 and entered into force in 1990. It contains the minimum entitlements and freedoms for children to be respected by both governments and civil society. The Convention covers the full range of human rights – inclusive of civil, cultural, social, economic and political and also recognises that children are entitled to special care and assistance. Its preamble notes that "the child, by reason of his physical and mental immaturity, needs special safeguards and care, including appropriate legal protection, before as well as after birth".

The UN Convention respects the worth and dignity of every child equally, regardless of race, colour, gender, language, religion, opinions, origins, wealth, birth status or ability and the United Nations Committee on the Rights of the Child monitors the performance of governments which have signed and ratified the Convention on its implementation.

However, governments are sometimes challenged on issues of implementation, and therefore general comments on the various articles in the convention are developed in order to give guidance on how the article can be optimally applied in the development and implementation of the domestic legislation of countries which have signed and ratified this Convention.

Although all articles in the Convention are considered non-negotiable standards and obligations, the obligations of governments relating to Article 19 of the Convention, dealing with the development of child protection systems, received specific attention in the recommendations that were made in the World Report on Violence Against Children. A number of the recommendations related to the development and maintenance of child protection systems in order to respond appropriately to, and prevent, violence against children.

The first recommendation of the World Report on Violence Against Children called upon States to strengthen national and local commitment via the development of a multifaceted and systematic framework to respond to violence against children, and to integrate this into national planning processes. The recommendation included the formulation of a "national strategy, policy or plan of action on violence against children with realistic and time bound targets, coordinated by an agency with the capacity to involve multiple sectors in a broad based implementation strategy." The recommendation stated further "National Laws, policies, plans and programmes should fully comply with international human rights and current scientific knowledge. The implementation of the national strategy, policy or plan should be systematically evaluated according to established targets and timetables, and provided with adequate human and financial resources to support its implementation. However any strategy, policy, plan or programme to address the issue of violence against children must be compatible with the conditions and resources of the country under consideration."

Article 19 of the unconvention on the rights of the child clearly relates to this recommendation and states the following

"State parties shall take all appropriate legislative, administrative, social and educational measures to protect the child from all forms of physical or mental violence, injury or abuse, neglect or negligent treatment, maltreatment or exploitation, including sexual abuse, while in the care of parent(s), legal guardian(s) or any other person who has the care of the child.

Such protective measures should, as appropriate, include effective procedures for the establishment of social programmes to provide necessary support for the child and for those who have the care of the child, as well as for other forms of prevention and for identification, reporting, referral, investigation, treatment and follow-up of instances of child maltreatment described heretofore, and, as appropriate, for judicial involvement."

Article 19 is embedded in the context of a much broader child rights policy that focuses on the child from a holistic perspective and therefore this article should be understood in the context of all other rights and it follows that Child Protection systems will embody all provisions in the United Nations Convention on the Rights of the Child.

The general comment 13

Effective Child Protection systems are complex and involve multiple role players, the activities of which must be coordinated to protect the best interests of the child. The General Comment 13 was therefore developed to provide guidance to governments on the development, functioning and maintenance of these complex systems. The General Comment was adopted in March 2011 by the UN Committee on the Rights of the Child.

Fundamental assumptions on which the general comment is based

The General Comment 13 is based on nine fundamental assumptions:

- No violence against children is justifiable and all violence against children is preventable

- Child protection systems must be embedded in a child rights approach
- Every child should be treated with dignity, recognised, respected and protected as a rights holder
- The rule of law should apply fully to children as it applies to adults
- Children have the right to be heard, and consulted and to have their views given due weight must be respected systematically in all decision-making processes, and their empowerment and participation should be central to child caregiving and protection strategies and programmes
- The best interests of children should be the primary consideration in all matters and decisions affecting them
- Primary prevention of violence against children is of paramount importance
- The family is recognised as the first child protection system—however it is noted that violence occurs in the context of the family and that families may need help and support
- Violence in state institutions and by state actors is also recognised.

The General Comment identifies the need to ensure that its content is disseminated—not just to governments, but also to parents, caregivers, professional organizations, communities—and children in order that the rights conferred by Article 19 are fully understood and implemented. The need to use a variety of channels of communication for this purpose, translate the General Comment in multiple languages and develop a child friendly version is also emphasised.

The objectives of the general comment are to

- Provide guidance to States parties in understanding their obligations with respect to Article 19 of the Convention to prohibit, prevent and respond to all forms of physical or mental violence, injury or abuse, neglect or negligent treatment, maltreatment or exploitation of children, including sexual abuse, while in the care of parent(s), legal guardian(s), or any other person who has the care of the child including those who work for or on behalf of the state;
- Outline the legislative, judicial, administrative, social and educational measures that States must take;

- To overcome isolated, fragmented and reactive initiatives to address child caregiving and protection which have limited impact on the prevention and elimination of all forms of violence;
- To promote a holistic approach to implementing Article 19 based on securing children's rights to survival, dignity, wellbeing, health, development, participation and non-discrimination when these are threatened by violence;
- To provide States Parties and other stakeholders with a basis on which to develop a coordinating framework for eliminating violence through comprehensive child rights-based caregiving and protection measures;
- To highlight the need for rapid fulfilment of obligations.

The General Comment 13 recognises the impact of violence against children in both the long and short-term, and how survival and development are compromised by a failure to protect children from violence and respond appropriately once violence has occurred. It emphasises the enormous human, social and economic costs of not preventing and dealing with violence against children.

Unpacking the meaning of article 19 of the unconvention on the rights of the child

The General Comment 13 unpacks each element of the Article fully, via defining, emphasising and explaining each concept. In unpacking the concept of all forms of violence the principle of "no exceptions" and the need for human and child rights-based definitions and approaches is noted.

Numerous forms of violence are listed and defined

- Physical violence
- Mental violence
- Neglect and negligent treatment
- Corporal punishment
- Sexual abuse and exploitation
- Torture and inhuman or degrading treatment or punishment
- Violence among children, including bullying
- Self-harm
- Harmful cultural and child raising practices
- Violence in the media
- Violence through information and communication technologies

- Institutional and system violations of child rights.

The definition of caregivers and care

The General Comment 13 notes that, while the evolving capacities of children are recognised, all children under the age of 18 years should be in the care of someone. The definition of caregiver used in the General Comment 13 is very broad and extends beyond parents, foster parents and adoptive parents, to include caregivers in the school and community environment. Where a child is an unaccompanied minor, a street child, or a child in a child headed household, the state is held to be the child's caregiver.

Likewise, the definition of care settings is broad and extends to all settings in which children live, learn, play, work and worship or observe their religion. It is inclusive of medical facilities, refugee camps and settlements, and whether the setting provides permanent or temporary care for a child or children.

The injunction: "shall take all appropriate legislative, administrative, social and educational measures"

The General Comment 13 notes that the phrasing used in this section of the Article gives States Parties no discretion and places them under obligation to fully implement this right for children.

The phrase "appropriate measures" refers to a broad range of activities and obligations, cutting across all spheres of government. It is noted that an integrated, cohesive, interdisciplinary and coordinated system is required to protect children, and that children themselves should participate in the development, monitoring and evaluation of this system.

The measures described in the General Comment 13 include:

1. Legislative measures which focus on the development and review of appropriate and comprehensive legislation and policy, extending from the ratification of all international conventions and treaties that relate to the care

and protection of children, to the development and review of all domestic legislation and policy. It is also noted that developing law and policy is not adequate in and of itself, and budget allocation, implementation and enforcement is essential.

2. Administrative measures which include the development of an independent national structure that protects children's rights; the establishment of policies, programmes, with monitoring and oversight of these at every level of government; the establishment of a national data collection system in order to monitor and evaluate the impact of services, programmes; and the development of indicators in order to measure the success of law, policy, programmes and activities.

3. Social measures inclusive of:

    a. Social policy measures which are broadly described and include the integration of child protection measures into mainstream social policy inclusive of identifying and preventing the factors and circumstances that contribute to the vulnerability of children to victimisation. Relevant social policy areas encompass poverty reduction, public health, safety, housing, employment, education, access to health, social welfare and justice services, child friendly cities planning, reduced access to alcohol, drugs and weapons and policies relating to media and the ICT industry.

    b. Social programmes to support the child individually and to support the child's family and other caregivers to provide optimal and positive child rearing. This section of the General Comment gives recognition to the fact that families do not rear children on their own, but also draw upon institutions and facilities in their communities to assist in child care.

4. Education measures that deal with attitudes, traditions, customs and behaviors that condone and promote violence against children. Educational measures should extend to all stakeholders, including children, families and communities, professionals and institutions that provide any services to children. It is noted that training should be formalised, especially for those that work with children as part of their professional and occupational duties.

The range of interventions to address violence against children

A range of interventions to address violence against children are described in detail in the General Comment 13. These include:

Prevention

This is often neglected as an activity, intervention and focus in child protection. Responses to violence against children appear prioritised by this neglect, whereas if more attention was given to prevention, this would reduce the resources directed at appropriate responses to violence against children. The General Comment 13 notes that prevention measures should be directed at all stakeholders, children, families and communities, professionals and institutions in both Government and civil society, and should include a broad range of activities such as:

- Changing attitudes which perpetuate violence;
- Promoting the United Nations Convention on the Rights of the Child;
- Developing partnerships with all sectors of society;
- Birth registration of all children;
- Educating children on their rights;
- Empowering children;
- Mentoring children who require extra support;
- Supporting families and caregivers to facilitate positive child rearing and positive discipline;
- Providing specific supportive services, respite opportunities to families who are vulnerable or facing especially difficult circumstances;
- Strengthening the links between services that work with families and children;
- Providing shelters and crisis care when appropriate to children and families.

Identification

The General Comment 13 notes the importance of identifying risk factors that feed into violence against children to enable prevention and early intervention strategies to be applied. All who come into contact with children should be educated on and trained on the recognition of risk, and children should be given opportunities to alert parents, caregivers and authorities when they are aware of risk to enable early intervention, with special attention to ensuring that marginalised children, such as children with disability, are not excluded from opportunities to give these alerts.

Reporting

The United Nations Committee on the Rights of the Child strongly recommended to all States Parties that all children should have access to safe, well publicised and accessible support and reporting opportunities to report violations of rights and acts of violence. This was further reinforced in the World Report on Violence Against Children, which recommended the use of 24 hours toll free helplines and/or other free Internet Communications Technologies.[5] The right of children to be heard is and the promotion of reporting mechanisms are stressed. Universal mandatory reporting is not recommended in the General Comment 13; however mandatory reporting by professionals who work with children is motivated, as well as protection processes and mechanisms for those who report violence against children in good faith.

Referral

Reporting must be followed by referral to an appropriate service or services. It is recognized that violence against children may require a multi-sector and multi-disciplinary response. The General Comment 13 identifies the need for protocols and training for interagency cooperation and collaboration in order to effect appropriate and effective referrals. Initial assessments are recommended during this intervention phase, in which both the child and family participate, and after which feedback should be given to both the child and family, and appropriate services, based on the assessment of need, offered.

Investigation

Trained and qualified professionals should conduct investigations during this activity, and a child rights and child sensitive approach, in which the child participates, should be adopted. Sensitivity to the possibility of secondary trauma (further harm) is promoted.

Treatment

May cover a wide range of services needed to "promote physical and psychological recovery and social reintegration". The General Comment 13 recommends that during this process attention should be given to

- Inviting and giving weight to the child's views
- The child's safety
- The need for a safe placement
- The predictable influences on interventions on the child's holistic well-being.

Treatment must also take into account the ecology of the child.

This action may also include treatment of the perpetrator of the violence, especially children with violent behavior, and it is noted that this behaviour is often driven by inadequacies and deficits in the offenders own history.

Follow-up

The General Comment 13 acknowledges the complex processes that children experience after victimization, and recommends that a professional be allocated to the child as a case manager to follow and support the child (and family) through all activities and intervention processes, as well as to coordinate and provide continuity. Delays in providing services should be avoided and monitoring and evaluating progress is emphasised, as well as the participation of the child in all aspects of the process.

Judicial involvement

Children have the right to due process, but the best interests of the child should determine all activities, including judicial process. The General Comment 13 also establishes the principle of providing the least intrusive intervention.

The following precepts should also be observed with regard to judicial involvement:

- Children and parents should be informed about judicial involvement
- The justice process should be child friendly and sensitive and adjusted to the developmental and other needs of the child
- The judicial process should be preventive and support positive behavior while prohibiting negative behavior, as well as support an inter-sector, interdisciplinary approach
- This process should adopt the celerity principle to ensure that judicial action is speedily completed
- A number of judicial interventions are described, criminal prosecution of the perpetrator

of the violence being only one of several possibilities. Other options include alternative responses such as family group conferencing and other mediation possibilities with the focus on restorative justice, care proceedings for children to ensure their safety, proceedings which enable compensation for children who have suffered violence that can contribute to their treatment and well being, and also disciplinary and administrative proceedings against child protection professionals and workers who fail in their care and protection of children.

Special courts and processes are recommended for children to ensure that children receive child friendly and appropriate justice, and which enable their participation. Training of justice and other participating professionals and confidentiality is motivated.

Effective procedures

All interventions and measures should have proven effectiveness. To achieve this there should be intersector coordination supported by protocols and/or memoranda of understanding, data collection and analysis that is systematic, ongoing, a developed and implemented research agenda, with measureable objectives and indicators, which focus on the positive well-being and optimal development of children.

The General Comment 13 is based on a broad interpretation of Article 19 of the Convention and links this to other core provisions, namely reinforcing a child rights approach to the development and implementation of child protection systems and services, emphasising the right to non-discrimination, the consideration of the child's best interests, the right to life, survival and development, the right of the child to be heard, and the right of children to receive direction and guidance consistent with evolving capacities.

National coordinating frameworks on violence against children

Many countries have national plans of action for children. However, the General Comment notes that these are considered inadequate on their own, and that in addition to national plans of action, national

coordinating frameworks should be developed to enable the specific protection of children against all forms of violence. The coordinating framework should bring together all sectors of government, non-profit organizations and civil society to collectively address the prevention and response to violence against children. Such a framework should promote flexibility and creativity, as well as have a clear focus on prevention.

No standard national coordinating framework is proposed by the General Comment 13, as it is recognized that different countries have different resources, legal, administrative and service delivery infrastructures, customs and profession working in child protection.

However, the inclusive involvement of all sectors and stakeholders in developing such a structure is advised, in order to ensure participation and ownership. The planning, finalization and implementation of the framework should be accessible and understandable to children and adults, costed and adequately financed and included in a national child budget.

The General Comment 13 identifies the following factors that should be integrated into the national coordinating frameworks:

- A child rights approach which recognises children as rights holders and not as the receivers of charitable activities. Children should therefore be involved in the development of national coordinating frameworks, taking into account age and evolving capacities;
- The gender dimensions of violence against children ensuring that the different risks facing boys and girls must be recognised. Imbalances of power, gender stereotypes, discrimination and inequalities should be addressed in every context in which violence against children can potentially occur, including the home, school, work, community and institutional care. Respect between the genders must be fostered and men and boys recognized as partners and allies, with women and girls, in order to prevent and address violence against children;
- Primary prevention should be recognized as vital in addressing violence against children;
- Families, including the extended family, should be recognized as having the primary position in child protection, and their potential to protect children and prevent violence supported. It is recognized that violence against children often occurs in the home, and that prevention and

early intervention strategies should strengthen and support families and that families should encourage, support and empower children to participate in their own protection, as the capacity evolves;

- Protective and resilience factors should be identified and supported. The General Comment 13 gives examples of protective factors such as stable families, child rearing practices that are nurturing and which meet the holistic needs of children, positive discipline, attachment to at least one adult, supportive relationships with peers, a social environment that promotes prosocial, nonviolent and non-discriminatory attitudes and behaviors, social cohesion and supportive networks in the child's community;
- Risk factors must also be recognised reduced. Although all children below the age of 18years should be considered vulnerable, babies and young children are considered more so because of their immature development and dependency on adults. Risk factors associated with parents are identified and inclusive of substance abuse, mental health problems, unemployment, marginalisation;
- Children in potentially vulnerable situations are a necessary focus of a national coordinating framework as they may require provisions specific to their vulnerability. The list of potentially vulnerable situations in the General Comment is extensive and inclusive and recognises that vulnerability can be located in the situation and/or characteristics of the child, family, community, or more broadly in society as a whole;
- Resources: the national coordinating framework must have provisions that ensure the adequate allocation of available resources to the prevention of violence and include monitoring mechanisms that ensure the resources are appropriately and optimally used;
- Coordination must occur at national, regional and local levels, across all sectors, inclusive of the research community and civil society;
- Accountability mechanisms much be cooperatively and proactively developed and applied, using norms and standards, indicators, tools for collecting information and monitoring, measurement and evaluation to ensure that the child protection systems do fulfil the obligation and commitment to protect

children. The Committee on the Rights of the Child recommends, through the medium of the General Comment 13, that countries publish annual reports and submit these to their Parliaments, and encourage discussion on and responses to such reports.

Resources for the implementation of child protection systems

Although the General Comment 13 recognises the differences in resources across countries, it urges governments to apply what resources they have to child protection systems. It is recognized that a country's national and decentralized budgets should be the primary source of funds, however international cooperation and assistance may be called upon to assist with shortfalls. The Committee on the Rights of the Child motivates international donor institutions such as the World Bank and private donors, the United Nations agencies and other international and regional bodies and organisations to work with the Committee to advance the cause of child protection.

Regional and international cross border cooperation

The General Comment 13 recognises that there is a need for cooperation across borders and regions due to child protection issues such as international trafficking and the cross border movement of children, both alone and with family members. It is noted that specific legislation, policies, programmes and partnerships are needed to deal with these cross border child protection issues, as well as the allocation of human, financial and technical resources.

Conclusion

The General Comment No. 13 (2011), which unpacks Article 19 of the United Nations Convention on the Rights of the Child, and which elucidates "the right of the child to freedom from all forms of violence", provides country parties and all involved with the protection of children, with a comprehensive guide for the development, implementation and evaluation of child protection systems. It systematically clarifies the challenges that children face in relation to violence, the consequences of such violence during childhood, as well as the mechanisms required in order to prevent and address violence against children.

The General Comment 13 should be read by all who contribute to the development of law, policy, and the implementation of law and policy relating to child protection. The grounding of child protection systems in a human and child rights foundation is central to its theme and approach.

The full text of General Comment 13 on Article 19 of the United Nations Convention on the Rights of the Child can be found on the following website: http://www2.ohchr.org/english/bodies/crc/comments.htm

15

Child Protection: Assigning Responsibility

Rajeev Seth

Introduction

The UN Convention of Rights of Child (UN CRC) (1989) is the most widely endorsed child rights intrument worldwide, which defines children as all persons aged 18 years and under.[1] In the UN CRC, Article 19.1, Child Protection has been defined as "States Parties shall take all appropriate legislative, administrative, social and educational measures to protect the child from all forms of physical or mental violence, injury or abuse, neglect or negligent treatment, maltreatment or exploitation, including sexual abuse, while in the care of parent(s), legal guardian(s) or any other person who has the care of the child.[2] Failure to ensure child right to protection adversely affects all rights. Child protection is critical to the achievement of Millennium Development goals (MDG). These MDGs can't be achieved unless child protection is an integral part of program and strategies to protect children from child labor, street children, child abuse, child marriage, violence in school and various forms of exploitation.[3]

Several well-developed countries of the world have well-developed child protection systems, primarily focused at mandatory reporting, identification and investigations of affected children, and often taking coercive action. The burden of high level of notifications and investigations is not only on the families, but also on the system, which has to increase it's resources.[4] In these contexts, the problems of child protection in Asia and many other developing countries, with huge populations, and additional socioeconomic constraints, needs serious and wider consideration.

Developing country experiences and magnitude of problem

In developing countries, the number of children needing care and protection is huge and increasing. Uncontrolled families, extreme poverty, illiteracy result in provision of very little care to the child during the early formative years. Even services that are freely available are poorly utilized. The urban underprivileged, migrating population (a very sizable number) and rural communities are particularly affected. In large cities, there are serious problems of street children (abandoned and often homeless) and child labourers, employed in menial work. Children in difficult circumstances such as children affected by disasters, those in conflict zones, refugees, HIV AIDS need appropriate care and rehabilitation.[5]

For example in India, there are about 440 million children; about 40% of them are vulnerable or experiencing difficult circumstances. 27 million babies are born each year. A large majority these births are among the underprivileged section of the population, mostly unplanned and where the parents cannot provide proper care to their children. The situation of the newborn and the periods of infancy and early childhood are particularly critical and the morbidity and mortality rates continue to remain very high. Maternal under nutrition, unsafe deliveries, low birth weight babies and poor newborn care, lack of adequate immunizations, poor nutrition, neglect of early development and education are major issues that need to be appropriately addressed. Child rearing practices reflect social norms and very often adverse traditions are passed from one generation to the next, especially in illiterate and poorly informed communities, and are extremely resistant to alter. As per Government of India (2007) survey, the prevalence of all forms of child abuse are extremely high (physical abuse (66%), sexual abuse (50%) and emotional abuse (50%).[6] In these contexts, every developing country must also seek its own insights and way forward plans to protect their children.

Wider implications of protection

The term "protection" readily relates to protection from all forms of violence, abuse, and exploitation. However, from a developing country perspective, the Indian Child Abuse Neglect and Child Labor (ICANCL) group has strongly propagated the view that "protection" must also include protection from disease, poor nutrition, and illiteracy, in addition to abuse and exploitation. The 9th ISPCAN Asia Pacific Conference of Child Abuse and Neglect (APCCAN 2011) conference outcome document "Delhi declaration" re-confirmed and pledged a resolve to stand against the neglect and abuse of children and to strive for achievement of child rights and the building of a caring community for every child, free of violence and discrimination. It urged and asserted the urgent need to integrate principles, standards and measures in national planning process to prevent and respond to violence against children.[7]

Effective child protection systems

Whose responsibility is it to ensure the safe, protective and caring environment that every child deserves? The UN CRC does not absolve either family or community or society at large. But it firmly puts the onus on the State. Governments are the ultimate duty bearer. In developing countries, the State should ensure that all vulnerable children have access to school, basic health care, nutrition, besides social welfare and juvenile justice systems.[8] These child protection systems can contribute to break down cycle of intergenerational poverty and exploitation.

Experiment models of child protection

Child protection for urban poor

In developing countries, rapid urbanization is a challenging problem. The present urban population of India is close to 285 million. Preventive social services are abysmal, with high prevalence of abuse and neglect. It is estimated that every year about 2 million children are born amongst urban poor, all needing care and protection. The ICANCL group members volunteer their services for health care and rehabilitation to these vulnerable children at drop in centers (DIC) managed by PCI, a NGO in various slums of the New Delhi. The group also looks after health of street children at one short stay home (Shelter home) in outskirts of the city.[9] The group has served more than 14000 street children since year 2000. A shelter home was started in year 2005, where 347 children have been rehabilitated; provided with formal education, vocational skills and job placement. Home repatriation has been achieved in 350 children.[10] The group assists in the following community services to protection of these vulnerable children:

Street and working children

In Urban metropolitan cities, street children are migrants from underserved states and have no formal education or job skills. They are subject all forms of abuse, including substance abuse & exploited as child laborers.[10] The DIC provide non-formal education, free medical care, vaccinations, counseling against substance abuse/HIV/AIDS, etc. mid day meals and vocational courses. Moreover, crèche and day care services are provided to these orphan and vulnerable children.

Education and health services for urban poor

The group runs an ongoing campaign to put "Every Child in School", to promote child protection and optimum development. Advocacy efforts made to retain children in school within the framework of Government programs, such as *Sarva Shiksha Abhiyan* and Right to Education (RTE) Act (2009). Health services were provided at DIC, as loss of daily wages and lack of transport prevents them to go to avail facilities at government hospitals. Health education and monitoring, nutritional screening, vaccinations, basic sanitation, hygiene and counseling services were provided.

Protection of children in underserved rural village

The I CANCL Group has developed a model for protection of children in an underserved village Bhango, district Nuh-Mewat, Haryana, which is primarily focused on provision of primary education and basic health care. Village Bhango is situated about 70 km from New Delhi; has a Population 1300. [Adults: 592 (male 311 and female 281) and Children 708]. Before the group started work, the only Government Primary School had low enrolment rate, high school drop outs, poor infrastructure, no toilets, teacher absenteeism and irregular administration of mid day meals.[11]

For the past 6 years, the ICANCL group volunteers have monitored the school program on an ongoing basis with the help of local village *panchayat* (local self-government) education committee, which comprised of sarpanch (head man) and some senior community members. An extra english remedial teacher was hired. Repair of building, safe water and regular mid day meals were administered. The government administration was approached to report teacher absenteeism and effective implementation of their program. The group managed health care clinic for sick children and immunization at the village chawpal (meeting point). In a period of 2years, the school had enhanced enrollment, no drop outs, and improved school performance. The key to the success of this initiative was due to a clear responsibility and accountability of *Panchayat* officials, teachers, community ownership and participation.[12]

What did we learn?

In the process of voluntary service in underserved regions of our country, our group learnt some important lesions from the vulnerable families and communities. The most important lesson was that public awareness about child abuse and neglect has to be raised and society attitudes have to change. Children should have knowledge regarding life skills, child rights and participation. Moreover, Governments should encourage public discussions on child maltreatment. The media has an important role to play in this regard. Legislation alone will not bring sufficient impact unless awareness and public attitudes are changed! Nevertheless, adequate Legislative framework and their consistent implementation and enforcement are very important. Beyond rationalization of existing laws, the main challenge in India remains their enforcement and the fact that there is a certain degree of impunity for those violating the law. For instance, if one compares the prevalence of child marriage in India (43% of women aged 20–24 years were married before they were 18 years) and the numbers of people prosecuted for violating the anti-child marriage law (a few hundred per year, at best), it is evident that the law is not enforced.[13]

Assigning responsibility

Ideally, the parents should be responsible for proper care and protection of their child. Every birth should be planned and all births registered. However, the child must not suffer in case the parents can't provide care and protection. It is the duty of the proximate community and the Government at large to address the issues of care and protection.

Education and empowerment of families

The magnitude and seriousness of the problems of underprivileged children are too great to be tackled through "external" measures. The child must be the responsibility of the parents, the family and the proximate community. The families and the community must be educated, informed and empowered so that they can provide care and protection to their children. Parenting skills, alternative forms of discipline and basic support to vulnerable families must be expanded. In developing countries, States cannot afford to separate children from their vulnerable families and place them in institutions. Such approaches are also being challenged in more developed countries as well. What most families need is some extra support to cater for their children, in the form of sponsorship schemes, social protection programs. Awareness of their rights and information about governmental assistance would ensure proper utilization of various "schemes".

Role of the community

Wherever the parents are unable to take care and protect the child, the proximate community and their elected representatives must take up that responsibility. Thus, in the village, panchayat officials (local self-government) and in the urban areas, the elected members must ensure that every child is in school, receives basic health care (particularly immunizations, nutrition) and protection from child abuse and neglect.[14]

Role of Non-government Organizations (NGOs)

A large number of NGOs are working in the field of child welfare and child protection. However, because of the huge numbers of children requiring protection, their efforts can make only a marginal impact. However, they should coordinate their child welfare activities and need to work together. They also need to oversee implementation of various government measures that are already in place. The crucial ones include basic right to health, education, infant and young child development and prevention of child abuse and neglect.

Role of Government

The ultimate responsibility to protect its nation's children lies with the Government. By ratification of International instruments such as UN CRC & UN General comments #13, the Governments should commit appropriate legislative, administrative, social and educational measures to prevent and protect children from maltreatment. In 1992, India accepted the obligations of the UN Convention on the Rights of the Child (CRC). In the last two decades, the government has taken several steps toward publically advance children's rights. These include the Juvenile Justice (Care and Protection) Act 2000 (Amended in 2006).

Prohibition of Child Marriage Act (2006), the formation of the National Commission for Protection of Child Rights (2005), a National Plan of Action for children (2005), Right to Information (RTI) 2005, the Goa Children (amendment) Act 2005, the Child Labor (Prohibition and Regulation) Act, 1986 (two notifications in 2006 and 2008), expanded the list of banned and hazardous processes and occupation), Integrated Child Protection Scheme (2009) and advancing various legislations such as Right to Education Bill (2009) to protect, promote and defend child rights in the country.[15] However still, there is a wide gap

between policy and implementation/practice and outcome, and millions of children fall through the gaps.

The Juvenile Justice (Care and Protection) Act 2000 (Amended in 2006)

The Juvenile Justice (Care and Protection) Act 2000 (amended in 2006) was a key step in the right direction by Government of India. It established a framework for both children in need of care and protection and for children in contact with the law. However, further harmonization is needed with other existing laws, such as the Prohibition of Child Marriage Act 2006, the Child Labor Prohibition and Regulation Act 1986 or the Right to Education Act 2009. Important contradictions exist among these laws, starting with the definition and age of the child. Conflict with personal laws should also be addressed, ensuring universal protection of children, regardless of the community they belong to.

National Commission for Protection of Child Rights (NCPCR)

National Commission for Protection of Child Rights (NCPCR) was established by the Government of India in March 2007 by an Act of Parliament, with a wide mandate and considerable powers. The Delhi Commission for Protection of Child Rights was started in July 2008. Similar bodies at State level have been pursuing various matters concerning child rights and protection. Telephonic help lines (CHILDLINE 1098) and Child Welfare Committees (CWC) have been established, where reports of child abuse or a child likely to be threatened to be harmed can be made and help sought.

Integrated Child Protection Scheme (ICPS)

The Ministry of Women and Child Development, Government of India has launched an Integrated Child Protection Scheme (ICPS) (2009), which is expected to significantly contribute to the realization of State responsibility for creating a system that will efficiently and effectively protect children. It is meant to institutionalize essential services and strengthen structures, enhance capacity at all levels, create database and knowledge base for child protection services, strengthen child protection at family and community level and ensure appropriate inter-sectoral response at all levels and raise public awareness. *The guiding principles recognize that child protection is a primary responsibility of the family, supported by community, government and civil society.* The document "The integrated child protection scheme (ICPS)—A centrally sponsored scheme of Government—Civil society partnership" gives detailed accounts of this scheme.

Public health approach

Given a large population and socioeconomic constraints in developing countries, a public health approach/system response to primary, secondary and tertiary prevention of child maltreatment is urgently needed. More vulnerable groups with greater poverty, unemployment, migrant workers, parents with mental health problems, substance abuse, domestic violence, children with chronic health problems and disabilities are at greater risk. In order to make a social and public health impact, the Government should integrate its social welfare policies and child protection scheme; ensure their proper implementation and effective convergence at the grass root levels. Universal prevention services also need to have the ability to identify vulnerable families early enough to change risky behavior and pathway to abuse.[4] Use of maternal and child health (MCH) services, integrated child development schemes (ICDS) can broaden the pediatric surveillance role of community workers in the community. The children subjected to maltreatment should be quickly assessed and provided treatment and appropriate secure placement to avoid further damage in situation where it is unsafe for children to remain at home.[16]

In developing countries, there is also a big need for appropriately trained human resources and adequate child protection budgets. The analysis of Indian child budget data revealed only 0.3% of child budget is allocated to child protection. The officials should also ensure that Governmental funds are properly utilized.[17]

Role of professionals, corporate sector, religious institutions

The professionals, all educated persons, corporate sector and religious institutions must help in child protection and child welfare. A major attitudinal change in civil society is called for. The "child's voice" must be heard by the policymakers!

Attitudes, traditions, customs, behavior and practices

Attitudes, Traditions, customs, behavior & Practices refers to social norms and traditions that condemn harmful practices and support those that are protective.

Many protective traditions and practices exist, such as strong family values. However, certain stereotypes, attitudes and social norms that violate the rights of the child also persist, such as the use of corporal punishment as a way to discipline children or the social acceptance of child labor. Other harmful practices associated to gender roles, such as child marriage or gender-biased sex selection, are deeply rooted and manifest a patriarchal and hierarchic attitude toward girls and women, who are still seen by many as a liability or as *parayadhan* (*someone else's wealth* or property of the marital family). A better understanding of those norms and attitudes, are necessary to promote social change in the best interest of the child.[13]

Monitoring, data collection, research and evaluation

Monitoring effective systems of data collection, routine monitoring, research and evaluation are necessary to assess progress in the protection of children. In most countries, as well as in India, there is limited data on child protection. Existing national census and surveys can give data on birth registration, child marriage, child sex ratio, etc. However, Data is difficult to find in many forms of violence, such as sexual abuse, exploitation, trafficking, etc. which thrive on secrecy. It is important to have reliable data in order to promote intersectoral and regional strategies and best practices in child protection and their evolution over time.

Recommendation

In developing countries, child rights, protection and exploitation (street children, child labor, trafficking, etc.) are intimately linked to poor socioeconomic conditions in a large population base. Survival, early child health care, nutrition, education, development and child protection are most crucial child rights. Illiterate parents are ignorant of their children rights. They must be made aware of child rights, must demand and fight to obtain them. Multidisciplinary child professionals should work together and monitor the government efforts in protection of child rights. They should be able to collate available national child health indicators, address key issues and concerns in their region, involve children in research and facilitate their participation in projects and policy development. There is an urgent need to assign responsibility and accountability to Government, elected representatives, policy makers, proximate community and education and empowerment of families. In any case, a child must not suffer, if the parents can't provide care and protection.

References

1. UN Convention on the Rights of the Child (with optional protocols),available from www.unicef.org/crc

2. Committee on the Rights of the Child, 56th session General Comment No. 13 (2011) Article 19: The right of the child to freedom from all forms of violence

3. Child protection : millennium development goals (2010)

4. O'Donnell M, Scott D, Stanley F Child Abuse & neglect –is it time for public health approach? Australian & New Zealand Journal of Public Health 2008; 32(4):325–330.

5. Srivastava RN. Child protection: whose responsibility? CANCL NEWS 2011; 11(1):4–5.

6. Study on Child Abuse: India (2007). Ministry of Women and Child Development, Government of India, available from www.wcd.nic.in/childabuse.pdf

7. Delhi Declaration. http;www.indianpediatrics.net/delhideclaration2011.pdf.

8. Srivastava RN. Child Abuse & Neglect: Asia Pacific Conference and the Delhi Declaration. Indian Pediatrics 2011; 49:11–12.

9. Seth R, Banerjee SR, Srivastava RN. National Consultation on Urban Poor. CANCL News 2006; 6(2):12–15.

10. Seth R, Kotwal A, Ganguly KK. An ethnographic exploration of toluene abusers among street and working children of Delhi, India. Substance use and misuse 2005; 40:1659–1679.

11. Seth R. Care of the Rural Child. CANCL News 2008, 8(1):9–13.

12. Mody RC, Seth R. Progress report of village Bhango: Education and health of rural children. CANCL News 2008; 8(1):23–24.

13. Bergua J. UNICEF India. Child Protection Basics 2011, 1–8.

14. Srivastava RN. Child health & welfare, *panchayats* & rural development. CANCL News 2008; 8(1):3–4.

15. Third & Fourth Combined periodic report on the Convention on the Rights of the Child 2011, available from www.wcd.nic.in

16. Aggarwal K, Dalwai S, Galagali P, Mishra D, Prasad C, Thadhani A, et al. Recommendations on recognition and response to child abuse and neglect in the Indian setting. Indian Pediatr 2010; 47:493–504.

16

Developing Disaster Preparedness for Child Protection

Tufail Muhammad

Introduction

Every year, natural and man-made disasters kill hundreds of thousands of people and inflict great sufferings on million others. Natural disasters devastate whole regions without warning, as the December 2004 Asian Tsunami, the August 2005 hurricane Katrina the October 2005 Pakistan's earthquake and super floods 2010 have demonstrated. A disaster tend to create a catastrophic situation in which the day-to-day patterns of life suddenly get disrupted and people are plunged into helplessness and suffering. These extreme events influence a society so strongly that it is overwhelmed and cannot cope using its own resources. Besides deaths and injuries, the effects of a disaster on a community include collapse of infrastructure, hampered communications, loss of electricity, potable water and sanitation. Community cohesion is destroyed and the weaker sections of society become more vulnerable to abuse and exploitation. Population movements and other environmental changes may lead to increased risk of disease transmission, e.g. diseases caused through the fecal contamination of water and food and inadequate protection from the climatic elements. Similarly, closer human contact as a result of overcrowding in relief camps and temporary shelters may increase the potential of airborne diseases. The disruption of the public health program may result in increased vector-borne and vaccine preventable childhood diseases.

Effects on children

Each type of disaster has the capacity to cause long-term suffering and long-term trauma. A catastrophe such as an earthquake, hurricane, flood or violent acts is frightening to children and adults alike. Events of the greatest significance with respect to children include death or physical injury to a family member, a loss of home or possessions, loss of school, relocation of home and/or school, parental disorganization or dysfunction and experiencing absolute destruction and an uncertain future.

Direct risks for children in natural disasters include; deaths and injuries, vulnerability to malnutrition and infectious diseases, acute and long-term psychological trauma and all types of abuse, neglect and exploitation. Psychological trauma occurs in a child when an event is sudden, unusual and unexpected and disrupts the usual frame of reference with respect to family and environment. Such an event overwhelms the child's perceived ability to cope and be in control. All these traumatic experiences have a sustained impact on children's development. Several factors will affect a child's response to a disaster including perceived or actual life threat, duration of life disruption, familial and personal property loss, parental reaction and extent of familial disruption, child's pre-disaster state and probability of recurrence. The way children see and understand their parents' responses are very important. Children are aware of their parents' worries most of the time, but they are particularly sensitive during a crisis. Seeing a parent, who represents security and protection, being victimized and helpless leaves children fearful with an acute feeling of insecurity. Parents should admit their concerns to children, and also stress their abilities to cope with the disaster. Following a disaster, people may develop Post Traumatic Stress Disorder (PTSD), which is psychological damage that can result from experiencing, witnessing, or participating in an overwhelmingly traumatic event. Children with this disorder have repeated episodes in which they relive the traumatic event. Children often relive the trauma through repetitive play. In young children, upsetting dreams of the traumatic event may change into nightmares of monsters, or of threats to self or others. Post-traumatic stress disorder rarely occurs during the trauma itself. Though its symptoms can occur soon after the event, the disorder often surfaces several months or even years later. Given their vulnerable position generally and the fact that their principle carers may be missing or dead, children are at increased risk of harm, like trafficking, sexual abuse and commercial sexual exploitation. For this reason it is essential to ensure that measures are put in place both to protect children from further harm and abuse, and to ensure that the effect of the trauma itself and the further consequences of it are minimized.

Developing response

The Convention on the Rights of the Child (CRC) provides the guiding principles for child protection and psychosocial recovery and well being of children. Article 39 of the CRC states that State parties should take all appropriate measures to promote physical and psychosocial recovery and social reintegration of a child victim of:

- Any form of neglect, exploitation or abuse;
- Torture or any form of cruel, inhuman or degrading treatment or punishment;
- Armed conflict

Such recovery and reintegration shall take place in an environment that fosters the health, self-respect and dignity of the child.

In shaping our response to a disaster, we need to address the fundamental needs of children: basic necessities for living—shelter, warmth, food and water, establishment of a routine, security and protection from abuse and exploitation. We would need a rapid assessment of the child's rights and protection situation. The facts that would need to be found and explored are:

- Situation of violation of children's rights at before the origin of traumatic events
- The community's normal mechanisms to respond to and deal with psychosocial distress
- What is being done to enable the families to live in dignity and provide care and protection for their children?
- Are children being provided appropriate opportunities to talk about concerns and questions they have?
- Provision of educational and recreational activities for children
- Are systems in place to identify and assist children experiencing psychosocial distress?
- Are there unaccompanied children and who is looking after them?
- Are system in place for tracing and reunification of separated children with their families?

The effect of a disaster on a child population produce a variety of reactions that are specific for each survivor, depending on a group of variables. Hence the interplay of the type, extent, and proximity of the impact on a child within a family living in a geographical area has to be conceptualized based on the child's psychology and disaster experiences. Of all these variables, the quality of attention given to the child's subsequent needs and the parental reactions emerge as particularly significant.

In the face of emergency and disasters, children and young people can become separated from their parents and carers. Such children have long been recognized as being particularly vulnerable to exploitation and abuse and need special protection measures. It is crucial that such children are quickly identified and registered. A coordinated tracking system should be established immediately so that children should be reunited as soon as possible with their families. The unaccompanied children should be provided quality substitute care that should be community based, wherever possible. Institutional type care should generally be avoided, except in some special circumstances and on interim basis. Documentation of social histories must be done as soon as possible and active tracing initiated for parents or other surviving family members or relatives.

Child friendly spaces

Regardless of where children live, there needs to be a system in place to ensure that they are being looked after adequately and that people know where they are. The most efficient way of ensuring that the needs of children and young people are met is to establish "Child friendly Spaces" at convenient locations. Similar safe places may be established for young can be established in existing facilities and can be open according to demand and available resources. The participation of Young people is essential in creating and running Safe Places in order to help create adolescent/youth-friendly environments. Professionals managing Safe Places should be skilled in supporting the participation and leadership of young people. The Core activities at such places should include provision of information, non-judgmental listening, discussion, education and social and recreational activities. A sense of routine and safety should be provided through activities like daily classes, play and other recreational activities, and set meal times, together with family members or other children from the same community. Maintaining connections with people from life before the disaster, such as family members, neighbors, schoolmates and friends can be reassuring and comforting for children.

Psychological support

Many children would need psychosocial support to cope with the trauma and distress. Psychosocial programming should consist of structured activities designed to advance children's psychological and social development and to strengthen protective factors that limit the effects of adverse influences. The program should promote activities for children to talk about painful experiences or express their feelings. Beyond reaching individual children, the emphasis of psychosocial programs should be on strengthening children's social supports, mainly the family and the community.

Role of media

The role of media vis-à-vis children is of crucial importance at the time of disasters. Media has a key role to play in informing people and international community on the true extent and damage of the disaster, dispel rumors, mobilize support, and inform the victims on how and where to get emergency services. On the other hand, showing images of horror and devastation may heighten children's feelings of fear and stress. We should work closely with the media, so that they are sensitive to the needs of children and transform its outcome to work for the well-being of children, at the times of disasters. We also need to strengthen the capacity of families, communities, faith-based organizations, local NGOs and others to become active partners in the promotion and protection of child rights. And finally, all countries and communities need to have their own emergency preparedness plans that consider logistics, supplies, infrastructure, human resources, media plans and interorganizational coordination for all phases of a disaster.

17

Corporal Punishment: Movement to Prohibit and Eliminate all Corporal Punishment of Children

Peter Newell

Introduction

Corporal punishment of children is a universal, global problem. Children identify such punishment as the most common form of violence they face in their every day lives. Violent and humiliating punishment is still the daily experience of children in most countries of the world. It would continue unless prohibited completely and systematically challenged by awareness-raising and public education over a long period.

Corporal punishment is defined by the Committee on the Rights of the Child in its General Comment No 8 on the child's right to protection from all corporal punishment. The Committee defines 'corporal' or 'physical' punishment *as any punishment in which physical force is used and intended to cause some degree of pain or discomfort, however light…".* Most involves hitting children, with the hand or with an implement – a whip, stick, belt, shoe, wooden spoon, and so on. The Committee goes on to list many other ways adults have devised to hurt children deliberately. And it concludes: "In the view of the Committee, corporal punishment is invariably degrading. In addition, there are other non-physical forms of punishment that are also cruel and degrading and thus incompatible with the Convention. These include, for example, punishment which belittles, humiliates, denigrates, scapegoats, threatens, scares or ridicules the child."

Children—including young children—are increasingly speaking out themselves—in Asia and elsewhere - about the hurt caused to them by the acceptance and legality of this violence disguised as discipline, by their parents and teachers—by people they want to love and respect. There are many studies now in all regions. In March 2011, a major UNICEF report was launched in Geneva, called rather coyly "Child disciplinary practices at home", covering interview research in 37 low and middle income states. It mentions that on average across all the states, three in four children between the ages of 2 and 14 years were subjected to some kind of violent discipline. 17 per cent of children faced the most severe forms of physical punishment. And the experience is no different in high income states. The first recommendation in the report is unequivocal: "Ensure legal prohibition of all forms of violence against children in all settings, including within the home, and provide support for effective enforcement measures." And this study involved self-reporting by mothers or primary caregivers—so it is undoubtedly an under-estimate of the actual experience of children.

All states have criminal laws on assault which protect people from being hit and hurt deliberately. But when it comes to children, in most countries the law still draws a protective circle not around the child victim, but around the adult perpetrator. So prohibiting all corporal punishment requires the removal of all justifications and defences of "reasonable" punishment or "lawful" correction. Thereafter children will have the same protection as adults from assault—whether or not it is disguised as discipline.

The purpose of banning all corporal punishment must be to transform attitudes and practice, to move parents, teachers and other caregivers on from violent punishment to positive forms of discipline that work. The purpose is not to punish more parents, because that of course would not be in the interests of children. So the law needs to deliver a very clear and explicit message, that it is no more lawful or acceptable to hit or deliberately hurt a child, than to hit anyone else. This is not an issue on which compromise is useful or acceptable. We do not compromise in condemning and prohibiting all violence against women or elderly people—so why children? Some suggest that law reform to ban corporal punishment, especially in the home, should wait and only follow a change in social attitudes. Nobody would make that argument now in relation to violence against women – that one should wait to prohibit domestic violence against women until a change in men's lives and attitudes, universal anger management courses, full employment has been achieved. It is equally unacceptable to wait in attitudinal changes toward violence against children. As long as the law states that it is acceptable to hit children or hurt them deliberately, attempts at promoting non-violent parenting and teaching are going to be hopelessly undermined. *Legal reforms alone can achieve little, and must be linked to comprehensive awareness-raising and education about the law and children's rights to protection, and the dangers of corporal punishment, together with promotion of positive, non-violent relationships.*

Prohibition of corporal punishment is an immediate human rights obligation. In all of the 30 countries which have achieved a complete ban on corporal punishment, majority public and parent opinion was against the ban, often massively so, when it was enacted. In these states, politicians and parliamentarians have been persuaded to act, as they often have to act on social issues, on the basis of their human rights obligations and professional opinion, ahead of public opinion. The law should surely be seen first and foremost as an educational tool, a preventive tool.

The scale of deliberate punitive violence against children, in their homes and families and also in many countries in alternative care, schools and penal systems—has only become visible quite recently. That is a big step forward, because once visible, it becomes very difficult to defend hitting and hurting children deliberately. With visibility has come recognition, across regions and systems, that the legality and social acceptance of corporal punishment and other forms of cruel or degrading punishment of children are human rights violations, condemned now by international and regional human rights monitoring bodies. The Convention on the Rights of the Child has been ratified almost universally, by 193 states including all in Asia Pacific. The Convention requires States to protect children from "all forms of physical and mental violence" and as the Committee on the Rights of the Child emphasises in its General Comment No. 8: "There is no ambiguity: 'all forms of physical or mental violence' does not leave room for any level of legalized violence against children. Corporal punishment and other cruel or degrading forms of punishment are forms of violence and States must take all appropriate legislative, administrative, social and educational measures to eliminate them".

The Committee has recommended prohibition of all corporal punishment to more than 160 States globally, including most across Asia; it has recommended this three times to my country and a number of others. Other United Nations human rights Treaty Bodies now consistently echo the Committee on the Rights of the Child, including the Committee against Torture. Also, when states overall human rights record is examined in the new Universal Periodic Review process in the Human Rights Council in Geneva, there have been constant recommendations to ban all corporal punishment of children. The issue was raised in the review of over 110 states, and more than 30 accepted other states' proposals that they should prohibit.

Regional human rights systems, in the Americas and in Africa have also condemned all corporal punishment and recommended prohibition.

In 2008, the Council of Europe became the first major inter-governmental organization to launch an explicit campaign for prohibition across its 47 member-states. 22 of the 47 member states have achieved complete prohibition, and the fact that the Council houses the strongest human rights mechanism, the European Court of Human Rights, has a lot to with that.

The Governing Body of the South Asia Initiative to End All Violence against Children, a project of SAARC, which comprises government and civil society representatives and two child representatives from the eight states, has agreed as a priority to launch a regional campaign for prohibition and elimination of all corporal punishment, and also endorsed a regional report on progress across the region. During the process of the UN Secretary General's Study on violence against children, regional consultations were held in Islamabad for South Asia and in Bangkok. At both, children were actively involved and spoke out strongly for prohibition of all corporal punishment. In South Asia, the states made commitments to proceed with law reform, repeated at a follow-up meeting, also in Pakistan, the following year. There has been some progress in banning corporal punishment in some settings across the eight countries, in schools and care and penal institutions in India; in schools in Bangladesh by order of the Supreme Court last year. Hopefully the SAIEVAC initiative will speed things up. It is encouraging to see that India's periodic report just delivered to the Committee on the Rights of the Child does make a clear commitment to prohibition in all settings. If India achieves complete prohibition for its 420 million children, it will of course transform the global statistics and add real momentum to the campaign.

The harmful impact of corporal punishment on children is well-researched now, with more than 100 studies reviewing its developmental outcomes. Their findings are strikingly consistent. Corporal punishment is associated with higher levels of aggression and antisocial behavior in children, and this association continues into adulthood. There are no research findings demonstrating that physical punishment leads to positive long-term outcomes; all findings reveal negative effects on children's development. In arguing for prohibition of violence against women, we would not look for research into its effects... it would be insulting to women. And it is equally insulting to children to suggest we have to prove harm in order to condemn this deliberate violence. It is a human rights violation. *We really do not need more research, although research into children's real experiences remains valuable for advocacy.*

Why is challenging and ending corporal punishment so important, given the extreme breaches of children's rights and the extreme forms of violence that children in India and so many states are still facing? We are not just challenging a particular form of violence—though it is the most common form of violence against children. As the Committee on the Rights of the Child asserts in its General Comment, ending it is an essential strategy for ending all forms of violence against children: the idea that breaching a child's human dignity and physical integrity is acceptable, or even

as some still suggest "in their best interests", makes every other sort of extreme abuse, including sexual exploitation, more likely and easier. No state can pretend that it has an effective child protection system while its laws and social attitudes still authorise and accept violent punishment of children. Ending all legalised violence against children is the only safe foundation for child protection.

It took more than 10 years of fairly systematic lobbying to get ISPCAN to sign up in support of the aims of the Global Initiative. And I have found it extraordinarily hard to get child protection practitioners, in the UK and elsewhere, to see what a difference it would make to their work, to the safety of children, if they could deliver an unambiguous message to parents: that it is as unlawful and unacceptable to hit or deliberately hurt children as to hit anyone else. Instead they have to say you mustn't hit too hard, avoid the head, avoid bruising and so on.

Corporal punishment really does seem to me to be the elephant in the room of child protection. Physical abuse is corporal punishment; may be a tiny proportion of it is administered by psychotic, sadistic parents for the pleasure of it... But more or less all is in the context of punishment, control or discipline. I believe the concept of child "abuse" has served children very badly. In the context of describing and challenging violence against women, there is no parallel; there is no attempt to draw lines and define a distinction between "abuse" and discipline... Although once there was of course and our law had the rule of thumb to define the thickness of cane that it was permissible for a husband to beat his wife with. With children, the distinction lingers on, and many child protection workers like to try and keep child abuse and physical punishment in two separate boxes.

Each year, corporal punishment kills significant numbers of children in all regions and seriously injures many thousands more, including babies and small children in their homes. But beyond the obvious child protection context for outlawing it, the acceptance and legality of this daily punitive violence is highly symbolic of children's low status in our societies, as possessions not people.

Just as challenging routine domestic violence has been a fundamental part of women's emancipation and protection, so it is with children. When we challenge all corporal punishment, however light, we are pursuing children's equal right to respect for their human dignity and physical integrity. This is as fundamental as anything can be to improving children's status and gaining recognition and respect for children as rights holders alongside the rest of us.

When we use parallels with the campaign to end violence against women, people respond: "But children are different". And of course they are different: the babies and small children, whom research suggests are the victims of most corporal punishment in the home, are different in that they are very small and very fragile. Children's vulnerability, their developmental status, their dependence on adults and the huge difficulties they in particular face in seeking protection for themselves: all these differences suggest that they should have more, not less legal and other protection.

This is a transformative issue for children. Attitudes to children can be changed and violence against children rapidly reduced if we can convince governments and parliaments to accept their human rights obligations and professional advice and move quickly to implement explicit prohibition. And also link law reform to using all the points of contact with families and children to transmit the basic messages about the law and children's rights to protection, about the dangers of corporal punishment and the principles of positive, non-violent relationships with children—they are not very complicated.

Most parents, once they are given space and time to think and talk, know what works in encouraging acceptable behavior and responsibility in their children. When I speak about building this educational process into all the state's contacts with parents and children. I always suggest that birth registration could be a moment to transmit very basic and simple messages about children's rights—including the right not to be hit. There are antenatal and postnatal contacts, all sorts of contacts by all elements of the health service; immunization—and one could perhaps use the slogan that immunizing your child against violence means not hitting them and not transmitting the message that you see violence as a way of sorting out conflicts. Other contacts in the pre-school sector, at school entry, in the school curriculum for future parents – and so on. NGO initiatives to promote positive parenting, and positive behavior management in schools are of course very welcome trail blazing—but the task of transforming traditional attitudes demands government engagement in taking it to scale and universalizing the educational process—and sustaining it over quite a long period.

It is essential to emphasise *that the first aim of banning corporal punishment in the family is educational, not punitive, to move parents on from violent discipline.* Prosecuting and sentencing more parents, sending them to prison or fining them, will not help children. So there needs to be a clear emphasis, either in the law itself or in guidance to all those involved, that charging and prosecuting parents should only be pursued when it is judged necessary to protect a child from significant harm, and to be in the best interests of the victim child. The Committee on the Rights of the Child provides detailed guidance on this in its General Comment No. 8.

Globally, there is real progress and the context has been the developed human rights consensus. The UN Secretary-General's Study on violence against children, led by Professor Paulo Pinheiro, highlighted prohibition of all corporal punishment as a key recommendation. The Secretary-General's Special Representative on violence against children, Marta Santos Pais, has adopted prohibition of all violence—including all punitive violence—as a key priority within her mandate as global advocate.

The human rights consensus and the follow-up to the UN Study is leading to accelerating law reform: across the world 30 states have implemented a complete ban on all corporal punishment, including in the family—the most recent are Poland, Kenya, Tunisia and the newest UN member state—South Sudan. Brazil is poised to be the first large state, with 69 million children, to achieve this reform, hopefully before the end of this year. It was in 2007 that New Zealand became the first state in this region, and perhaps more significantly, the first English-speaking state to ban corporal punishment in all settings. The Philippines has a Bill in its Assembly which could prohibit in all settings, or had last time I heard.

A significant majority of states globally—120—have achieved a ban in schools. It has been prohibited as a disciplinary measure in penal institutions for children in 113 states. But at least 42 states—including some across Asia Pacific—still authorize the sentencing of child offenders (in some cases as young as 8) to corporal punishment—caning, whipping or flogging. And in alternative care settings of all kinds, just 37 states have achieved clear prohibition. Our website—www.endcorporalpunishment.org includes full details on progress and individual reports on every state in the world, and much else.

The biggest challenge everywhere is that for most people, most of us, this issue has a strong and often painful personal dimension: most adults were hit by their parents in their childhood. Most parents have hit their own growing children. We do not like to think badly of our parents, or of our own parenting, and that makes it much more difficult to move on to see this issue as one of equality and human rights.

People often respond to me, in all regions "But corporal punishment is part of our culture"—as if it wasn't part of the culture of my country. The UK in its colonial past did much to promote the use of corporal punishment, in the context of slavery and armed occupation, in the development of school and penal systems for young people and in some missionary teaching. The traditional English common law defence of "reasonable chastisement" has existed in the laws of more than 70 states worldwide, including many across the Asia Pacific region. It's a deeply shaming legacy.

Another challenge, in UK and many other countries, is that some adults believe their religion gives them a right or even a duty to use corporal punishment. The international human rights instruments uphold the right to freedom of religious belief. But belief cannot lead to practices which breach others' rights, including their right to respect for their human dignity and physical integrity. Violence of any kind cannot be dignified or justified by reference to religion; increasingly this is accepted in relation to violence against women, and it must be accepted in relation to children. Now, respected leaders of all faiths, including Christianity and Islam, Buddhist and Hindu scholars are increasingly speaking out against all violence against children, and supporting the prohibition and elimination of all corporal punishment.

Achieving rejection of violent and humiliating punishment of children is needed not simply for children but for the development of more peaceful, non-violent human societies.

Resources

The Global Initiative to end all corporal punishment was launched in 2001 by Thomas Hammarberg, now the Council of Europe's Commissioner for Human Rights and myself, to emphasise and use the human rights consensus against corporal punishment and to support regional and national campaigns with technical assistance. An e-newsletter is distributed about every two months (available from< info@endcorporalpunishment.org>)

18

Child Abuse and Neglect: Influence of Context, Culture and Timing on Resilience

Michael Ungar, Jerry Thomas

Introduction

A growing interest in the term resilience is occurring among mental health practitioners and policy makers concerned with children who have experienced physical, emotional and sexual abuse and neglect. This interest represents a shift from a focus on psychopathology and disorder following exposure to violence to the many ways that individuals, their families and communities protect themselves and continue to grow in positive ways.[1,2] The emphasis when studying resilience is on what people are doing to maintain well-being, rather than the discovery of the roots of disorder. This shift is potentially very useful to policy makers and those designing mental health interventions as there are lessons to be learned from those who are already managing to succeed despite their disadvantage. In this chapter, we will present a social ecological definition of resilience that emphasizes the influence context, culture and timing have on a child and how protective factors help children overcome adversity related to maltreatment.

The most common understanding of resilience is to imagine a child who bounces back from maltreatment and either: (i) returns to age-appropriate normative behavior (the child stays in school, maintains attachments to a caregiver, avoids risky behaviours, shows the absence of mental health problems); or (ii) exceeds expectations and demonstrates post-traumatic growth.[3,4] At first glance, both pathways to coping are evidence of positive adaptation under stress. Research suggests that children who adapt well are likely to function normally.[5]

A few problems exist, however, with this way we commonly understand resilience. First, there is the risk that we see resilience as solely a quality of the individual. Studies of personal hardiness, and the ability of individuals to bounce back because of temperament or other personal quality, reinforce the myth of the rugged individual as resilient. The danger with conceptualizing resilience as the ability of the individual to survive and thrive independent of help from others is that there is the potential to blame those who do not do so well for their failure. Emphasis on the individual also excuses those mandated to support children (child welfare workers, police, policy makers) in higher risk environments from designing and implementing effective interventions to remove the risk factors to which children are exposed. After all, if the argument is that resilience is an individual quality, then there is no need to shape the child's environment to facilitate the child's well-being.

Instead, as we will show, resilience is the result of the interaction between the individual and his or her environment, with the quality of the environment playing as large, and often larger role, than personal qualities like intelligence or personality in determining the resilience of an individual.

The second problem with the study of resilience has been its lack of cultural embeddedness. There are now many studies published that identify a set of protective mechanisms known to improve child developmental outcomes.[6] Increasingly, these studies are being done with racial and cultural minorities to document whether patterns of coping under stress show heterogeneity (differences) or homogeneity (sameness) across populations exposed to different forms of adversity. We know, for example, that a mother's education protects a child from early school leaving, and that the trauma that follows physical abuse during childhood can be either prevented or treated through a secure attachment to a primary caregiver.[7] These protective factors, like others such as the development of self-esteem, personal efficacy, and access to a mentor, originated from the work of resilience researchers in the west, principally the United States and Britain. What is not known is whether there are as yet unnamed protective processes that are relevant to other populations around the world that have not been studied because of the Eurocentric bias of resilience researchers. In other words, are there types of resilience that are powerful predictors of positive development under stress which have not been identified by western researchers because they were not meaningful to them or because they do not exist in the contexts in which the research has taken place? Furthermore, if the flow of knowledge was reversed, and emerging scholars in lower and middle-income countries set the resilience agenda, would we identify new protective mechanisms among children in higher income countries that have so far been overlooked?

Case study: Ang

Ang is a young man from a tribal community in Manipur, India, near the border with Myanmar. He describes his village and the surrounding area as a "battleground" for the many insurgent and militant groups that operate in Manipur. The violence has deepened the impact of the poverty that characterizes the region.

As a child, Ang lived with his parents and five siblings. His father farmed the small paddy field they owned and was a respected man in the community. With the little income he had he helped pay for other children in the village to get an education. Ang was told that his father believed that education was the way out of poverty and perhaps, a way to end conflict. When Ang was five years old his father died suddenly. Ang says that if it were not for his mother's courage and hard work the family would not have survived. She took upon herself the financial burden of the family, working as a vegetable vendor and sourcing vegetables

from the neighboring villages and selling them in a nearby town. When there were no vegetables to sell, Ang's mother sold chickens. She would leave home early in the morning and return late in the night. Sometimes Ang would accompany her.

Ang's elder brother left school to work in the paddy field. Ang thought that he too would have to drop out of school, except he reasoned that, "My father helped the village children to go to school. And here I am, his son, about to drop out of school." Ang's mother and other adults in his village made it possible for him to continue going to school. Today Ang is completing his Masters degree in Social Work and making plans to work with the youth of his community. He says, "I realize every adversity is a challenge, an opportunity to create good. My mother is living proof of that."

The need for cross-cultural understandings of resilience

A story like Ang's helps demonstrate the need for cross-cultural research on resilience. There are many scholars who have noted that more contextually diverse research will help to reveal patterns of coping that are not yet well documented. Kagitçibasi,[8] who has looked at differences in the way parents cope in what she terms Majority World (people living in low and middle income countries and aboriginal peoples) and Minority World (people of European descent) contexts, writes, "What appears to be lacking are studies conducted within the cultural context that reveal functional/ adaptive links among phenomena that may, in turn, repeat themselves in different contexts, thus pointing to some fundamental causal relations" (p.16–17). The advantage to looking across cultures is that we are better able to see causal mechanisms in action. We can see what is occurring "naturally" in different contexts, cultures, and sociohistorical periods without the blinders that come with seeing the world from the vantage point of just one set of assumptions. In Ang's case, it was both his mother's ability to support the family financially, and Ang's access to the support of other adults, that made it possible for him to continue his education. It is this facilitated access to education which is at the root of Ang's description of his resilience.

To illustrate similarly diverse patterns to resilience that are revealed through observation in different cultural contexts, Bamba and Haight[9] studied orphans in Japan who are frequently housed in group home settings where their caregivers provide a model of care that might be considered mildly neglectful in the United States, Canada and Britain. For example, children are encouraged to resolve their own conflicts with their peers, with adults seldom intervening to change children's behavior:

Mimamori is a socialization practice through which Japanese adults support children's attainment of developmental goals, not primarily through targeted individual interventions as may be more common in the United States, but by providing a rich social and physical ecology in which they may learn and flourish "naturally," including recover from maltreatment. Mimamori is primarily indirect support, through which adults may create an accepting and positive social-emotional ecology that provides the children with opportunities for exploration, self-expression, and peer relationships (p. 190).

Observation of children's interactions inside group home settings shows that staff intervene less during disputes than staff in other countries. Instead, staff who work with children apprehended from their parents see it as their job to create *ibasho*, a sense of acceptance and security inside their institution, a resource to the children that was likely absent in their lives before removal from their families of origin. There is, therefore, a tension between staff promoting children's independent problem-solving skills and providing them with a stable holding environment that nurtures their emotional well-being. It is this specificity in the way resilience is promoted in different contexts which is emerging as a focus of many new researchers to the field.

A second example of this specificity in the way resilience is shown is the ability of ethnoracial minorities to demonstrate resistance to oppression. At the level of the individual child, what this means is that children are taught by their parents, and supported by their peer groups, to resist the imposition of cultural hegemony that would cause them to devalue their culture or race. A child who is taught to be proud of his cultural identity and who is given opportunities to display that identity through language, dress, and other behavior is likely to experience greater well-being[10, 11].

In these examples, the protective mechanisms that make children resilient are specific to the context in which they are shown. Why, though, are children in these countries evaluated with concepts imported from higher income countries, but children in the economically well-developed countries never assessed based on criteria for well-being developed in middle and lower-income countries, or countries with populations that do not share a European ancestry. One could, for example, speculate that children with *mimamori* and *ibasho* might fare better than children placed in foster care and cared for in ways typical of nations with an Anglo-European history.

By engaging in this transcultural debate over resilience, we open ourselves to much less certainty in regard to what children need developmentally. For example, in different countries, and frequently across social classes, we see differences in the level of entitlement children experience. The overly indulged or "spoiled" child in a safe community with no responsibilities for others is likely to develop few coping skills that he can use should he experience a traumatic event.[12] Another child's story reveals this pattern, in this case challenging stereotypes of the child laborer.

Case study: Binus

Binus grew up as a child laborer after both his parents died when he was four years old. He belongs to one of the most economically and socially deprived communities in Assam in the northeastern part of India. In order to survive following his parents' deaths. Binus was placed into the household of a farmer where he was expected to work and denied education. Nevertheless, his employer had a daughter who was the same age as Binus and who eventually went to school. Binus recalls sneaking up next to her to see what she was writing and hear what she was reading. It was that passion to study that made him run away from his employer's house when he was 8.

Fortunately, his determination to learn and his willingness to continue to earn money while studying resulted in him being admired by the adults who got to know him, including his next employer. Today he has a degree in social work and works as a manager for UNICEF in the eastern districts of Assam.

Defining resilience

Many children who encounter significant adversity maintain normal levels of functioning, or do better than expected. These patterns of coping, known as resilience, are more than a quality of the individual. Resilience is a set of interactions that are nurtured rather than indicative of a child's personality, intelligence or other quality alone. The more facilitative the social environment, the more likely children are to be resilient. This social ecological definition of resilience means that:

In the context of exposure to significant adversity, resilience is both the capacity of individuals to navigate their way to the psychological, social, cultural, and physical resources that sustain their wellbeing, and their capacity individually and collectively to negotiate for these resources to be provided and experienced in culturally meaningful ways.[13]

This definition encourages a view of resilience as the result of successful navigation and negotiation. People experiencing adversity do better when there are resources made available that they value and exercise control over.

The concept of resilience, therefore, suggests a need for flexibility with regard to which resources are provided and how. Models of intervention, for example, to address childhood maltreatment need to reflect the values of the children and families they are meant to serve.

Negotiating the meaning of resilience across contexts, cultures, and time

How children like Ang and Binus navigate and negotiate for the resources they need to be resilient is always a function of how well individuals and their environments interact. The emphasis is as much on the environment as it is the child. Miller[14] wrote that "For most of its history, psychology has been a culturally grounded discipline that has recognized the constitutive role of collective meanings and practices on the development of self" (p.217). And yet, the tendency has been to seek universal laws akin to the physical sciences for rules across cultures. Psychological processes have naively been thought of as culture free. Instead, the semiotic view of culture, as Geertz[15] expressed it, shows that what we accept as truth (i.e., which child is resilient and which is not) is more correctly understood as the result of meaning systems that are embodied in symbols. What that means is that we accept as resilient the abused child who

continues to attend school and has no nightmares. However, as research is beginning to show, the child who withdraws from school, and who manifests symptoms of disorder like nightmares may be coping actively with past-trauma, albeit in ways that we judge as maladaptive.[16] Long-term, these more active strategies may protect the child from the long-term psychological consequences of early victimization. Viewing resilience as a social construct in which the meaning of behavior is negotiated between people and institutionalized, we can see that resilience is different for different children in different contexts and cultures.[17]

This pattern of negotiation is discussed by Miller[14] in her look at the implications of a more culturally based sense of self. Models of attachment, e.g. work poorly to describe positive ways of behaving in India among Hindu families. Models of attachment, she says, are "premised on a tension between too much autonomy, with its threat of isolation, and too much connection, with its threat of self" (p.227). But is such an idea really salient, she wonders, in a culture where isolation is unlikely, and selflessness not so problematic? In other words, the broader forces of interaction and social rules shape a concept like attachment. Even though the concept relates to an observable phenomenon globally, symbolically, what we envision as healthy attachment is likely to vary by context.

This variation will occur as a consequence of a number of different factors, including time. As Schoon[18] shows, the sociopolitical period in which one grows up will influence not only one's access to resources (like education and health care) but also the values one holds. This point is easier to see when we look across contexts. Different contexts support different definitions of resilience just as different historical periods have placed value on different social behaviors. The process is not, however, simple, and there is frequently conflict between the values of individuals as societies change.

For example, a study of Bedouin teachers-in-training showed that individuals in a traditional society that is in transition culturally may seek accommodation to new norms without assimilation.[19] The teachers remained very connected to their families (a traditional value) but wanted a middle class life associated with western styles of consumption. Their education was not valued for its content, but instead seen as a tool forsocial advancement and economic security: "Schools represent institutions trying to spread modernity among a traditional society, but the emphasis on achievement is viewed as contrary to tribal loyalty and social status" (Para 14). It is these competing value systems that can make defining resilience complex. Is a successful Bedouin the one who acculturates to the values of non-Bedouin or the one who holds fast to his traditional cultural practices? Modern economic behavior with its emphasis on individual financial independence does not characterize the lifestyle of traditional Bedouin.

Furthermore, they do not seem to regard Western education, which is the main content of their studies, as having any revolutionary significance for them. The students describe the education they are acquiring mainly as a tool in the achievement of their ambition to improve their standard of living, quality of life, and social standing. Even their vocation as teachers, in so far as they relate to it, is seen as a way of helping other Bedouin children make similar progress. We can sum up by saying that our students coexist in two worlds. They identify with the tribal world but also turn to Western values in an effort to get a better life. Managing these two lifestyles simultaneously is the secret of their success (Para 83).

These coping strategies are, therefore, responsive to context, culture and time. The child's developmental phase, like socio-historical period, will also determine which protective processes are most likely to predict better outcomes, with different strengths exerting a larger influence at different developmental periods. Cultural adherence among immigrants, e.g., may vary by the age of the child, with children who immigrate younger being more likely to remain attached to their family's cultural values (like filial piety), whereas teenagers who immigrate may quickly shed the dominant values they held in efforts to get along with peers.[20] Likewise, the age at which a child experiences physical or sexual assault is associated with the likelihood that she experiences trauma afterwards, as well as which protective factors are most likely to help developmentally.[21]

Navigating toward protective resources

While the specific way in which people define resilience may be negotiated differently based on the person's context, culture and time period, there is remarkable similarity to the types of resources people need to protect themselves against risk. In work by Ungar and his colleagues around the world, at least seven factors emerge that are predictive of resilience. Each factor, or what has been termed "tension," is a resource that individuals in adverse environments seek that help them cope. These include:

1. Relationships with peers and adults, both primary caregivers and others in one's community.
2. A powerful identity resulting from others acknowledging an individual as special and her talents as valuable.
3. Experiences of power and control, such that the person is able to feel in control of what happens to him and attribute his success in some part to his own actions, or those of his social group (in more collectivist societies).
4. Experiences of social justice, in particular the feeling that one is being treated fairly in her family and community.
5. Access to basic material resources like clothing, shelter and safety when outside one's home.
6. A sense of cohesion, life purpose, spirituality or belonging when a part of one's family and community.
7. Cultural adherence that comes from feeling an attachment to one's culture over time.

Each of these seven aspects of resilienceare, as the example of the Bedouin discussed earlier show, negotiated inside contextual, cultural and temporal spaces. While the themes are common in people's narratives of resilience around the world, the actual patterns they use to achieve all seven are always reflective of where they live and the social discourses that define what is and is not successful coping under stress.

Discussion

As this chapter has shown, resilience is not generated under spectacular circumstances; rather it is the result of everyday interactions between individuals and their environments in circumstances where deprivation and hardship are realities. Yet when someone from such environment succeeds our tendency is to attribute causality to some exceptional quality of the individual alone, rather than to the quality of the interactions between the individual and his environment. When understood ecologically, resilience is the result of effective but everyday navigations and negotiations with family and community.

Both case studies suggest that there is potential for children to grow in their capacity to deal with stress through exposure to adversity. Arguably, Binus is fortunate to have had the opportunity to work and learn how to survive on his own rather than being institutionalized or abandoned altogether. In this case, we could say that the exposure to the risks associated with work and the trauma of losing his parents may have caused Binus to experience posttraumatic growth.[3] For children, PTG is the opportunity to develop their capacities following dangerous life events. The experience becomes a platform for skill development that would otherwise have not occurred.

While child labor is exploitive and should be stopped, there is evidence that Binus' experience is typical of many. Working children may gain some benefit through their work when their environment provides no other reasonable opportunities to support them. Work can help children develop personal assets such as a sense of personal power that comes with contributing to one's family's welfare and hopefulness for the future because of the training that is received.[22,23] Over-protective parenting may be more of a threat to children's psychosocial development than the child who is forced to do domestic work or work in a family business where she develops skills that will make her much more resilient when confronting future stress. As the example of Binus illustrates, our notion of what constitutes risk, and the nature of protective processes, is biased by a particular worldview. Discursively, the better we are at engaging people with diverse values in debates over resilience, the more likely we are to identify universal protective processes. Therefore, if we are to help protect children from abuse, there is a need to look at both emic (local, indigenous) and etic (foreign, culturally homogeneous) patterns of coping under stress.

Both Ang and Binus *The authors wish to acknowledge the support of the International Development Research Centre of Canada and the Social Sciences and Humanities Research Council of Canada for their support of an International Community University Research Alliance which made this article, and the research upon which it is based, possible.

The authors wish to acknowledge the support of the International Development Research Centre of Canada and the Social Sciences and Humanities Research Council of Canada for their support of an International Community University Research Alliance which made this article, and the research upon which it is based, possible developed survival skills because the responsibilities that were placed on them required them to take initiative. While such talent makes both young men stand out, neither would have succeeded without assistance from others. Their resilience depended on both the material resources of others who helped them obtain education and the necessities of life and the symbolic resources of a value system that defined goals that were protective. Concern for their family, a positive attitude toward work, and a sense of community cohesion in which they felt a part of the lives of others are all generic factors that make resilience more likely. As Ang explained, from the age of 11 years he recalls the sadness he felt when he assumed responsibility for cooking for the family in the evenings while his friends played football in a nearby field. However, the recognition he received from his family for his contribution and the very real skills he developed as a consequence were in part the reason for his success.

Such examples show that the factors that are most protective will always reflect local value systems, the nature of the risks an individual faces and the resources that are close at hand. In both Ang and Binus' lives, education played an important role mitigating the impact of their poverty and neglect. However, both young men were also forced to work which was approved of socially. Binus worked on construction sites and did odd jobs to finance his education. Ang was a bright student that was noticed by his teachers. In fact after he cleared the class 8 examinations, one of his teachers encouraged him to appear for the class 10 public examination and complete his high school education. This education, though, came at a cost. Ang's mother could contribute only so much so he worked in a rice mill before and after school. Later, to pay for Higher Secondary school, he worked as a helper in a government officer's house, looking after cows and selling the milk in the evenings. Finally, he worked as a teacher in a private school to pay for the rest of his college studies.

The question still remains, though, why these two individuals have survived so well when others do not. Arguably, in both cases there were community elders who noticed the young men and helped them succeed. When Ang was in school and college his progress was discussed in community meetings and in his church. The community came together to provide him with some of the supplies he needed to study. Such support counter balanced the wider corruption and poverty that would have made Ang's success practically impossible without the support of his community.

Narratives such as these help explain the nature of resilience and how the successful individual takes advantages of opportunities, finding ways to access all seven factors discussed earlier. The family and community that want its children to be resilient ensures that opportunities are available in ways that children themselves value. From a social ecological point of view, resilience is a facilitated quality of individual and environment interactions that help people to realize their abilities in contexts of adversity.

Acknowledgement

The authors wish to acknowledge the support of the International Development Research Centre of Canada and the Social Sciences and Humanities Research Council of Canada for their support of an International Community University Research Alliance which made this article, and the research upon which it is based, possible.

References

1. Rutter, M. (2012). Resilience: Causal pathways and social ecology. In M. Ungar (Ed.), *The social ecology of resilience: A handbook of theory and practice* (pp.33-42). New York: Springer.

2. Ungar, M. The social ecology of resilience. Addressing contextual and cultural ambiguity of a nascent construct. *American Journal of Orthopsychiatry*, 2011; 81:1–17.

3. Klasen, F.,Oettingen, G., Daniels, J., Post, M., Hoyer, C., & Adam, H. Posttraumatic resilience in former Ugandan child soldiers.*Child Development*, 2010; 81(4):1096–1113.

4. Tedeschi, R. G., & Calhoun, L. G. The Posttraumatic Growth Inventory: Measuring the positive legacy of trauma. *Journal of Traumatic Stress*, 1996; 9:455–471.

5. Luthar, S. S. The culture of affluence: Psychological costs of material wealth. *Child Development*, 2003; 74(6):1581–1593.

6. Luthar, S. S., Cicchetti, D., & Becker, B. The construct of resilience: A critical evaluation and guidelines for future work. *Child Development*, 2000; 71(3): 543–562.

7. Bus, A. G., &Van Ijzendoorn, M. H. Mothers reading to their 3-year-olds: The role of mother-child attachment security in becoming literate. *Reading Research Quarterly*, 1995; 30:998–1015.

8. Kagitçibasi, C. (2007). *Family, self, and human development across cultures: Theory and applications, 2nd Ed.* Mahwah, NJ: Lawrence Erlbaum.

9. Bamba, S. &Haight, W.L. (2011). *Child welfare and development: A Japanese case study*. Cambridge, MA: Cambridge University Press.

10. Beckett, C., Maughan, B., Rutter, M., Castle, J., Colvert, E.,Vedder, P. (2006). Immigrant youth: Acculturation, identity, and adaptation. *Applied Psychology: An International Review*, 55(3):303–332.

11. Juang, L. P., & Nguyen, H. H. (2009). Misconduct among Chinese American adolescents: The role of acculturation, family obligation, and autonomy expectations. *Journal of Cross-Cultural Psychology*, 40(4), 649–666.

12. Ungar, M. (2009). Overprotective parenting: Helping parents provide children the right amount of risk and responsibility. *American Journal of Family Therapy*, 37(3), 258–271.

13. Ungar, M. (2008). Resilience across cultures.*British Journal of Social Work*, 38(2), 218–235.

14. Miller, G. (1997). Systems and solutions: The discourses of brief therapy. *Contemporary Family Therapy, 19*(1), 5–22.

15. Geertz, C. (1973). *The Interpretation of Cultures*. New York: Basic Books.

16. Bonanno, G.A. & Mancini, A.D. (2012). Beyond resilience and PTSD: Mapping the heterogeneity of responses to potential trauma. *Psychological Trauma, 4*(1), 74-83.

17. Ungar, M. (2004). *Nurturing hidden resilience in troubled youth*. Toronto, ON: University of Toronto Press.

18. Schoon, I. (2006*). Risk and resilience: Adaptations in changing times*. Cambridge, UK: Cambridge University Press.

19. Kainan, A., Rozenberg, M., &Munk, M. (2006).Change and preservation in life stories ofBeouin students.

Forum: Qualitative Social Research, 7(1), Art. 7. Retrieved from: http://www.qualitative-research.net/fqs-texte/1–06/06–1–7-e.htm.

20. Roopnarine, J. &Gielen, U.P. (Eds.)(2004). Childhood and adolescence: Cross-cultural perspectives and applications. Westport, CT: Praeger.

21. Chartier, M. J., Walker, J. R., & Naimark, B. Separate and cumulative effects of adverse childhood experiences in predicting adult health and health care utilization. *Child Abuse & Neglect*, 2010; 34:454–454.

22. Liborio, R. & Ungar, M. Children's perspectives on their economic activity as a pathway to resilience. *Children and Society,* 2010; 24:326–338.

23. Liebel, M. (2004). *A will of their own: Cross-cultural perspectives on working children.* London, UK: Zed Books.

19

Public Health Approach to Child Abuse and Neglect: From Grass Roots to Public Policy

Vandana Prasad

Introduction

While 'civil society' has traditionally played a critical role in articulating and struggling for child rights, ultimately, child rights can only be actualized at scale through programmes that are supported by State Policy and legal mechanisms. However, it is well understood that it takes an intensive process of civil society engagement and pressure to firstly achieve such State action, and then ensure it functions well. Such civil society engagement takes many forms and is necessary at every level; from grassroots work such as service delivery and community mobilisation, to research and documentation to policy advocacy and campaigning. Unfortunately, if these various elements remain unconnected, while they may assist individual children, they rarely achieve the public health objective of creating systems for the overall population of children in need.

Thus, a route map needs to be established from grassroots experience to public policy that is able to synthesise theoretical learning that is grounded in experience in order to achieve favourable changes in public policy. Practitioners in the arena of child survival, development and protection, need to understand the skills this complex process requires.

Unfortunately, the advocacy processes that have led to important changes in public policy related to children are poorly documented in formal published literature; they are to be found relegated to the minutes of various committees and consultations held in the echelons of power and policy making, or in campaign documents.

Nonetheless there is a growing interest in trying to understand the complex civil society processes; actors and factors that impact policy-making (Pelletier et al, 2012)

This chapter will discuss why it is important to link grassroots work to policy advocacy and vice versa, how this can be achieved, what difficulties /complexities are encountered in this process and how these can be circumvented and overcome.

Case Study I

Action for creches on construction sites: Mobile Creches (MC)

Children of construction workers living or accompanying their parents on construction sites are the victims of gross neglect and also abuse. Mobile Creches is an organization that has been providing comprehensive services such as care, nutrition, health and holistic education for children on construction sites for over 40 years. Simultanously, it has learnt the art and skills of policy advocacy with a degree of success using the framework demonstrated in the diagram below.

The battle for children's rights has not been an easy one for MC. It includes interventions at national and state levels on the policy, programme and legal fronts, alliances with partners and working with communities amid their daily battle for survival, to build pressure from the ground up. Mobile Creches works with other NGOs, academic institutions, women's organizations, trade unions and all concerned citizens to sharpen thought and broaden a common platform, for joint advocacy with the Government.

At Mobile Creches, action centers around the following issues: Universalized and Quality Integrated Child Development Services (ICDS); Nutritional support for children under three; Pre-School Education (PSE) and hot, cooked meals for all children in the age group of 3–6 years; Creches and Universalized Maternity Entitlements. Policy advocacy is targeted at the Planning Commission, Ministry of Women and Child Development (WCD), senior officials overseeing the ICDS and the Delhi Commission for Protection of Child Rights (DCPCR). Campaign partners include the India Alliance for Child Rights; Right to Food Campaign; National and Delhi chapter of Forum for Creche and Childcare Services (FORCES). Advocacy tools used are action research, signature campaigns, rallies, press meets and public hearings (Fig. 1).

As a result of these efforts, MC has made an impact on the following laws, programmes and schemes, either in terms of their intitiation or reform:

1974—Scheme for Creches for Ailing and working Mothers

2002—National Creche Fund

2005—Rajiv Gandhi National Creche Scheme for the children of working mothers

1996—Building and Other Construction Workers Welfare Cess Act

2010—Public Interest Litigation (PIL) Filed in Delhi High Court on non compliance of workers rights on CWG sites as per the Building and Construction workers Act

2011—Extension of provision of ICDS Scheme to children of migrant laborers/temporary Residents, Inputs in 12th Five Year Plan, National Plan of

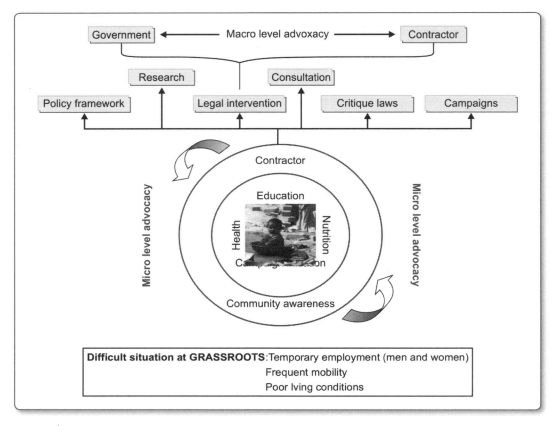

Figure 1 Mobile Creches approach at construction sites

Action for Children, Curriculum Framework for ECCE and IGMSY

2012—Inputs into the proposed National ECCE Policy

It has also been able to influence many contractors and builders to comply with the law and provide creches on site for children accompanying their mothers. However, there is still a long way to go before a situation is reached that all construction sites containing children provide creches by default and in compliance with the law.

Case Study II

Action for street children: Dil Se

Dil Se is a campaign coordinated by Centre for Equity Studies (CES) which was founded in August 2000. CES is an autonomous institution engaged in research and advocacy on issues of social and economic justice and equity. It seeks to enquire into the nature and causes of social injustice and inequity and to find ways to collectively move toward a more equitable, humane and peaceful world. To this end it seeks in particular to help influence and shape public policy and law in favour of people who are most disadvantaged. It attempts this through law and social policy design and advocacy; research into the interface of disadvantaged people with government, law, policy and programmes; and also grassroots engagement to help develop alternatives to existing policy, programmes and law. It provides methodologies and opportunities to people of diversity and across the development spectrum, including academics, civil servants activists and marginalised people.

The Centre also plays a direct grassroots implementation role in certain related areas such as homes for street children and health clinics for the homeless.

The Dil Se Campaign for street children was conceived as collaboration between government and diverse civil society interventions to secure the rights, dignity and future of the urban poor, specifically children who live and work on the street. This experience was taken into government policy-making through strategically placed senior individuals and has resulted in the formation of the Indradhanush Academy in 2010 with the purpose of becoming a resource centre for in-depth understanding of the approaches, functioning and nuances of work around the urban street child, with specific focus on the non-custodial residential care approach. This is being done by extensively studying, reviewing and analyzing the models of residential care that exist across the country as well as initiatives worldwide, and documenting, designing and recommending the best, scalable service practices.

Meanwhile, as a result of many years of advocacy, the Ministry of Human Resources Development has announced a National Scheme for Residential Care of Urban Street Children, which has placed an even more urgent responsibility on the Academy to ensure that its relevant materials reach as many state governments and NGOs as possible and are put into practice across the country.

Thus, the organization has been in the forefront for converting direct grassroots action and experience to policy in issues related to street children.

Case Study III

Lobbying and advocacy for elimination of child labor through realization of right to education; MV foundation[3]

MV Foundation (MVF) works to create child labor free zones/panchayats through an area-based approach and has determinedly campaigned and mobilized for changes in government systems and policies. Its strategy comprises of drawing up specific plans to withdraw children from all forms of work and making arrangements to prepare such children to be enrolled/re-integrated into schools. Meanwhile, the state government was running Non Formal Education centres (popularly known as night schools) for working children in the evenings legitimized the continuation of child labor.

In the year 1997, MVF conducted a campaign throughout the state against this system with government school teachers which resulted in converting them into day time schools. Further, the State government took a clear stand to abolish all forms of child labor and it defined "any child out of school" as a "child laborer".

The organization also contributed to many related policy issues such as simplifying admission

Table 1 Government Orders issued to encourage Children to attend Schools	
Go Number/Date	**Details**
No. 454/BS-3/97 dated 20-10-97	The NFE centres are expected to function for two hours in the moring hours in the school premises only.
No. 4990/DEEP/B4/2000 Dated 2-8-2000	Keeping in mind that the insistence on transfer medical and other certificates, detention on lack of attendance was pushing children out of schools, the rules were relaxed in all these cases.
6536/DEEP/B5/2000 Dated 24/2002	It was instructed that attendance monitoring of teachers and pupils will be done regularly and fortnightly.
G. O. Ms. No. 53 Dated 20/4/2001	Moreover, the minimum attendance prescribed shall be calculated from the date of admission of the child in the school.
No. 272/B4-1/2001 Dated 19/4/2001	The Headmaster of the primary school concerned will first prepare a list of all children in class V due to go to class VI and will communicate this list personally to the headmaster of the nearest UP school or High School.
272/B4-1/2001 Dated 20/4/2001	No. child will be detained in the same class merely on the grounds that he/she has not achieved the appropriate standard. The Headmaster of the concerned school will be held responsible for any wrong detention of a child in the same class.
G. O. Ms No. 300 Dated 21st May, 2002	keeping in mind that the community, demanded minimum levels of learning/ quality education in school where they have taken up the initiative to motivate all children to enter and remain in schools, a programme of learning guarantee was introduced.
G. O. Ms. No. 163 Dated 17-11-2001	Children who have studied in the RBCs and NRBCs and willing to write the 7th class and 10th class examinations are exempted from payment of attendance exemption and examination fee.

procedures, ensuring learning guarantee in schools, making the government provide residential bridge course camps and intervening in the national Right To Education Act, 2009 (Table 1).

Apart form its influence at State level, the organization was able to have one of its leaders in a important policy making body for child rights at national level by dint of its work in the area of child labor.

Case Study IV

Child protection; Haq centre for child rights[4]

Legal aid and counselling have been the road to monitoring the criminal and juvenile justice system and the functioning of implementing agencies dealing with children who come in contact with law. HAQ has therefore always been clear in the mandate to take a few cases as test cases, and while providing them the service of legal aid and/ or counselling, use the information generated for purposes of research, training and advocacy the child protection work of HAQ has concentrated on monitoring the judiciary and other statutory mechanisms set up to deal with children who come in contact with law. Although part of HAQ's overall work on children and governance, child protection also forms a distinct programme with a team dedicated to it.

Providing legal aid and counselling, visits to a children's home run by the Delhi Government, interaction and trainings with police, public prosecutors, probation officers, members of the Child Welfare Committee and Judicial Magistrates, development of training materials for Delhi Police and active participation in other activities of the monitoring committee on juvenile justice set up by the Delhi High Court, litigation and drawing attention of media to sensitive child protection issues, campaigning against child trafficking and hosting CACT (the national Campaign Against Child Trafficking) have been some of the major areas of work.

The experience and insights gained by HAQ through its child protection interventions and attempts at monitoring state performance led to a publication—Blind Alley: Juvenile Justice in India which drew upon all the cases that HAQ has undertaken as well as information that the team has collected in the course of its trainings with major stakeholders, and visits to other states. This was circulated amongst important stakeholders, including members of the judiciary and law enforcement agencies responsible for dealing with children. Simultaneously, research work was undertaken for the International Development Law Organization (IDLO) as part of their 'Girls Count' project carried out in Kenya, Ethiopia, Bangladesh and India in order to assess the situation of girls in these countries, the legal protection frameworks, exposure to risk, and access to justice.

As a result of these processes, HAQ has also been able to contribute to the monitoring role of the Committee on Juvenile Justice set up by the Delhi High Court as well as to the training and capacity building initiatives of Delhi Police, the Delhi Judicial Academy, NGOs and other actors. HAQ is an important partner with Delhi police on the issue of child rights and is part of the Special Juvenile Police Unit of the Central District, New Delhi, thereby providing assistance to the police in better of handling cases involving children. HAQ attends the meetings of the Supervision Committee set up by the Delhi High Court on the basis of an order of the High Court in W.P.(C) 9680/2009 dated 12 December 2009 as a member.

Why it is important to link grassroots work to policy advocacy and vice versa?

Scale

While many of us may have entered the domain of social action for children out of humanitarian or philanthropic concerns, it becomes clear after just a little experience that our efforts as individuals or even single organizations are too small to make an impact at scale. The 'State' remains the only organization with the means and powers to create systems that can provide large scale improvements to the situations of child abuse and neglect. Not only that, from the rights perspective, it is the responsibility and mandate of the State to do so.

Complexity

Our experience also tells us that many complex actors and factors have to be impacted simultaneously to create change in favour of child rights. Only the government has the powers to tackle all these

together. To take a small example, an intervention in favour of child nutrition necessitates action on food security systems, water and sanitation, health facilities, social security programmes etc. This multisectorality can truly only be achieved through the will of the government.

Costs

It is self-evident that these complex interventions at scale are expensive and beyond the means of individuals or NGOs. Thus, the State must take responsibility for costs.

However, it does not prove to be meaningful for the State to take unilateral action that is not informed by the experience of civil society for reasons discussed below.

Depth of understanding and quality

It is only grassroots work that allows the depth of understanding that is necessary to inform laws, polices and programmes related to child protection survival and development. This grassroots work provides different contextual frames within which programmes and schemes are expected to work, and is able to suggest both challenges and solutions. Thus, incorporating and learning from the experience of grassroots practitioners enhances the quality of theory and also provides nuances related to different contexts. More importantly, people know their problems best and have a right to articulate them. It is the States duty to give this articulation some primacy in policy making. In ideal circumstances, a complementarily can be achieved between the processes adopted by the State (such as appointing committees or experts to assist policy making) and the independent processes of non-governmental players and stake holders who have a more direct experience.

Credibility, testing grounds and model building

Grassroots work provides credibility to the recommendations being made toward policy since it is based on real-life experience. Thus, even organizations with the primary agenda of advocacy, research or academics in the area of child protection must engage with grassroots organizations to test their recommendations, though ideally the process should be 'bottoms-up' rather than 'top-down'. Civil society organizations play the vital role of providing 'laboratories' for the models they are advocating. For example, the organization 'Dil Se' had been running institutions for street children for a number of years and were able to demonstrate the infrastructural, human resource and financial implications for running such services. Through various processes of advocacy through demonstration, they were able to convince the government to launch a nation wide scheme based on their model. Similarly, the work of the organization SEARCH[1] (Society for Education, Action and Research in Community Health) lead by doctors Abhay and Rani Bang on Home Based Neonatal Care has led to learnings for the national health worker programme. The experience of HAQ; a resource group for child rights with legal action informed many positive amendments to the Indian Juvenile Justice Act.

However, these influences upon policy were far from serendipitous. They required a great deal of effort to engage with policy makers and policy making for a. These processes are further detailed below.

Collaboration

No single agency can provide all the skills and resources (including time and energy) to convert grassroots experience to impact on policy at National or International or even State level. The skill sets for this include legal expertise, issue based expertise on child development, child psychology/ psychiatry, health, gender, economics, social work, public policy, programme planning, research (qualitative and quantitative) and evaluation of complex interventions. Further, it is required that the grassroots agency engages with broader campaigns that are working either directly for child rights or determinants such as health, right to education, livelihoods, gender, etc.

This can be noted in the MC case study wherein the grassroots organization deputed a senior founder leader to participate in Working Group for Children Under Six constituted by Peoples' Health Movement-India (Jan Swasthya Abhiyan) and the Right to Food Campaign. This Working Group then concertedly worked toward legal, policy and programme reforms related to ECCD and had a significant impact as a result of being able work with members of the campaign who were placed in important policy making for a such as various

Committees of the Ministry of Women and Child Development, the Planning Commission as well as the National Advisory Council.

Meanwhile, the campaigns also allowed contact with large numbers of grassroots organizations to build consensus and understanding of issues related to issues such as malnutrition through mass events such as the various national conventions. Thus, a clear process of horizontal and vertical networking was adopted by the champions of child nutrition and development for achieving impact on related public policy.

Evidence building

The background to this approach lies in effective documentation and research to build the evidence that backs the policy advocacy. Generally, this requires further collaborations with resource organisations who can either build the documentation and research skills of grassroots organizations or assist them directly.

Difficulties and complexities

While many practitioners and organizations would accept the need to reach toward policy changes on the basis of their grassroots work, the actual process is fraught with difficulties and complexities.

Effort and time

Concerted follow-up of policy advocacy requires much effort and time and is a full time task requiring multiple skills and leadership. Most grassroots organizations are thin on human resource and the leadership might have to choose between guiding the grassroots work and keeping it on track with sufficiency of funds, quality, etc. or leading the policy advocacy. Their is thus a risk of dilution of leadership and reduction in quality to the grassroots work policy advocacy. The skill sets for both are also different since the stakeholders are of different nature.

Geographical and temporal separations

Both sets of work occupy different geographical spaces: much of the policy work requires presence at national or state level while the grassroots work is located closer to the ground. This makes communication between the two difficult. Temporal phase lags may exist between the urgent requirements of policy work; such as the need to urgently respond to a government draft, and the ability of a grassroots organization to receive and respond to such a demand.

Contradictions and ideological dilemmas

The short-term objectives of grassroots work are often at variance with policy work, leading to dilemmas and conflicts. Grassroots work has to respond to the immediate needs of the community while policy must take into account larger issues and balance the needs of more than one stakeholder. For example, a grassroots organization may facilitate the government pulse-polio programme while the campaign may be challenging the immunization policy of the pulse programme. A grassroots organization may be grateful for donations of baby food tins for severely malnourished and very poor children, while the campaign or broader network may be in opposition to such interventions and may be demanding more long-term measures of food security,

The challenge of maintaining a focus on prevention while tackling immediate crises programatically is also a part and parcel of such dilemmas.

How these can be circumvented and overcoming difficulties

These case studies demonstrate the critical steps and strategies that maximize the possibilities of achieving impact on policy that is derived from grassroots action.

An important common factor, considering the fact that this is arduous work requiring much time, effort and patience is to consciously select the focus issue, prioritise and commit to action upon it. While identifying this niche is very important, it is also important to recognize its inter linkages with other issues to be able to build solidarity. This can only be done by engaging with larger networks and campaigns around social determinants that are allied with our chosen focus issue. A long-term working relationship with other organizations can only be built upon common principles and values, and it is important to make an assessment of common non-negotiables through processes such

as defining charters, vision-mission statements or positions.

Networking with like-minded organizations and persons to achieve policy impact requires vertical and horizontal networking; networking with other persons working on the same issue and at the same level (sub district/district/state/national) or across issues strategies and levels. For example, a grassroots organization working in villages on the issue of child labor is likely to benefit from alliances with campaigns on the right to education, groups of human rights lawyers, child rights agencies etc. as part of vertical networking, and groups of industrialists, district administration, other rights-based organizations working in the same area etc as part of horizontal networking. Geographical and financial constraints are mitigated in part by the use of E groups and internet communications. However, it is critical to also use other forms of communication such as snail mail and regular meetings and this is specially important to keep grassroots organisations in the communication loop. Critical meetings and decisions must be given due notice time even if there are policy imperatives that are external to the group.

This approach needs dedicated personnel and since the skill sets are diverse and the requisite core team should be built that can perform various communication and advocacy functions. This team needs to consistently facilitate a two-way communication loop between the 'grassroots' and the policy—advocacy work for the reasons outlined in the previous sections. Experience from child protection shows us that the skills required relate to legal expertise, expertise on child development, child psychology/psychiatry, health, gender, economics, social work, public policy, programme planning, research (qualitative and quantitative) and evaluation of complex interventions.

Conclusion

This chapter highlights the importance and processes of linking grassroots experience to policy advocacy with the intention of making an impact, and also discusses the challenges of doing so. While these issues have been illustrated through case studies of micro-processes, studies at country level echo the issues that have been presented here.

A constant dialogue is also required with the unconverted with genuine respect for differences of opinion and efforts to resolve them. Thus, a constant process of sharing, learning, consensus building and documentation is critical to be able to pursue a course of policy advocacy.

Experience from studies in Bangladesh, Bolivia, Guatemala, Peru and Vietnam which sought to identify the challenges in the policy process and ways to overcome them, with respect to commitment, agenda setting, policy formulation and implementation of nutritional interventions showed the following findings:

".... (a) high-level political attention to nutrition can be generated in a number of ways, but the generation of political commitment and system commitment requires sustained efforts from policy entrepreneurs and champions; (b) mid-level actors from ministries and external partners had great difficulty translating political windows of opportunity for nutrition into concrete operational plans, due to capacity constraints, differing professional views of under nutrition and disagreements over interventions, ownership, roles and responsibilities; and (c) the pace and quality of implementation was severely constrained in most cases by weaknesses in human and organizational capacities from national to frontline levels".

The study used a 12-point framework for analysing the factors that determined success in policy-making and these include finding emphasis for the issue in high level political speeches, the existence of public campaigns, promotion with all levels and concerned departments of government, establishment of specific goals and targets, presence of laws, policies, programmes and coordinating structures for the issue, the existence of national staff for the agenda, concrete operational plans by government, sufficiency of financial investments by government and donor agencies and regular reviews by politicians and civil servants.

It is a challenge for committed grassroots organizations to consider these findings as opportunities and meet the requirements to convert micro gains at grassroots levels to gains in macro policy that can impact children's status at scale. The process takes consistent steady hard work and faith, optimism and doggedness in our pursuit of a better world for children.

Acknowledgement

This article is based on the master class of the same title that was held on 6th October, 2011 during the Asia pacific Conference on Child Abuse and Neglect in New Delhi, India. The author is grateful to Mr. Harsh Mander (Dil Se), Ms. Enakshi Ganguly (HAQ Centre for Child Rights). Ms Amrita Jain (Mobile Creches). Mr. R. Venkat Reddy (MV Foundation) and Dr. Shanti Raman (Community Paediatrician) for their contributions to the master class.

References

1. Pelletier, A Gervais L.Honey, P Menon, Tien Ngo, J Stoltzfus, A.M. Ahmed, T. Ahmed (2012) Nutrition agenda setting, policy formulation and implementation: lessons from the Mainstrearning Nutrition Initiative.

2. Jain A.2011 Mobile Centre.org, Personal Communication.

3. http://www.myfindia.in/.

4. http://www.haqcrc.org/

5. http://www.searchgadchiroli.org/

20

Monitoring and Evaluating Community-Based Interventions for Children and Families in the Asia-Pacific Region

Emma Williams, Adam M Tomison

Introduction

In the first half of the 20th century the patronage of eminent practitioners and academics was commonly seen as sufficient to ensure the development and funding of interventions to improve health and well being and/or to reduce social ills (Crouch 1998). The 1960s heralded not only the modern 're-discovery' of child abuse via Kempe and colleagues' work on the 'battered child' syndrome (Kempe et al. 1962), but also the first empirical tests of the effectiveness of health and welfare programs (Tomison 2000). These studies heralded the dawn of the program evaluation era, and with it, the expectation that public sector programs should be able to objectively and scientifically demonstrate program success and client satisfaction (Rist 1997).

Program evaluation provides a systematic method for the collection, analysis and use of information that enables:

- A determination of what is and is not working in a program or intervention, enabling modifications to enhance a program's effectiveness;
- Evidence for funding bodies and stakeholders of what a program does, its level of effectiveness and the benefits for participants; and/or
- New knowledge about the most beneficial approaches that can be used when adopting programs of a similar type, and when dealing with similar participants (Tomison, 2000).

However, applying program evaluation techniques to community-based interventions is not simple, particularly when the community is of a different cultural and linguistic background to the researcher/evaluator. Drawing on the authors' experience in undertaking and supporting community-based research in Australia with populations such as migrant, rural and Indigenous (Australian Aboriginal or Torres Strait Islander) peoples, some examples are provided of culturally and contextually-informed approaches for monitoring and evaluating community-based interventions. Special emphasis is placed on describing evaluation methods that have been designed to involve various sections of the community, including children and young people, so that their voices are heard, and their contribution to monitoring and evaluation can lead to meaningful change.

While Asia-Pacific communities have their own heterogeneous cultural and community contexts, it is contended that the principles and approaches described here can be considered and potentially applied when developing evaluations of community-based interventions in the wider Asia-Pacific region.

In the Australian context, four factors are repeatedly referred to as foundations for effectively engaging and working with Indigenous communities (e.g. Tomison 2003; Tomison 2004). It is contended that these can apply to working with a range of culturally and linguistically diverse communities and also underpin effective community-based evaluations. The factors are:

1. Developing culturally secure (culturally appropriate) practice
2. Ensuring community support or ownership for interventions and evaluations
3. Active participation and engagement of community members

4. Infrastructure—Providing engaged community participants with adequate training and support to enable them to participate actively in evaluation research and the use of its findings.

The authors' intention is not to provide a series of absolute rules and regulations for undertaking community-based evaluation, but to identify and consider issues that might be at play in evaluating community programs and to describe some ways that these may be addressed.

Context

This chapter is not focused on evaluation theory, although there are obvious links to aspects of empowerment evaluation approaches (Fetterman 1994, Fetterman 2001, Fetterman and Wandersman 2004) and of utilisation-focused evaluation (Patton 2008). Instead, by presenting examples where different methods have been implemented in specific cultural contexts, the intention is to demonstrate how even sound, theory-informed approaches must be customised to the contexts in which they operate.

For instance, empowerment evaluations are based on ten principles:

1. Improvement
2. Community ownership
3. Inclusion
4. Democratic participation
5. Social justice
6. Community knowledge
7. Evidence-based strategies
8. Capacity-building
9. Organizational learning, and
10. Accountability Wandersman et al. 2004).

These are not culturally neutral concepts; the cultural context in which programs operate needs to be understood to apply such evaluation approaches successfully. Taking the fourth principle of 'democratic participation' as an example, in some Australian Aboriginal communities select members such as 'elders', 'law people' and/or 'traditional owners' may be particularly entitled to present community views, while other community members may not feel that they have equal authority to speak on these topics to evaluators. Treating every community member as 'equal' and disregarding the special role of elders may be perceived as culturally disrespectful and lead to a refusal by the community to participate in programs or evaluation research.

Even in the wider or 'mainstream' Australian culture, some groups may struggle to have their voices heard. For example, the members of some cultural minorities may not speak or write fluent English, whereas the women in some religious and cultural groups may not readily participate in mainstream public life. As the interventions discussed here were chosen for their potential impact on children, it is worth noting that children's own views are often not taken sufficiently into account, typically for logistical as well as cultural reasons. The examples below demonstrate approaches used to include the views of such groups, often marginalized in standard evaluation procedures.

Key factors

Perhaps the most critical contextual factor is the nature of the evaluation, its scope and the purpose for which it was initiated. Chelimsky (1997) distinguishes between evaluations intended for development, for accountability and for knowledge. Each entails different priorities, but in practice it is common for evaluations to be multi-purpose.

Questions that may be useful in determining the nature of a proposed evaluation include:

- What are the objectives and intentions that sit behind the evaluation?
- Is the evaluation top-down (i.e. framed by external stakeholders, such as governments, health services or researchers) or bottom-up (driven by the community's identification and focus on particular issues)?
- What are the parameters or restrictions on what the evaluator can achieve (e.g. a lack of available data; community access is limited and can only be achieved by researchers when in company with senior community members)?
- What resources, in terms of time and money, are available to conduct the evaluation?
- Who are the main intended audiences (e.g. policy makers, program staff, other professional or community participants)?
- Does the evaluator control how the results will be used and disseminated?
- How does the funder of the evaluation (if there is one) intend to use the evaluation results? For example:
  - to improve knowledge;
  - to understand the process of development;
  - to prove success or impact;

- as part of government financial accountability requirements;
- to justify government spending; and/or
- as support for a predetermined course of action (i.e. to cease, increase, or maintain a program or policy).

Each of these questions has important implications for evaluation design and particularly for community participation in the evaluation. Some contextual factors may pose a danger for community participation. It is quite common for an evaluation to be developed without in the provision of sufficient time and funding that would enable appropriate participation by the community.

'Bottom-up' evaluations, framed around the community's expectations and the active participation of community members, will clearly facilitate active community participation. In contrast, ' top-down' approaches are driven by external stakeholders who wish to determine the effectiveness of a particular program and typically the parameters of the research are more firmly defined before the community is consulted. These externally derived parameters may support or constrict the ability of community members to be involved or to shape the nature of the research.

Occurring less frequently but of concern, the funder of an evaluation may intend that the evaluation will provide support for a pre-determined course of action such as terminating a program, or the continuation of a program. In such cases, pressure may be placed on the evaluator to modify their results to align with the funder's pre-determined decision, particularly if the evidence collected for the evaluation points to a different outcome (Markiewicz, 2008). Community participation in such an evaluation would most likely prove to be a disempowering experience, making the development of trust with community members and their willingness to participate in future evaluations more difficult. This issue is not restricted to, but is particularly evident when looking at the history of researching and evaluating with Australian Aboriginal communities (and some other indigenous communities around the world), where a history of unethical research, or research that has been perceived as being used to harm Aboriginal people has meant that many communities are now wary of participating in research. As a result developing the trust and engagement of such communities can be slow

and difficult to achieve (e.g. Stanley, Tomison and Pocock, 2003).

The community's own expectations of participation in research or an evaluation will also impact on the evaluation process. Does the community, or elements of the community have preconceived views of what evaluation is, and of the findings that will result from an evaluation? Is there a community expectation that the evaluation will ensure the continuation of a program, an obligation the evaluator will not usually be able to meet? Further, does the development of a relationship (engagement) with an evaluator cause the community to develop other expectations that the evaluator is expected to meet, even if these are not possible?

For example, communities may expect that an evaluator granted access to the community will return to the community to explain the findings of their research. (This is also often a requirement of ethical approval for such research and while it should be a part of the research process it is not always completed). Of greater difficulty in meeting expectations, some groups may expect that the evaluator will continue to maintain contact and work with the community even after the evaluation research is complete. The limitations of what can be undertaken as part of the research process must therefore be clearly explained, as part of the informed consent of the community and to avoid the development of mistrust and disappointment. As Scougall notes:

The expectations placed on an evaluator working in an Indigenous context are often great. The ideal is someone in close relationship with the community, employing culturally sensitive methods, fostering broad community involvement, transferring evaluation skills and contributing to a process of empowerment and positive social change. The hard reality is that evaluators are most often outsiders with limited resources and precious little time to spend in the field (2006: 49).

The evaluation process

Each evaluation should be tailored to fulfil the specific purpose for which it is required and to meet the needs of the various stakeholders involved. Often there are multiple reasons to evaluate and multiple stakeholders whose needs must be considered. Different stakeholders will often have disparate interests and may well require different evaluation 'products' and styles of communication (Williams 2010; Williams et al. 2010b).

In order to establish the key questions, measures and resources for programs and evaluations, many evaluators use a variant of a 'program logic' or 'theory of change' framework. (See Clark and Anderson 2004 for a brief discussion on these approaches, or Funnell and Rogers 2011 for more detailed discussion). These frameworks are influenced by those who are involved in their development; frameworks developed in isolation by the evaluator and the staff of an intervention or program may lack the depth, rigour and ecological validity that can be achieved if a wider group of stakeholders, including community participants, are involved in the framework development process. This is particularly important where there are cultural or language differences between the evaluator/researcher, community members and other stakeholders. Ensuring there is a shared understanding of key concepts and intentions between the evaluator(s) and the range of stakeholders for the evaluation is critical to the evaluation's success.

The research question(s) and the level of explanation required determine the methodologies and research tools used and the degree of experimental rigour that is desired and/or possible (Tomison, 2000). Not infrequently, interventions to prevent child abuse and neglect operate in areas where there may be limited statistical data or records, and where what is available may not capture the reality of life or the issue under consideration. Nevertheless, funding bodies and other external stakeholders often require quantitative measures, 'hard data', to ensure the methodological rigour of any findings, and to enable comparisons over time and between programs and/or communities. The challenge when undertaking work in applied community settings, particularly when working with local communities of different cultural and language backgrounds, is creating evaluation evidence that is meaningful to funding bodies and other stakeholders in contexts where traditional research methods such as surveys, individual interviews, focus groups and pre/post tests may not be suitable. The use of multiple methods and data sources to 'build a picture' over time typically improves the ability of the evaluation to demonstrate program success (Tomison 2004). Community members' views are more likely to be a component of a multi-method approach, while

they may be discounted or shut out of a purely quantitative evaluation approach.

The nature of the intervention is also an important contextual element; initiatives that are locally-initiated and managed (i.e. where the community feels a sense of ownership) often make it easier to build an evaluation partnership with the community than may be the case with 'imported' programs that have been brought into the community by government services, non-government agencies or other external stakeholders and enacted without strong community partnership or engagement. Such programs are often introduced by external decision makers as a result of a desire to replicate or 'scale up' successful programs developed elsewhere. (See Pawson and Tilley 2004 for issues that need to be taken into account in evaluations in such cases.)

There are both benefits and challenges in evaluating in partnership with communities; identifying relevant stakeholders and what the role of each should be in the evaluation is one of the first challenges. Fetterman (2004) notes the importance of including funders, even in 'empowering' evaluations. However, the role of different community members may be more complex to establish. The impact that cultural differences can make was noted above, with researchers needing to understand and accept the special role of elders or traditional landowners in many Australian Aboriginal communities. Researchers may also need to develop and modify their research methods to take into account the special needs of groups such as: children, cultural minorities speaking a different language from the dominant culture and where literacy may be an issue, or those who may have concerns about engaging with 'public' processes, such as women from some religious and cultural groups.

Further, in some cultures the western research practice of individual interviewing or surveying does not fit with cultural practices where most information sharing is done via group interactions. Much Australian Aboriginal knowledge is based on personal accounts and stories, passed on through repeated sharing and confirmation by many people. Indigenous perspectives can therefore be seen as similar to some of the qualitative methodologies (e.g. focus groups) increasingly being used by non-Indigenous researchers (Stanley et al. 2003).

Involving community members in evaluation

Engaging with the 'right' stakeholders, and in the 'right order' according to the community's protocols or norms, is vital for culturally respectful evaluation practice. In communities of diverse languages, interests and backgrounds, some may have little interest in westernised research processes and may even experience discomfort with standard research and evaluation techniques such as interviews, surveys, written pre and post-tests (e.g. Stanley et al. 2003). The involvement of community members in monitoring and evaluation therefore often requires traditional research methods to be tailored or modified to ensure a meaningful process for the participants, while still enabling the collection evidence of program or intervention outcomes relevant for a wider stakeholder audience. This is particularly the case where communities are suspicious of any 'research' because of previous negative experiences and the sometimes unwelcome outcomes that have resulted from previous evaluations (Stanley et al. 2003).

The following examples of evaluation practice demonstrate various ways that the four foundational factors for engaging and working with Indigenous communities can be successfully applied across various communities, ensuring the participation of community members of varying ages and genders, while respecting cultural norms. Further, they demonstrate approaches for positive community engagement and participation that have enabled communities to lead and evaluate their own programs with the support of external researchers 'walking alongside' them, and that have enabled them to influence decisions taken by governments or agencies from outside the community.

Case Study 1

The fire tool

The 'Fire tool' evaluation method (Williams and Cummings, 2009) was developed for use in remote Australian Aboriginal communities where westernised evaluation techniques such as surveys and individual interviews are inappropriate, but where governments and other funding bodies still require quantitative measures of community issues

that can compare change between communities and over time. Developed and piloted over three years with remote Aboriginal community men and women from different language and cultural groups, the Fire tool provides communities with an opportunity to identify issues in their community, and to assess if these issues were worsening or improving over time and for specific sections or elements of the community.

However, the Fire tool is also able to translate assessments of community strengths and problems that are meaningful for the community into quantitative data that is also acceptable and meaningful for Government funders and mainstream agencies working in the communities. In essence, the 'Fire tool' is a culturally-grounded version of a Likert scale, with ratings elicited from community groups rather than individuals. Although ideally suited for accountability evaluations and external monitoring of community progress by agencies and government stakeholders, it inevitably also produces rich qualitative data (community assessments and explanations) that provide context for the community's view of local problems or issues.

The process

Before employing the tool, the evaluators needed to ensure that cultural and community protocols were met. After agreement with critical stakeholders, the evaluators (one a senior Aboriginal woman elder known to members of the community, the other an outsider) entered the community and commenced the evaluation process. The Fire tool process was flexible enough that the tool could be used separately for discussions with men and with woman and/or for people of different ages. Community members were able to identify what was most appropriate practice locally for collecting the community's views; group work with different segments of the community began after these details were negotiated.

The Fire tool is based on the centrality of fire in Aboriginal community life. Fire as a symbol was found to be meaningful to traditional and semi-traditional Aboriginal communities throughout the Northern Territory of Australia. Even in the more tropical areas of the Northern Territory, a fire was seen as a place togather. Community members interpreted 'closeness' to the fire positively as a metaphor for physical and psychological closeness to the community group, while 'distance' from the fire was readily seen as a symbol of problems and/or isolation from the community. Thus, people abandoning traditional cultural practices, neglecting or abusing their children, and causing problems in the community due to gambling or fighting were perceived to be 'further from the fire' than those participating in traditional ceremonies and other cultural elements of tribal life, and caring responsibly for children and families ('close to the fire'). Similarly, the presence and misuse of alcohol in a community could be seen as a force pushing people away from the central fire (and community), while engagement with tribal ceremonies, or program interventions directly targeted to prevent child abuse and neglect, could be seen as factors helping people 'back to the fire'.

The Fire tool is made of readily available materials so that it is cheap, light, and capable of use outdoors under various conditions; it is essentially a large piece of fabric (of an Indigenous art design) which represents the community and which has a cloth 'fire' stitched into the centre. A number of figurines representing local Australian animals are provided to the community participants. These can then be selected by community members or groups to represent the factors and/or programs being evaluated, or used to represent specific sectors of the community.

Use of the tool begins by asking community members to select the physical symbols (animal figurines) for the different groups within the community (e.g. children, young men, women). The choice of the symbols acts as an introduction to the tool but also elicits participants' views as they discuss together why each symbol is emblematic of a particular group, issue or program. After a brief explanation of the tool, discussion moves to identifying the community's strengths; once this is done the facilitators quantify the impact of each strength. This is achieved by the facilitator (evaluator) moving each animal figure closer or further away from the symbolic fire until participants reach consensus on the placement of the symbol.

For example, the community may identify that having ready access to productive employment for young people is an important strength they have, placing the chosen animal symbol for 'youth employment' quite close to the fire on the fabric world. There may not be initial agreement; different participants' reasons for placing the symbol closer or further from the fire are captured as they provide valuable insights. For example, older women may feel youth employment is a very important community strength, while young men may not see it that way. These ratings can be recorded using the Fire tool and monitored over time.

Finally, once agreement has been reached on the placement of the animal symbols, a tape measure is used to quantify the distance of the symbol from the fire on a scale (in centimetres). In this way the facilitator can measure how each community strength changes over time—increasing its positive impact or having a reduced impact over time as interventions are introduced, or other elements of the community environment change. The distance from the fire is then translated into a score from zero (close to the fire) to 100 (furthest away from the fire). These data can be recorded and used in a quantitative sense to demonstrate the role of particular strengths on a community—as judged by the community (consensus view) or as the views of various segments of the community – over time.

Once the community has identified and rated the effect of the community's strengths, the exercise is repeated, this time with a focus on identifying the risks or negative forces present in the community that are 'pushing people away from the fire' (e.g. women leaving their children alone to visit a nearby city, alcohol abuse, violence, or children not learning their ceremonial responsibilities). The third stage of the process is framed to assess the impact of specific interventions intended to reduce local rates of child abuse and neglect or other social harms, in order to quantify the degree to which each intervention is perceived to be successful or 'bringing people back towards the fire'.

When the Fire tool was used to assess community safety (and the prevention of child abuse and neglect), community members were also invited to talk about their community and the improvements they most wanted to see to 'keep children safe and families strong'. This resulted in rich qualitative data that helped to explain the community's ratings, and often indicated that the programs offered to communities did not necessarily target the issues that community members saw as the most important.

As many of the communities are multilingual (with English a third or fourth language, and

Monitoring and evaluating community-based interventions for children and families in the Asia-Pacific region *Chapter 20*

165

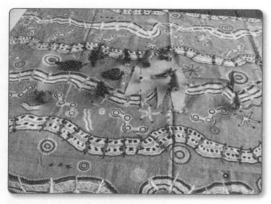

Figure 1: The 'Fire Tool' – capturing Aboriginal community views and measuring change.

often not spoken fluently), a key process for using the Fire tool was to spend a considerable amount of time ensuring that discussions were translated into the relevant local Indigenous languages and that everyone developed and shared a common concept or understanding of the terms under discussion before the next steps in the evaluation were taken. For example, terms such as 'marital rape' or a concept such as the 'sexual abuse of children' can be conceived and expressed differently by individuals; the groups participating did not necessarily understand or accept the Anglo-Australian meanings used by the evaluators. It was therefore vital to take the time to explore these issues in all of the languages used locally to resolve differences in understanding before any assessment was undertaken using the Fire tool. It is to be hoped that ongoing training and support for local researchers and evaluators will address these issues more effectively over time; although the material aspects of the tool are cheap and easy to replicate, the cultural and conceptual infrastructure require substantial time and resources to achieve.

Case Study 2

'Painting the elephant'—bridging cultural differences in an evaluation

The Remote Aboriginal Family and Community Worker (RAFCW) Program (Williams et al. 2010a), was a Northern Territory government program that employed local people from remote Aboriginal communities to act effectively as bridges or liaison points between their community and the Northern Territory statutory child protection services. To protect their safety, the workers were not to be involved in any removal of children from their families by child protection services, but they did provide support to at risk or vulnerable families, and assisted child protection workers with local and cultural information as well as building local community members' knowledge of child development and child protection issues.

The program was evaluated in 2009–2010 using a multiple methods evaluation that was comprised of a review of program documentation, interviews with workers and a range of stakeholders, community observations, and site visits to four remote communities, each with a different Aboriginal cultural group and language (Yolngu, Warlpiri, Anmatjere, and Tiwi). The Fire tool was used to elicit community views on the program's progress and impact. The resulting evaluation report was quite detailed and divided into multiple products, some designed for policy-makers, some for the remote community participants, some for RAFCW program staff, etc.

Over a 12 month period, the evaluators followed up with the various stakeholders to identify which evaluation elements had led to practice improvements and policy outcomes, and which elements of the evaluation proved of most value for each group of stakeholders (Williams et al. 2010b). The Program Manager at the time of the evaluation noted that the 'painting the elephant' exercise was the most important component for her, outweighing every other aspect of the evaluation. The Program Manager noted that if the non-Aboriginal stakeholders carefully read and understood the results of this exercise, they would understand exactly how the program had to operate differently in its remote Indigenous ommunity context, even if they did not engage with any other aspect of the evaluation.

The exercise was conducted as part of a 'theory of change' workshop conducted several months into the evaluation, with the participation of remote RAFCW staff, as well as their Aboriginal supervisors and the Program Manager. The 'painting the elephant' name for the exercise came from two sources. One was the Indian fable of the blind men and the elephant, where each man perceived the elephant differently based on the part of the elephant they touched—one who grasped the leg thought it was like a pillar, one who grasped the tail thought it was like a rope, etc. The other source was the phrase 'the elephant in the room', denoting a critically important issue that is not talked about.

The exercise was designed to share participants' perceptions of the heretofore unspoken cultural context of their work, making it visible to the non-Aboriginal evaluation stakeholders, who were often unaware of what was very obvious to the Aboriginal evaluation participants—so much so that it hardly seemed worth elucidating to the participants. Although simple, the exercise proved powerful in ensuring that culturally embedded maxims (such as what sorts of activities did or did not put workers at risk, and what was required to care for children at risk in remote community contexts) shaped the evaluation and later helped to reshape aspects of the program.

1.5 Case Study 3

The community as researchers— The stronger families learning exchange action research model

The following case study describes a model of support for community members—professionals and laypeople—who had devised and were running community-based programs. In this case the community owned their interventions but were provided with external research and evaluation experience to assist them to assess their programs and to enhance their overall success. it was very much a 'walking alongside' model of support.

The Stronger Families Learning Exchange (SFLEX) was set up within the Australian Institute of Family Studies. Part of its purpose was to contribute to the formation of an evidence base from which to inform policy, practice and research in strengthening families and communities. This was achieved through the development of a 10-person Training and Support Team that supported community-based, community-run projects funded under the national Stronger Families and Communities Strategy. From 2000-2004 the SFLEX research team provided training and ongoing support to teams of local community members and professionals to assist them in running and evaluating various family support and antiviolence projects they had developed in 46 different communities across Australia that had been identified by the Australian Government as

being of 'high need' (Tomison, 2003). Half of these projects involved Indigenous communities, while a number of others were based around recent migrant populations.

A key element of effectively supporting the projects was therefore to ensure that a culturally respectful process was developed that was flexible enough to be used with a range of diverse community groups—some operating in urban environments, with others operating in remote areas of the country. Each community was assisted with training to develop and carry out evaluations of their projects using participatory action research methods. SFLEX also gathered data across projects and identified key learning's for the wider field, focusing on both process and outcomes. (For free resources and publications, see http://www.aifs. gov.au/sf/)

Given the diversity of programs and desired outcomes, Participatory Action Research (PAR) was chosen as the foundation methodology for the SFLEX Team (Wadsworth, 2011). PAR is cyclical in nature, with iterative cycles of Planning, Acting, Observing and Reflecting. Such an action research approach allowed projects to develop their own evaluation frameworks and ways of working, enabling project teams to take the time to write down their observations and reflect on them—in essence it is a continuous improvement methodology.

PAR is based on the development of a partnership between the evaluator, funding body and participants, with participants taking an active role in developing and informing the evaluation, i.e. the project teams 'owned' their projects and the evaluation. PAR is expressly designed to be participatory and collaborative, with evaluators in the role of 'walking alongside' and 'doing with' rather than 'doing to' a project. While PAR is most often used with qualitative research, it fits with a multiple methods approach and is flexible enough to underpin many evaluation models and approaches, and to operate in a range of cultural contexts, enabling culturally secure evaluation practice (Wadsworth, 2011). However, there may be a trade-off in terms of methodological rigour and PAR may not meet the expectations of funders anticipating quantitative data collected under a classic pre or post-test experimental method based on a consistent application of program guidelines.

PAR also requires a significant commitment of time and resources. The approach would not have succeeded without the involvement of the ten SFLEX researchers, who trained and supporting project teams or communities to participate and undertake their own evaluations in their communities. As part of the skills development of the local community teams, SFLEX also brought representatives from all of the projects together to share learning's and to develop a network of support for the communities. The 'skilling up' and capacity-building for local people was aided by the iterative nature of PAR, which allowed for relationship-building to occur over time, as well as by the principles of PAR, which seek to promote partnerships, while empowering people who may be shut out of other evaluation approaches to have a real voice.

Overall, PAR can be a very useful approach for such human service evaluations, particularly where the focus is on program and service improvement rather than accountability (Crane and O'Regan 2010; see the range of SFLEX publications). While it was a successful approach for the SFLEX-supported projects, individual project funding ceased after three years, and the SFLEX team also had to cease operations. As a result many of the programs and program teams subsequently ceased to operate and the skills that had been developed in the communities dissipated over time. This was despite many of the programs having made demonstrable positive change in their communities through their programs, as evidenced through the evaluation process. The SFLEX experience demonstrated clearly the importance of longer-term support for community-based programs, and the professionals and community people who are asked to run them, if the benefits accrued through engaging communities in action are to be maintained.

1.6 Case Study 4

Children influencing community decisions through evaluation

There are many techniques that build community members' *participation* in evaluations, but evaluation techniques that enable community members to have an *impact on decision-making* are less frequently discussed.

The City of Wyndham is a local government area near the city of Melbourne in the Australian state of Victoria that was seeking to build more community-engaged decision-making processes and a more 'child and family friendly' community. The use of local land was one of the areas where this 'child and family friendly' approach was to be reflected.

The Wyndham local government area had many areas of undeveloped land. It was proposed to sell some pieces of land in order to raise money to develop the remaining pieces of vacant land and to make them more suitable for children and families to use. Children were likely to be most affected by these changes as they typically used the existing undeveloped land for play. It was therefore decided that children aged 7 – 12 years should be asked to assess each piece of vacant land and its relative worth to them, before the decision to sell or retain the land was made. Importantly, the adults in charge of the sale process agreed to take the children's views into account in deciding which pieces of land should be sold off and which should be retained and improved.

Children's views were gathered through the use of large laminated photos showing the patches of land, as they might look from a child's point of view. As the photos had been laminated (and were therefore difficult to damage), the children were able to handle the photos as much as they pleased and to pass them to each other as they met in one of the several groups that participated in the assessment. Children identified the particular areas of land much better than adults were able to, confirming the validity of involving them in the decision-making process. Where adults might see just a few trees and some dirt that they passed by occasionally, the children often recognized areas they used for a particular type of play or activity.

Children's opinions differed by age and gender, with girls typically preferring spaces they could walk and talk in, or sit safely together, relatively close to their homes. In contrast, boys typically wanted areas for active play, and were willing to travel further from home. Younger children's views also differed in some cases from older children's views. However, enough consensus emerged that some areas could be identified as of special value to children, with others were identified as being of relatively little worth.

When the children's views were communicated to the adults in charge of the process, the adult group had already decided which parcels of land should be sold and which should be retained—and their decision did not match the children's assessment of the lands' worth. However, when the evaluator presented the children's views, the group reversed their original decisions and made their final decisions based on the children's input as to which land should be preserved and not sold or developed.

In this case, those with the decision-making power honoured their commitment to be guided by the views of those with less power (children), as expressed though the finding of the evaluation. It is vital that such commitments are made and honoured, or even the most participatory evaluation may not result in better outcomes for the evaluation participants, and communities may no longer trust or agree to participate in further research and evaluation processes. This has been the experience of many Indigenous Australian communities, where research has not been seen as benefiting the communities who have participated in it.

1.7 Case Study 5

The wyndham community report card

The final case perhaps represents the ultimate in community members' participation in evaluation. Using a 'community report card' method, community members can choose what should be evaluated in their community and how it should be measured; they are in control of the entire process. For an interesting although not entirely accurate discussion of such 'report cards' from an international perspective, see materials and articles developed by the World Bank (2005).

In the case of the Wyndham Community Report Card (the most recent version of which is available at http://www.wyndham.vic.gov.au/aboutwyndham/planspolicieslocallaws/qcp/2008) the report card was based on a long-term strategic vision for the local government area (Wyndham City Council 1997, 2002, 2007) developed with the input of over 2,000 community members, who identified the community priorities they wanted addressed by public officials and others, and which also sets out the measures the community wanted to use each year to determine if their vision was on track (see Green at al 2000 for further discussion of community visioning). In each case, community perceptions formed

one part of the measures chosen, but there were other measures such as the proportion of public commitments to the community that were met on time, and special measures identified by community members, such as how children were faring at school or whether they were able to find jobs when they left school.

A variety of techniques in addition to more traditional survey exercises and focus groups were used to ensure that marginalized groups within the community had equal opportunities to identify their vision for the future of the community and how they wanted it to be evaluated (Williams 2001, 2003). For example, peer interviewing (adequate training and support was provided) was used to reach women in religious and cultural groups who were less comfortable participating in public spaces and public research processes. A variant of a 'snowballing' technique was used to reach difficult-to-reach teenagers, and many other engagement techniques were used for newly arrived community members speaking languages other than English.

Two techniques are worth discussing in greater detail as they were designed not just to increase marginalized community members' participation in evaluation but also to increase the impact of their involvement. The first was a 'rippling' technique, which required that the views of the most marginalized groups be collected first, and then presented to the next most marginalised group to form part of their basis for discussion.

For example, when looking at child and family issues in the community, it was found that most decisions were being taken by a relatively small group of adults in influential, policy-making positions. There was also a small group of engaged parents who were consulted frequently, and who could be accessed relatively easily at public meetings. However, there was a larger group of parents who were less engaged, due to issues of language, education or simply due to them being so busy with work and family that they had little opportunity for public participation.

Importantly, it was also identified that children's views were rarely sought. Thus, child and family issues were overwhelmingly being determined through the input of 'experts' and a small number of parents. As the local government wanted to develop 'textured' policy (i.e. policy that takes gender, age, culture, etc. into account), the engagement of other groups was critical.

Monitoring and evaluating community-based interventions for children and families in the Asia-Pacific region *Chapter 20*

169

Given the hierarchy of historical influence (see above), the engagement process for the evaluation of the community visioning commenced by eliciting the views of the most marginalised first. Thus, the initial focus was on collecting children's views—using art and discussions in schools for younger children and a wider range of techniques for older children. When the children's views had been collated, they were presented as initial input to groups of 'less-engaged' parents. Again, a range of engagement techniques was used to reach these parents. The views of the 'less engaged' parents were then collated; the views of the children and the initial round of consultations with less-engaged parents were then presented to the 'more engaged' parents and experts to act as the initial basis for their discussions. This method resulted in much more widely grounded decision-making, with the views of those previously marginalized from most evaluation discussions now made central to them.

The second significant technique used to ensure that community participation in the evaluation had a real impact on public decision-making was the Wyndham local government's '3 + 2' principled approach. In essence, this was an iterative process of information collection that also involved enabled community members to make more informed decisions over time. The '3' denoted clear communication of the nature and extent to which community members could influence decisions. Specifically, the model was founded on ensuring that before commencing evaluation input community members were made aware of:

- What program and policy elements were fixed and could not be altered through their evaluative input (such as rapid population growth in the Wyndham context);
- What program and policy elements could and would be altered through community members' evaluative input (such as the location where programs would operate); and
- What program and policy elements could *potentially* be influenced through community members' evaluative input, but the final decision would be made by people outside the community (such as substantial changes in budget priorities).

The '2' section of the principles was equally important, standing for 'choice' and 'consequence'. Every community choice has

one or more consequences. They could be as simple as recognizing that money spent on one program element (e.g. better street lighting) would require funding cutbacks elsewhere; more subtle consequences – such as the interaction between housing density and transport costs – required substantial community education. The evaluators committed to community education as part of the iterative evaluation process, so that when community members proposed actions, the evaluators informed them of the range of consequences that could be expected, and asked the community members to change or confirm their views, based on that knowledge.

Conclusion

Four factors have been repeatedly referred to as foundations for engaging with Australian Indigenous communities:

1. Developing culturally secure (culturally appropriate) practice
2. Ensuring community support or ownership for interventions and evaluations
3. Active participation and engagement of community members
4. Providing engaged community participants with adequate training and support to enable them to participate actively in evaluation research and the use of its findings.

However, as the case studies presented here demonstrate, such principles may also be usefully applied to a range of culturally and linguistically diverse communities and underpin effective community-based evaluations in general. Clearly, it is important to tailor evaluation approaches to enable the participation by often-marginalized groups, including children, cultural minorities and others who may be left out of evaluation processes.

For all evaluation processes, clear, informed consent as to the nature of the evaluation and what the evaluation process (or evaluator) will deliver is vital. However, the response of decision-makers such as funders and governments to evaluation findings may also impact on community perceptions of the value of evaluation. History has shown that harm resulting as a consequence of participating in an evaluation, or the failure to deliver on key processes or outcomes, may seriously reduce a community's willingness to participate in future research and community-based evaluation. On the other hand, the cases presented here have shown the potential and value of community engagement in evaluation, and the techniques presented have demonstrated effectiveness in securing such engagement.

Bibliography

1. Chelimsky, E. The coming transformation in evaluation. In E. Chelimsky & W. Shadish (Eds), Evaluation for the 21st century: a handbook. Thousand Oaks, CA: Sage, 1997.

2. Clark, H. & Anderson, A. Theories of Change and Logic Models: Telling Them Apart. Presentation to the American Evaluation Association, Atlanta, Georgia, November 2004.

3. Crane, P. & O'Regan, M. On PAR: Using Participatory Action Research to Improve Early Intervention. Canberra: Department of Families, Housing, Community Services and Indigenous Affairs, Australian Government, 2010.

4. Crouch, R.A. The progress of experiment: science and therapeutic reform in the United States, 1900–1990. Book review, BMJ, 320(7137), 1101, 1998.

5. Fetterman, D. Empowerment evaluation: the pursuit of quality. In A.P. Benson, D.M. Hinn & C. Lloyd (Eds), Vision of Quality: How Evaluators Define, Understand and Represent Program Quality (Advances in Program Evaluation, Volume 7) (pp.73–106). Bingley UK: Emerald Group Publishing Limited, 2001.

6. Fetterman, D. Empowerment Evaluation Principles in practice: Assessing levels of commitment. In D. Fetterman and A. Wandersman (Eds), Empowerment Evaluation Principles In Practice (pp. 42–72). New York: Guildford Press, 2004.

7. Funnell, S. & Rogers, P. Purposeful Program Theory. San Francisco: Jossey-Bass, 2011.

8. Green, G., Haines A. & Halebsky, S. Building our future: a guide to community visioning. Madison WI: University of Wisconsin Extension (Report G3798), 2000.

9. Kempe, R. S., Silverman, F. N., Steele, B. F., Droegemuller, W. & Silver, H. K. The battered child syndrome. JAMA, 18(1):17–24, 1962.

10. Markiewicz, A. The political context of evaluation. Eval J Australas, 8(2), 35–41, 2008.

11. Patton, M.Q. Utilization-Focused Evaluation (4th ed). Thousand Oaks CA: Sage, 2008.

12. Pawson, R. & Tilley, N. Realistic Evaluation. London: Sage, 1997.

13. Rist, R.C. Evaluation and organizational learning: some international observations. Paper presented to the Australasian Evaluation Society International Conference, 1-3 October, Adelaide, 1997.

14. Scougall, J. Reconciling tensions between principles and practice in Indigenous evaluation. Eval J Australas, 6(2):49–55;2006.

15. Stanley, J., Tomison, A.M. & Pocock, J. Child abuse and neglect in Australian Indigenous communities, National Child Protection Clearinghouse (NCPCH) Issues Paper no.19. Melbourne: Australian Institute of Family Studies (AIFS), 2003.

16. Tomison, A.M. Evaluating child abuse prevention programs. NCPCH Issues Paper no.12. Melbourne: AIFS, 2000.

17. Tomison, A.M. Evidence-based practice in child protection: Building bridges to better inform practice. Paper presented at the 9th Australasian Conference on Child Abuse and Neglect 'Many Voices Many Choices', 24-27 November, Sydney, 2003.

18. Tomison, A.M. Current issues in child protection policy and practice: Informing the Northern Territory's child protection review. Darwin: NT Department of Health and Community Services, 2004.

19. Wadsworth, Y. Do it Yourself Social Research (3rd Ed). Melbourne: Allen & Unwin, 2011.

20. Wandersman, A. et al The Principles of Empowerment Evaluation. In D. Fetterman and A. Wandersman (Eds), Empowerment Evaluation Principles In Practice (pp 27–41). New York: Guildford Press, 2005.

21. Williams, E. & Cummings, E. Moving toward the fire: developing a tool to provide meaningful results to both government funders and to remote community members. Paper presented at the Australasian Evaluation Society International conference, 31 August - 4 September, Canberra, 2009.

22. Williams, E. A new way to engage with the 'silent community'. Paper presented to the Commonwealth Local Government Forum, October, Brisbane, 2001.

23. Williams, E. Engaging with 'hard to reach' stakeholders. Workshop presented to the Victorian Local Government Association, May, Melbourne, 2003.

24. Williams, E. Evidence, policy & practice: A long and winding road. Occasional seminar presented at the Crawford School of Public Policy, Australian National University, 16 November, Canberra, 2010.

Monitoring and evaluating community-based interventions for children and families in the Asia-Pacific region *Chapter 20*

171

25. Williams, E., Cummings, E., Guenther, J. and Arnott, A. (2010a).'I'm here to support you': updated formative evaluation of the Remote Aboriginal Family and Community Program, Unpubl report.

26. Williams, E., Cummings E. and Hussien, L. (2010b). The proof is in the pudding. Paper presented at the Australasian Evaluation Society conference, 30 August–3 September, Wellington, New Zealand.

27. World Bank Citizen Report Card and Community Score Card. http://web.worldbank.org/WBSITE/EXTERNAL/TOPICS/EXTSOCIALDEVELOPMENT/EXTPCENG/0,,contentMDK:20507680~pagePK:148956~piPK:216618~theSitePK:410306,00.html. Accessed 20 July 2012, 2005.

28. Wyndham Quality Plan Taskforce Our Vision for Wyndham in 2015: the Wyndham Quality Community Plan. Melbourne: Wyndham City Council, 1997.

29. Wyndham Quality Plan Taskforce Our Vision for Wyndham's Future: the Wyndham Quality Community Plan. Melbourne: Wyndham City Council, 2002.

30. Wyndham Quality Plan Taskforce Our Community Vision for Wyndham's Future: the Wyndham Quality Community Plan. Melbourne: Wyndham City Council, 2007.

31. Wyndham Quality Plan Taskforce Wyndham's Community Report Card. Melbourne: Wyndham City Council, 2008.

Section 4

Judicial Aspects

21

Enforcing Justice Through Law and Governance in the Context of Child Abuse

Ranbir Singh

Introduction

India is home to almost 19 percent of the world's children. More than one-third of the country's population, around 440 million, is below 18 years. According to one assumption 40 percent of these children are in need of care and protection, which indicates the extent of the problem. In a country like India with its multicultural, multi-ethnic and multi-religious population, the problems of socially marginalized and economically backward groups are immense. Within such groups the most vulnerable section is always the children. A large percentage of this population is subject to abuse, exploitation and neglect. Child abuse is a state of emotional, physical, economic and sexual maltreatment meted out to a person below the age of 18 years and is a globally prevalent phenomenon.

At the outset we must recognize that the child does not have an existence of its own under normal conditions. Although there may be children without parents, without homes and without food, shelter, education and even clothing, but normally children are with their parents and they live together in the family till they become adults and stand on their own feet. There are millions of children under the care of the parents, they get vaccinated against the more dangerous health hazards even when they are still infants, they are brought up with breastfeeding, nutritious foods, they go to play schools and onward into the best of educational facilities and have the opportunity to graduate, to specialize, to join professions, often of their own choice and become prosperous citizens with access to all the modern gadgets of civilization. There is nothing these children of India cannot get which is not available to other children in any part of the world.

But such children are born of families that constitute about 300 million of India. There are about 900 million who do not have these privileges. Among them there are those at the bottom about whose numbers there is an eternal controversy.

The practice of child protection has undergone a significant change. There has been a shift from the traditional approach of custodial care of child in an institution to recognizing that right to family is every child's right. With the adoption of the rights based approach, issues that were hitherto peripheral came to the forefront. What emerged was that on the one hand, there were enormous numbers of children needing care and protection, while on the other hand there were not enough schemes or sufficient budgetary allocations to deal with them. It was also observed that to carry the issue of child protection forward there was a need to create an enabling environment through a legislation to address issues of child abuse, make a policy on child protection, formulate interventions and outreach services and create an information base on child protection.

The Indian State has been quite prolific when it comes to meeting international standards. There is no reason to be worried as India is quickly mastering the Art of compliance with International Human Rights standards. After all, the first measure that is required for compliance is to pass a law that invokes the standards. Looked at from this point of view India has a fairly good track record. Constitution Indian and Rights of the Child.

The Constitution of India recognizes the susceptible position of children and their right to protection. Following the doctrine of protective discrimination, it guarantees in Article 15 special attention to children through necessary and special laws and policies that safeguard their rights. The right to equality, protection of life and personal liberty and the right against exploitation are enshrined in Articles 14, 15, 15(3), 19(1) (a), 21, 21(A), 23, 24, 39(e) 39(f) and reiterate India's commitment to the protection, safety, security and well-being of all it's people, including children.

Then there is also the juvenile justice law in India that contemplates the legal response with respect to two categories of children, namely those who are 'in conflict with law' (an individual under the age of 18 years who is accused of committing an offence); and those 'in need of care and protection' (children from deprived and marginalized sections of society as well as those with different needs and vulnerabilities). India has a progressive record on legislations relating to Human Rights including child rights and child protection.

India is signatory to a number of international instruments and declarations pertaining to the rights of children to protection, security and dignity. It acceded to the United Nations Convention on the Rights of the Child (UN CRC) in 1992, reaffirming its earlier acceptance of the 1959 UN Declaration on the Rights of the Child, and is fully committed to implementation of all provisions of the UN CRC.

Articles 34 and 19 are the key provisions that protect the child from sexual exploitation. Article 34 provides that countries have an obligation to eliminate child prostitution and child pornography within their borders.[1] Article 19 establishes measures for mandating that countries facilitate legislation against the sexual exploitation of the child. Both articles focus on punishment for patrons and parents of child prostitutes, as well as other measures to prevent child prostitution. The implementation mechanism of the Convention entails the monitoring and reporting of activities.[2] Article 39 discusses recovery and rehabilitation of children. It mandates that contracting states promote the recovery and social reintegration of children. Although India ratified the convention in 1992, a lot remains to be done.

In 2005, the Government of India accepted the two Optional Protocols to the UN CRC, addressing the involvement of children in armed conflict and the sale of children, child prostitution and child pornography. India is strengthening its national policy and measures to protect children from these dangerous forms of violence and exploitation. India is also a signatory to the International Conventions on Civil and Political Rights, and on Economic, Social and Cultural Rights which apply to the human rights of children as much as adults. India is also a signatory to many other Human Rights instruments which urge that the Human Rights of the people be protected and these apply to the Human Rights of Children as much as adult.

Contextualizing the topic

As soon as we won independence, we spent three years writing the constitution and gave onto ourselves the promise of a new India in which such inequality would not be tolerated and untouchability was banned outright. We promised that our children would be provided education and that their tender age would not be exploited. We explicitly banned child labor in the factories, mines and hazardous occupations and promised schooling up to the age of 14 years for all children within ten years of the constitution coming into force.

The Fundamental Rights and Directive Principles of the Indian Constitution provide the framework for child rights. Several laws and national policies have been framed to implement the commitment to child rights.

It is also established that it is utopian to address the problems of children, without addressing the problems of the adults. For instance, if adult households are breaking up, for whatsoever reason, then it is difficult to expect a life of dignity for the child. There are also children who live in squalor, in the slums and the shanties of urban India or in the ghettoes earmarked for the dalits-on the outskirts of literally every village.

What we have just now described is better referred to as the 'Root Cause' for the misery and penury of millions of children in India. The troubling question that we ask is whether we can afford to ignore the root cause while discussing the rights of children in India.

It is in this context that the State must turn its attention to ask what are its 'Immediate obligations', in relation to the children of India. Indian Human Rights Jurisprudence-thanks to our Supreme Court, has already made a breakthrough in this regard (especially through the Unnikrishnan case and the PUCL case on right to food).

The major policies and legislations formulated in the country to ensure child rights and improvement in their status include:

- National Policy for Children, 1974
- National Policy on Education, 1986
- National Policy on Child Labor, 1987
- National Nutrition Policy, 1993
- Report of the Committee on Prostitution, Child Prostitutes and Children of Prostitutes and Plan of Action to Combat
- Trafficking and Commercial Sexual Exploitation of Women and Children, 1998
- National Health Policy, 2002
- National Charter for Children, 2004
- National Plan of Action for Children, 2005

National legislations

National legislations for protection of child rights in the country are:

- Guardian and Wards Act, 1890
- Factories Act,1954
- Hindu Adoption and Maintenance Act, 1956
- Probation of Offenders Act, 1958
- Bombay Prevention of Begging Act, 1959
- Orphanages and Other Charitable Homes (Supervision and Control) Act, 1960
- Bonded Labor System (Abolition) Act, 1976
- Immoral Traffic Prevention Act, 1986
- Child Labour (Prohibition and Regulation) Act,1986
- Prevention of Illicit Traffic in Narcotic Drugs and Psychotropic Substances Act, 1987
- Prenatal Diagnostic Techniques (Regulation and Prevention of Misuse) Act, 1994
- Persons with Disabilities (Equal Protection of Rights and Full Participation) Act, 2000
- Juvenile Justice (Care and Protection of Children) Act, 2000
- Commission for Protection of the Rights of the Child Act, 2005
- Prohibition of Child Marriage Act, 2006: and also
- Protection of Children from Sexual Offences Act, 2012, for which Presidential assent is awaited.

Role of judiciary

The judiciary has played a key role in protecting the Child Rights. It can be illustrated with few instances. In preventing and combating trafficking by pronouncing some landmark judgments in "Public Interest Litigations". Prominent among them are the 1990 case of *Vishal Jeet v. Union of India* and the 1997 case of *Gaurav Jain v. Union of India*. In the former case, on the directions given by the Supreme Court, the Government constituted a Central Advisory Committee on Child Prostitution in 1994. Subsequently, State Advisory Committees were also setup by State Governments. The outcome of the latter case was constitution of a Committee on Prostitution, Child Prostitutes and Children of Prostitutes to look into the problems of commercial sexual exploitation and trafficking of women and children and of children of trafficked victims so as to evolve suitable schemes in consonance with the directions given by the Apex Court. These and subsequent case laws thereafter have influenced Government policies, programmes and schemes, as well as law enforcement.

Similarly in the case of Naz Foundation India Trust, a NGO, has moved the Delhi High Court, by a PIL asking that Section 377 be read down as not covering private consensual homosexual intercourse. The government delayed for two years before filing a response. It did so only after immense pressure from civil society organizations.[3] The reply of the Union Government[4] provides an interesting angle to the discussion on 'shame culture' raised earlier. The reply clearly shows that even the central government has an opinion on the subject of decriminalizing certain activities, and that the opinion is largely reflective of a cultural straitjacket of shame as a dominant social more.

The reply mentions the 42nd and the 156th reports of the Indian Law Commission as stating that society does not approve of homosexuality and that therefore there is a justification in retaining the section 377 IPC in the books of statutes, while conveniently ignoring to mention that the same Law Commission in a later report namely the 172nd report of the Commission has actually recommended that the rape laws be changed to (a) make it gender neutral; (b) make special provisions for child sexual abuse; and (c) repeal section 377 of the IPC.[5]

Therefore, if the argument put forth by the State is to be accepted, the State has not just a function to, but actually a *duty* to stop 'unnatural sex', or else the social order would break down, and law would lose legitimacy. The Government does not have any moral right to interfere in the private sexual activity of two consenting adults, regardless of its interpretation of what is natural or unnatural sexual behavior.[6] The values of a plural society demand decriminalizing homosexuality, and the recognition of child sexual abuse as a grave criminal offence. The government runs a risk of putting in jeopardy the gains that other such demands have yielded historically, e.g. the women's rights movement, or the movement for the upliftment of the *dalits* and other oppressed castes, the civil rights movement, the social gains that have been made over years of struggle in the seeking of a multicultural tolerant society. All of these movements have been conducted in opposition to some or the other prevailing majoritarian belief system and we stand to risk those gains, were the government's view to be deemed credible.[7]

Role of ministry of women and child development

Based on the Report of the Central Advisory Committee on Child Prostitution, the recommendations of the National Commission for Women and the directions of the Supreme Court of India as well as the experiences of various non-governmental organizations working in this area, the Ministry of Women and Child Development, the Nodal Ministry in the Government of India dealing with issues concerning women and children drew up a National Plan of Action to Combat Trafficking and Commercial Sexual Exploitation of Women and Children in the year 1998.

The Ministry of Women and Child Development has also undertaken a study in collaboration with UNICEF on Rescue and Rehabilitation of Child Victims Trafficked for Commercial Sexual Exploitation. The Report of this study was released to the public in 2005. The Ministry of Women and Child Development, in 2005, also formulated a Protocol for Pre-Rescue, Rescue and Post-Rescue Operations of Child Victims of Trafficking for Commercial Sexual Exploitation.

The Ministry of Women and Child Development in collaboration with UNICEF and various other organizations has developed three manuals – the "Manual for the Judicial Workers on Combating Trafficking of Women and Children for Commercial Sexual Exploitation", "Manual for Medical Officers for Dealing with Child Victims of Trafficking and Commercial Sexual Exploitation", and "Manual for Social Workers Dealing with Child Victims of Trafficking and Commercial Sexual Exploitation". The Manual for Judicial Workers has been developed in collaboration with the National Human Rights Commission.

Role of the national human rights commission

As a follow-up of a recommendation made by the Asia Pacific Forum of National Human Rights Institutions in a meeting held in Manila in September 1999, the then United Nations High Commissioner for Human Rights had requested each National Institution in the region to nominate an appropriate individual to serve as a Focal Point on Human Rights of Women, including Trafficking.

Accordingly, in the year 2001, the National Human Rights Commission designated one of its Members to serve as the Focal Point on Human Rights of Women, including Trafficking. The Focal Point undertook several activities, which included an Action Research on Trafficking in Women and Children in India and a National Workshop to Review the Implementation of Laws and Policies Related to Trafficking: Toward an Effective Rescue and Post-Rescue Strategy. National Human Rights Commission and National Commission for Women have decided to work in unison and draw up an Integrated Plan of Action to Prevent and Combat Human Trafficking with Special Focus on Children and Women.

The Government of India recognizes sale of children as an organized crime and has therefore accorded highest priority to combating sale and trafficking of children. The Government has adopted policies and plans, which reiterate its commitment to the rights of the children. These include the National Charter for Children (NCC), 2003, and the National Plan of Action for Children (NPAC), 2005. The NCC provides that children are not used in the conduct of any illegal activity, namely, trafficking, prostitution, pornography or violence. The NPAC has laid down specific strategies to protect children from sexual exploitation and pornography like setting up crisis intervention services and centres; sensitising police, judiciary and medical authorities toward victims; promoting public awareness on the harmful effects of such offences, etc. Indian has also ratified the Optional Protocol (OP) to the Convention on the Rights of the Child (CRC) on the Sale of Children, Child Prostitution and Child Pornography on September 16, 2005.

A communication strategy for prevention of trafficking has also been developed for specific target groups, such as parents, panchayat members, police, teachers and others. Issues related to sexual abuses and trafficking of children are broadcast through the electronic and print media. Initiatives taken by MWCD, in collaboration with UNICEF, to spread awareness include display of messages on trafficking on kiosk hoardings, and back panels of buses. *'Lalli'*, a 30-second spot on trafficking, was telecast on National and regional television networks and private channels in 2005.

The ICPS also provides for expansion of the Childline Service through the Childline India Foundation. With 20 new locations added in the current year, the Childline is now operational in 103 cities. This service started in 1996 with one location, i.e. Mumbai. Childline India Foundation is assisting 229 organizations for running Childline projects in 26 States and 3 UTs. Childline is a 24-hour toll free emergency outreach telephone service for children in distress.

There are a number of orphan, abandoned and surrendered children presently in the country. To facilitate their adoption and to ensure that parents desiring to adopt do not endure unreasonable delays, Central Adoption Resource Authority developed launched Child Adoption Resource Information and Guidance System (CARINGS), a web based management information system on 14th February, 2011. CARINGS is an online web-based platform under which prospective parents can register on-line, track the progress of their application and get information about availability of children, thus making the process more transparent.

National policies and programmes

Some of the existing child protection schemes and programmes include:

- A Programme for Juvenile Justice for children in need of care and protection and children in conflict with law. The Government of India provides financial assistance to the State Governments/UT Administrations for establishment and maintenance of various homes, salary of staff, food, clothing, etc. for children in need of care and protection and juveniles in conflict with law. Financial assistance is based on proposals submitted by States on a 50-50 cost sharing basis.

- An Integrated Programme for Street Children without homes and family ties. Under the scheme NGOs are supported to run 24 hours drop-in shelters and provide food, clothing, shelter, non-formal education, recreation, counseling, guidance and referral services for children. The other components of the scheme include enrolment in schools, vocational training, occupational placement, mobilizing preventive health services and reducing the incidence of drug and substance abuse, HIV/AIDS, etc.

- Childline Service for children in distress, especially children in need of care and protection so as to provide them medical services, shelter, rescue from abuse, counseling, repatriation and rehabilitation. Under this initiative, a telephone helpline, number 1098, runs in 74 urban and semi-urban centres in the country.

- Shishu Greha Scheme for care and protection of orphans/abandoned/destitute infants or children up to 6 years and promote in-country adoption for rehabilitating them.

- Scheme for Working Children in Need of Care and Protection for children working as domestic workers, at roadside dhabas, mechanic shops, etc. The scheme provides for bridge education and vocational training, medicine, food, recreation and sports equipments.

- Rajiv Gandhi National Creche Scheme for the Children of Working Mothers in the age group of 0–6 years. The scheme provides for comprehensive day-care services including facilities like food, shelter, medical, recreation, etc. to children below 6 years of age.

- Pilot Project to Combat the Trafficking of women and Children for Commercial Sexual Exploitation in Source and Destination Areas for providing care and protection to trafficked and sexually abused women and children. Components of the scheme include networking with law enforcement agencies, rescue operation, temporary shelter for the victims, repatriation to hometown and legal services.

- National Child Labor Project (NCLP) for the rehabilitation of child labor. Under the scheme, Project Societies at the district level are fully funded for opening up of Special Schools/ Rehabilitation Centres for the rehabilitation of child laborers. These Special Schools/ Rehabilitation Centers provide non-formal education, vocational training, supplementary nutrition and stipend to children withdrawn from employment.
- INDO-US Child Labor Project (INDUS): The Ministry of Labor, Government of India and the US Department of Labor have initiated a project aimed at eliminating child labor in 10 hazardous sectors across 21 districts in five States namely, Maharashtra, Madhya Pradesh, Tamil Nadu, Uttar Pradesh and NCT of Delhi.

International conventions

Under CEDAW, states parties are obliged to eliminate discrimination and must take all appropriate measures to suppress all forms of traffic in women (Articles 2(e) and 6).

India ratified the **Convention on the rights of child** 1989 (CRC). States parties are obliged to protect children from all forms of discrimination (article 2), to protect them from sexual exploitation and abuse, including prostitution and pornography (article 34) and to make every effort to prevent the sale, trafficking and abduction of children (article 35). Under article 39, states parties have an obligation to ensure that victims of exploitation receive appropriate treatment for their recovery and social reintegration.

The primary responsibility of protecting children from abuse and neglect lies with the families or the primary caregivers. However, communities and civil society and all other stakeholders are also responsible for the care and protection of children. The overarching responsibility is that of the state and it is the state that has to create a protective environment and provide a safety net for children who fall into vulnerable and exploitative situations.

Mandatory laws and detection of abuse

When the ways in which this form of abuse can be tackled is examined, there are a few pointers for the Indian context. This largely relates to how the legal discourse has operated to consistently make invisible the daily abuse that many children suffer. The question is; is there any legal mechanism to detect and prevent child sexual abuse? How does one conceptualize a response, which can detect and prevent it? Finally, what kind of legal institutions and processes can combat the deeply entrenched social and cultural beliefs regarding the sanctity of the family?

The United States has detailed statutory provisions to deal with the issue of detection and prevention.[8] All their states had enacted child abuse reporting statutes by 1967, with the following basic elements:[9]

- Best interest of the child
- Minimum punishment
- Bringing the perpetrators to book

Perhaps comparable to this would be the provisions of the Juvenile Justice (Care and Protection) Act, 2000, which lays down detailed procedure to bring a complaint before the authorities under the Act; the Act is child-friendly in the sense that an individual can approach the authorities directly. If a similar mechanism were to be adopted by the proposed legislation, that would be the ideal way to regulate the detection of abuse.

Conclusion

There is no lack of political will when it comes to building 'infrastructure' for 'growth.' But when it comes to the 'growth and development' of our impoverished children—there are ever so many excuses and so much 'poverty of thinking.' The real reason is that there is no 'political will' when it comes to the children of the 'others.' The 'others' being children of the excluded communities. For 'our own' children there are excellent schools everywhere in India! We know how to impart 'quality' education for 'our own'!

Above all when children of the excluded in India, who constitute the overwhelming majority of children in this sub-continent receive proper education-they will ask why the 'root causes' are not addressed by the powers that be. Only then will the 'Rule of Law' truly flourish in this part of the world.

Acknowledgement

I am thankful to Mr. Ketan and Prof Babu Mathew for their valuable inputs in preparing this article.

References

1. Youth Justice, Critical Readings, Ed. John Muncie Et Al, Sage Publications, New DELHI (2001) at 47.

2. Supra n. 6, at 223-52. From http://www.giveworld.org/naz/naz_profile.htm (accessed 17 February 2005), the Union of India's response to the Naz petition, 6 September 2003, Delhi High Court.

3. On 9th September, 2003, the Union Government filed an affidavit in response to a petition filed by the Naz Foundation (India) Trust before the Delhi High Court, asking the court to decriminalise private, consensual adult sexual behavior. The Government's response is cause for grave concern as its position is in contravention to its role as the upholder of the fundamental rights of all citizens. Para 24 of the reply says: "…deletion of the said section (Sec.377) can well open flood gates of delinquent behaviour and be misconstrued as providing unbridled licence for the same."

4. In paragraph 32 of the reply the government states: "In fact, the purpose of this section 377 IPC is to provide a healthy environment in the society by criminalizing unnatural sexual activities against the order of nature." And then goes on to add in Paragraph 33: "If this provision is taken out of the statute book, a public display of such affection would, at the most, attract charges of indecent exposure which carry a lesser jail sentence than the existing imprisonment for life or imprisonment of 10 years and fine. While the Government cannot police morality, in a civil society criminal law has to express and reflect public morality and concerns about harm to the society at large. If this is not observed, whatever little respect of law is left would disappear, as law would have lost its legitimacy."

5. Supra n.9, pp. 186-91

6. Martha C. Nussbaum, Platonic Love and Law: The Relevance of Ancient Greek Norms to Modern Sexual Controversies, Virginia Law Review 80, 1994, pp. 1515–1651.

7. Hank Estrada, Recovery For Male Victims Of Child Sexual Abuse, Red Rabbit Press, 1994.

8. See, US Statute on Children Related Offences, available at http://www.usstatelaws.childabuse/florida/101.pdf (last visited, September, 2006).

22

Juvenile Justice in India: Challenges and the Way Forward

Ved Kumari

Introduction

Juvenile Justice in India at present is in the state of flux. The legislation governing the subject, namely, the Juvenile Justice (Care and Protection of Children) Act, 2000 has been already amended twice in 2006 and 2011 and yet another committee has been appointed by the Government to consider further amendments. Each High Court has been directed to create a Juvenile Justice under the leadership of the High Court judge to supervise and improve the functioning of the JJA. In Delhi, members from the Delhi Legal Services Authority, the National Commission for Child Rights Protection and other NGOs working with children have been directed to visit homes running under the JJA and report on their functioning. Many skeletons are tumbling out and one is in a quandary to decide the next best course of action. My first introduction to the subject was in LLM, when I opted to study the course on Juvenile Delinquency in 1978 and since then there has been no other time when there was so much focus on juvenile justice and children in need of care and protection. Hence, it is a critical time to focus on the challenges juvenile justice faces today and which may determine the shape of things to come in future.

The phrase 'Juvenile Justice' is used in India usually in its juridical sense and refers to measures, systems, agencies that are involved in ensuring justice to children. This paper also uses the phrase in the same sense and hence, is limited to institutions and processes under and related to the JJA in India.

Historical analyses of legislations preceding the JJA shows that there has been gradual progression from care and protection being the exception to it becoming the rule in case of children committing offences. The first legislation to deal with children below the age of 15 years committing petty offences or found to be vagrants was the Apprentices Act 1850 and it provided for their binding over as apprentices instead of sending them to prison, if found appropriate. Under the Reformatory School Act 1998, children found to have committed offences and sentenced to imprisonment could be sent to Reformatory Schools instead of prison when found suitable. The era of Children Acts began with the Madras Children Act, 1920 and it brought a shift in the approach by making sending children to children homes as a rule but permitting keeping them in prisons in serious offences. The Children Act 1960, passed by Central Government introduced complete exclusion of prison in case of children. However, applicability of this Act was limited to only Union Territories and was in fact enforced primarily only in Delhi. Multiplicity of cut off age and differential rule regarding use or exclusion of prisons in case of children continued till the Juvenile Justice Act, 1986 was passed by Parliament for the whole country that brought uniformity in the cut off age and the approach of care and protection and no punishment to children charged with commission of whatever offence.

However, the JJA 2000 was needed to be enacted to bring juvenile justice administration in conformity with the obligations of the State to bring the local laws in conformity with the CRC, the

Beijing Rules and other International instruments signed by India. The JJA 1986 defined child as a boy below the age of 16 years and a girl below the age of 18 years while the CRC defines child as a person below the age of 18 years. Now, the JJA 2000 defines 'child' as a person who has not completed the age of 18 years. The JJA applies to children committing offences as well as children in need of care and protection. The nature and functioning of all the institutions and processes under the JJA are protective and non-penal.

Despite the gradual and complete shift from some protection to deserving children coming in contact with criminal justice to exclusion of punishment for these children, care and protection to children has not been assured for various reasons. The next part focuses on the obstacles and challenges that have inhibited provision of care and protection to children falling within the purview of the JJA.

Challenges that inhibit care and protection to children

Lack of funds

It is usual to assert that all these legislations were not implemented fully for paucity of funds. However, the first field work research done by me way back in 1980 on juvenile correctional institutions under the then applicable Children Act 1960 in Delhi showed that it was more the lack of awareness about the role and responsibilities of these homes that was responsible for the lackadaisical functioning of the Act. During the field work research, all the responding Superintendents of various Homes under study stated that they were granted the budget they asked for. However, analyses of the budget showed that 97% of the budget was spent on food, clothing, and maintenance of the homes including salaries of the personnel. The remaining three percent was spent on treatment, reformation and rehabilitation. This pattern was not limited to Delhi but was true at the national level too. So it seemed that it was more the lack of awareness and understanding of the purposes of Homes for children or apathy towards children's needs and importance of care, protection, provision of opportunities for development of one's abilities to the fullest, that resulted in the neglect of the crucial role and responsibility of such institutions.

This perception gathered in that research has only been reconfirmed and affirmed by my future exposure to juvenile justice across various countries of the world—the problem of attitude towards the 'other'—the divide between 'us' and 'them'.

'Us' and 'Them'

After my doctoral research on juvenile justice system in India, I concluded, rather naively, that the primary reasons for unsatisfactory state of affairs under the JJA in India were lack of resources (primarily funds), high rate of illiteracy, and the large number of children. However, I was forced to re-examine that conclusion after visiting the rich and powerful countries of the world, namely, USA, UK, and Russia, and not so rich country like Nepal, and seeing the functioning of juvenile justice institutions there. The treatment meted out to children in official residential facilities was not linked with how rich or poor the country was but with the attitude of personnel toward children. In the juvenile home in Nashville, USA, the child who bullied and the one who got bullied, both were kept in isolation—the former as part of punishment and the latter as protective measure against possible retaliation from the bully's friends in the institution. Nobody moved an eyelid when a child was brought to the juvenile court in handcuffs and fetters. The difference in the standard of living in children homes and middle class families in the US and UK was comparable to the difference in the living standards of children homes and middle class families in India. While the small scale pilot projects dealing with very small number of children requiring close supervision were very impressive, the big institutions having 200–300 children did not provide the promised individualized care. One third of the young offenders were 'banged up' in their rooms for the whole day every third day as the number of classrooms and vocational training facilities were not enough for all of them in the institution in Portland. In the children home in St. Petersburg in Russia, the military style walking by children moving from one classroom to another was in quite contrast with friendly atmosphere in their dormitories where children were allowed to have and play musical instruments and sing and their was ambiguity in the attitude toward children in those homes. While the big children homes in US. The US and Russia had high walls and barbed wire on top, the children home I visited in Nepal had no such trappings of a prison. The atmosphere in the children home was very friendly and inclusive and it was difficult to distinguish the teachers and taught as it employed its former inmates as teachers, and the inmates and the guards who were not dressed in official uniform and were playing with the children!

During trainings for judicial, police, and correctional officers, I have been told many a times, 'Poor parents are irresponsible.' 'They even do not know how many children they have.' 'Children living off the streets are smart and know the ways of the world while 'our' children are innocent and vulnerable.' 'We are encouraging others to exploit children by not providing any punishment to children for commission of offences.' All such comments reflect a negative view of 'them' and unless sufficient awareness and acceptance is generated about 'them', it is not easy to ensure the care and protection sought to be provided by the JJA.

As children in need of care are perceived as 'poor and unfortunate', they are treated with pity and sympathy. They are not seen as entitled to care as a matter of right. However, children alleged to have committed an offence pose additional challenges that hinder the care approach toward them.

Children vis-à-vis crime

Children alleged or found to have committed an offence are perceived as troublesome even by those who have sympathy for children in need of care and protection. During the national consultations prior to the enactment of the JJA 2000, there were serious differences among various groups about inclusion of the neglected and delinquent children under the same legislation. There was demand from groups dealing with neglected children that they should be completely segregated from children in conflict with law as their inclusion in the same legislation stigmatized children in need of care and protection. Delinquent children were perceived as violent and hardened whose behavior adversely affected the behavior and attitude of children in need of care and protection. As a consequence, the JJA 2000 completely segregated the two categories of children by providing separate homes for them even during pendency of proceedings. It suggests that the moment a child is alleged to have committed an offence, it is assumed that she is likely to adversely affect the other children, irrespective of the final outcome of the inquiry.

Children who are found to have committed an offence—specially a serious and violent offence, challenge the very notions that surround childhood. Children are perceived as innocent, pure, loving, dependent, vulnerable and hence, entitled to care and affection. Commission of serious and violent crime by them negates all these perceptions as it connotes a scheming mind and ability to harm others—an antithesis of all the notions surrounding childhood. The harm caused by the offence is visible to all to see but the fact that children grow in the world that the adults around them create and they have no control over the circumstances which may have led them to the commission of crime, is lost. There is expectation that criminal liability and punishment should be imposed on them as 'they knew the difference between right and wrong.' Section 82 of the Indian Penal Code 1860 further reinforces this notion by laying down seven as the age of criminal responsibility and presumption of doli capax.

There is little appreciation of the fact that the children's notions of right and wrong are not complicated by the complex classification of wrongs into civil and criminal wrongs and further sub-divisions in each in the legal system. Many children are motivated to knowingly commit a wrongful act just to test their newly acquired skills and abilities. From their perspective it may have been a fun and dare activity which went wrong.

Categorization of children as 'children in conflict with law' and others as 'in need of care and protection' and further sub-categories in the latter, also presents its own problems. First of all, children in conflict also are children in need of care and protection as it is the absence of care and protection that results in their involvement in crime. Rationale for their segregation is that the two groups require different kind of treatment. Going by that rationale, children covered under various sub-categories of children in need of care and protection also need to be segregated. By no stretch of imagination it may be argued that the range of categories in the definition of children in need of care and protection may be taken care of by a single programme or institution. The definition includes children who are neglected, victims of natural disaster, exploited and abused as well as seriously ill. Surely, each one of them need different kind of care and programme for their reintegration in society. However, there is very little focus on the individualized need of each of the sub-group included in the definition.

The negative attitude or the mindset towards children committing serious offences has led to their exclusion from juvenile justice in many jurisdictions in UK and USA. In India the judges face the dilemma of balancing the dictate of law and their own sense of justice and the perceived demand for punishment to those children by society the absence of the possibility of exclusion of any child alleged or found to have committed any offence and provisions of law that provide for only care and protection and complete exclusion of any punishment to children, the judges. Many judges took the escape route provided by silences in the law relating to many age related issues under the legislations preceding the JJA.

The silences in the law – the age related issues

Primarily four kinds of issues were raised before courts in relation to age in the absence of clear provisions in the law. First, how to determine whether the person before the court is below the specified age defining child? Second, what is the relevant date on which the person should be below the specified age to be covered under the JJA? Third, at what point of time the issue of juvenility may be raised? Forth, who has the obligation to raise the issue of age before the courts?

The judgments of the Supreme Court on these aspects may be classified primarily in two categories—inclusionary and exclusionary. Judgment of the Supreme Court in *Rajinder Chandra* adopted the inclusionary approach when it laid down that benefit of doubt up to one year in age determination should be given to children. In contrast is the approach adopted by Sethi J in *Ramdeo Chauhan* when he stated that there is no scope of providing benefit of doubt in case of age and also the way the age was determined by him by excluding the complementary evidences of age contained in the school register and the medical report. Similarly, the Supreme Court allowed the plea of child status being raised for the first time before it in *Gopinath Ghosh* on the ground of the then in force Children Act being a beneficial legislation. However, in *Sushil Kumar*, another Bench of the Supreme Court dubbed the late raising of the plea as an after thought. In *Umesh Chandra*, the Supreme Court laid down the date on the date of commission of crime to be decisive of applicability of the Children Act, in *Arnit Das*, it

held that it was the date of first appearance. The matter had to be finally determined by the five judge bench in *Pratap Singh* reiterating the date of commission as the determining date. In relation to cases pending at the time of enforcement of the JJA 2000 on 1st April 2001, the Supreme Court limited the applicability of the JJA 2000 to children who were below the age of 18 years on that date.

All these aspects have now been specifically addressed by clear language of the provisions of the Act and the Model Rules framed under it. Amended definition of 'juvenile in conflict with law' specifically mentions that the child should be below the specified age on the date of commission of offence. Newly inserted Section 7A specifically provides that the plea of child status may be raised at any time, *even after the final disposition of the case*. Rule 12 of the Model Rules 2007 lay down the hierarchy of the evidence and that the latter piece of evidence has to be sought only if the previous ones are not available. It also incorporates the principle of benefit of doubt up to one year in favour of juvenile laid down in *Rajendra Chandra*.

The limitation contained in *Pratap Singh* on applicability of the JJA to children to children above the age of 18 years on date of enforcement even though below the age of 18 years on the date of offence was specifically removed by the amendment of the JJA 2000 in 2006 by inserting an explanation specifically providing that the JJA will apply to all children who were below the age of 18 years irrespective of their age on the date of enforcement of the Act. Despite this amendment, many post-amendment decisions of the Supreme Court continued to follow *Pratap Singh*. It was only in *Hari Ram* that the Supreme Court took cognizance of the true position of law and held that the JJA applied to all those children who were below the age of 18 years on the date of commission of offence but may have crossed the age of 18 years on the date of enforcement of the law.

All interpretations of law that exclude or limit the application of the JJA to children below the specified age on the date of commission of offences due to one or the other reason are reflective of the discomfort with the beneficial and protective approach of law to children in conflict with law. The primary focus of those judgments is the offence committed rather than the child who committed them.

The above analyses of the law, practices, processes, and judicial decisions show that the biggest challenge to ensuring protection is the mindset of people who lay down the law, who implement it and those who interpret it. Hence, it is important to focus on the possible measure that may be taken to meet this challenge.

The way forward

Faced with the growing demand for further changes in the law from various quarter for better implementation of the law, the Government has appointed a National Consultation Committee to suggest further changes in the law and various amendments are being considered in its deliberations. It is my firm belief, however, that it is not the letter of law but the spirit and attitude of persons that determines the success or failure of legislation. Without denying the importance and function of legal language, it is submitted that we need to focus on the mental concepts that go on to determine our responses to the legal language and its scope, content, and implementation.

Understanding impoverishment rather than focusing on poor

Many training programmes are conducted across India various bodies—governmental and non-governmental to generate awareness about juvenile justice. However, most of these programmes focus on increasing the knowledge base of the trainee officers about various provisions of the Act. Exceptionally trainings address the question of bias and preconceptions about poor people. It is common to believe that poor people are poor because they do not want to work; they are lazy; and that they are burden on society. These beliefs are further reinforced by the occasional newspaper reports when thousands of rupees are found under the sack of the dead beggar; or when some of us offered the beggar a job in our house to work and she refused. It is assumed that beggars should not save for the rainy day; and they must trust our bona fide intentions while making the job offer even though they do not know us. Very little training focuses on causes of poverty and how many development programmes impoverish marginalized people by displacement. In addition, many are displaced due to famine, natural disasters, communal violence, fire, floods, pull from the cities, push from the villages, and many other similar causes beyond their control.

It cannot be expected that there will be empathy toward poor without understanding and accepting the contribution of all of us – the educated and the capable – in making them poor and that they continue to be human beings despite being poor.

Reconstructing childhood and criminality – including the children's world view

Another aspect that needs to be focused in trainings is conceptualization of childhood and children. The primary feature of childhood is the process of growth—mental and physical. Children discover every day their new capabilities and potential. They are focused and encouraged to do better. It is more a matter of absence of appropriate guidance rather their desire to do harm that leads them to commission of crime. Many a times they are roped in commission of crime by the adults around them. In criminal law, liability is imposed if the person had the necessary mens rea. Motive is not important. It is submitted that children jurisprudence should conceive criminality differently. We are likely to understand and accept children committing offence better if we inquired 'why they did it' rather than 'did they do it'. Children respond to the stimuli provided by their immediate environment spontaneously and they do not have the ability to plan on a long-term basis. The answer to the why question may bring to the fore their innocence of the reality of life rather than the criminal and calculating mind at work. Children living in difficult circumstances bear an outer shell of being hard and tough. It is important to break that outer covering to discover the children within who need love, affection, care, and protection like all children.

Involving community in juvenile justice – expanding the human resource base

Children in conflict with law need acceptance of not only the personnel working under the juvenile justice system but of the community at large for their ultimate rehabilitation and reintegration. The primary occasion for most of us have to meet with street children is on the red lights where they are found begging or selling cheap items. Some of us felt harassed when they tug at our sleeves around holy shrines, cinema halls, market places, and so on. We have also been victims of offences committed by them. None of these occasions allow us to believe that they are innocent and vulnerable like our children. Hence, it is important to evolve spaces for involvement of civil society to expose them to the real children hidden underneath the hard cover.

The JJA 2000 does provide for appointment of civil society members in the Child Welfare Committee and the Juvenile Justice Board but the number of persons involved is meagre. For example, in Delhi which is home to close to 160 million people, there are barely 36 persons from civil society appointed to these bodies[1] who have the real hands on experience of the lives and aspirations of children covered under the JJA at a given point of time. The civil society members of the CWC and JJB in Delhi are appointed on full time basis but without proper salaries. Young and professionals thereby are excluded by the very terms and conditions of service. It is the retired or others who have other means of livelihood who may accept to work on these bodies on full time basis without proper salaries.

In contrast is the system of lay magistrates in the UK and the system of Child Welfare Committees in Scotland with much less number of people and children in each jurisdiction in comparison to India. Lay magistrates in England and Wales deal with petty offences. Each year about 30000 lay magistrates or justices of peace impart justice at the local level. They commit minimum of 26 to the usual 35 half days in a year. They work without salary but are entitled to basis allowance to meet their expenses. It is incumbent on the government to ensure that they are chosen from different walks of life and represent their local community. The system has been working for 600 years in England. The child welfare committees work in the same fashion in Scotland. Children up to the age of 16 years are dealt with by these Committees. These children include those who may have committed an offence as the age of criminal responsibility in Scotland is 16 years and they are treated at par with other children in need of care and protection.

It is time that we examine our policies about appointing full time members without salaries to deal with children who we want to grow in to robust citizens of tomorrow.

Another good practice I found in the UK was that each day a member of an NGO was present in the institutions for children. It assured that the personnel in the institutions felt under supervision and the children felt secure in the knowledge that they can approach the volunteer if they had some complaint. NGOs in India have a long way to go to evolve networks among themselves to ensure presence of a volunteer every day in a residential institution to ensure protection of children.

Redefining 'care and protection' to increase community involvement

Currently, custody and care is given to members of community only if they can provide shelter, clothing and food to the child on a long-term and full time basis. It is submitted that the concept of care needs to be reconsidered. I have found better acceptability of street contact programmes among children than the children homes established to provide them round the clock care to children. Salam Balak Trust was running a 2–hour contact programme for children found on the New Delhi Railway Station and it only provided a mid-day meal but lot of bonding. Children who were part of that programme regularly reported the duration for which they were leaving the station and going somewhere else and returned as promised. Absconding of children from children homes, on the other hand, is a regular feature.

There is scope for inclusion of such programmes so that more children can be cared for. Provisions for placing children with 'fit person' and 'fit institution' are useful in expanding the scope of persons and institutions that may provide care to children in non-institutional setting. However, these provisions have remained mostly unutilized in the absence of appropriate understanding of their role and functions and identification of fit persons and fit institutions for various purposes.

Persons and institutions that are ready to provide care or training on part time basis should be identified to be used as fit persons and fit institutions. Programmes like weekend home-visits or taking children out during vacation, may offer opportunities to many who want to involve themselves in helping children but are not in a position to do that on a full time basis.

Evolving community based programmes

It is well established that institutionalization is only a time gap arrangement as all persons sent to an institution have to come out of it sooner or later. Longer the period of institutionalization, harder it becomes for children to return to mainstream. Even a short stint in the home may stigmatize the children and further marginalize them. Beijing Rules and the Convention on the Rights of the Child are categorical that institutions should be used as a measure of last resort and only for the shortest duration till suitable community programmes are evolved or found for them. However, institutionalization has continued to be the primary method of disposal of children's cases[2] when family is not found suitable. In order to change this, there is need to evolve newer and proactive community based programmes that may decrease the need to send children to institutions for providing care and protection.

Restorative justice is gaining ground in many jurisdictions as the most appropriate social integration option. It recognizes that the harm caused by an offence is not limited to the body or property. Each crime also destroys the social ties between the victim and the offender. Restorative justice seeks to remedy that by bringing the two face to face. Consent of both parties is essential for evolving a programme that will be acceptable both to the victim and the offender. Mediators and counsellor prepare the two sides to speak to each other and evolve a programme that will make the children in conflict with law understand the extent of harm caused by them beyond the harm to person or property. This interaction is also focused on making the victim understand that after all the offender is a mere child. It has been found that many offenders dread meeting the victim more than the punishment provided for the offence. Victims too, after their initial anger, tend to pardon the offender if they offer genuine apology and offer to amend the harm caused. This approach is far more successful in integration of children in society than any other.

Schools and school going children may be involved in activities like running children clubs; neighborhood sports meet; mentor programmes for children out of schools in their neighborhood. In appropriate cases children may be sent to an institution only on the weekends while they continue to carry on their normal activities during the weekdays. Community service programmes appropriate to the child's circumstance and aptitude need to be evolved so that children learn from their interaction with realities of life.

However, close supervision of community based activities is essential so that children are not humiliated or abused in those programmes. It is a welcome development that India is seeing the growing involvement of civil society in juvenile justice and more and more NGOs are coming forward to provide care to children. Hence, there is need to evolve mechanisms for close supervisions of the activities of all the NGOs and individuals involved in providing care to children through their residential and non-residential programmes. This is a real concern as there is report in the media about abuse of children in a home run by well recognized and committed child right activist. The JJA has made it compulsory to register all facilities that provide residential care to children in need of care and protection. However, it has been argued before the Delhi High Court that a residential institution established under the Sarva Siksha Abhiyan need not be registered under the JJA. These recent developments and have left the child right activists in quandary about the way forward for protecting children against exploitation and abuse.

Creating data base for appropriate policy, planning, and programmes

Most crucial for the success of any programme and planning is a solid data base. Unfortunately, this is missing in case of India. UNICEF reports that the total number of child population below the age of 18 years in India was 447309000 in the year 2010[3] but the source of that figure is not known. The Report of the Sub-groups on Child Rights 2012 of the Ministry of Women and Child Development mentions that there are 43 crore children in the 0–18 years age group on one page[4] and 44 crore children on another page.[5] As the Census of India collects figures for persons below the age of 14 years and above but not about the number below the age of 18 years, it is not clear whether these figures are estimates or projections. In relation to adolescents, the Report categorically acknowledges that "lack of reliable data and information on adolescent age-group is a major impediment in preparing the profile for adolescents."[6] UNICEF mentions 242,991,000 as the adolescent population constituting 20% of India's population in the year 2010.[7] If such basic information about child population is not available, it is a dream to find figures for the various sub-categories contained in the definition of children in need of care and protection.

It is, therefore, essential for the government and civil society to create appropriate data base so that appropriate programmes for each category of children may be created and sufficient resources allocated for them.

In conclusion, the only point that needs to be reiterated is that the biggest challenge to ensuring care to children falling within the purview of juvenile justice is our negative attitude and misconceptions about those other children. Acceptance of those children as our children is the first step required that will motivate and push us to secure the required resources and practices that will ensure care and protection to all children.

Bibliography

1. It has been in force 1st April, 2001.

2. More details are included in Ved Kumari, Juvenile Justice System: From Welfare to Rights (2nd edn, 2nd reprint 2011) Oxford University Press.

3. Except the State of Jammu and Kashmir that enjoys a special status under Article 370 of the Constitution of India.

4. S.2(k) of the JJA 2000 uses the terms ' juvenile or child' in the definition but this paper uses the term 'child' to the exclusion of the term 'juvenile' which has acquired a negative and stigmatising connotation in social usage.

5. S.1(4) read with s. 2(l) since the amendment of the JJA in 2006 provide that the JJA applies to all children, irrespective of the offences they may have been alleged to have committed, if they are below the age of 18 years on the date of offence.

6. As per s. 2(d), 'child in need of care and protection means a child who is found without any home or settled place of abode and without any ostensible means of subsistence, who is found begging, or who is either a street child or a working child,"who resides with a person (whether a guardian of the child or not) and such person has threatened to kill or injure the child and there is a reasonable likelihood of the threat being carried out, or has killed, abused or neglected some other child or children and there is a reasonable likelihood of the child in question being killed, abused or neglected by that person, who is mentally or physically challenged or ill children or children suffering from terminal diseases or incurable diseases having no one to support or look after, who has a parent or guardian and such parent or guardian is unfit or incapacitated to exercise control over the child, who does not have parent and no one is willing to take care of or whose parents have abandoned or surrendered him or who is missing and run away child and whose parents cannot be found after reasonable inquiry, who is being or is likely to be grossly abused, tortured or exploited for the purpose of sexual abuse or illegal acts, who is found vulnerable and is likely to be inducted into drug abuse or trafficking, who is being or is likely to be abused for unconscionable gains,who is victim of any armed conflict, civil commotion or natural calamity.

7. I got exposed to juvenile justice in these countries as Fulbright Fellow at Vanderbilt University in 1997, Commonwealth Fellow at Warwick University in 1998, and as part of sabbatical research in Russia in 2005.

8. I saw the children home in Kathmandu during a training programme on juvenile justice in 2006.

9. This was the expression used by the inmates as the doors of their cells were banged shut to lock them.

10. (2002) 2 SCC 287.

11. (2001) 5 SCC 714.

12. 1984 Cri LJ 168 (SC).

13. AIR 1984 SC 1232.

14. `AIR 1982 SC 1057.

15. (2000) 5 SCC 488.

16. (2005) 3 SCC 551.

17. S. 2(l).

18. Rule 12 (3)(b).

19. Explanation inserted in Section 20 of the JJA 2000 reads: In all pending cases including trial, revision, appeal or any other criminal proceedings in respect of a juvenile in conflict with law, in any court, the determination of juvenility of such a juvenile shall be in terms of clause (l) of section 2, even if the juvenile ceases to be so on or before the date of commencement of this Act and the provisions of this Act shall apply as if the said provisions had been in force, for all purposes and at all material times when the alleged offence was committed.

20. 2009 (6) SCALE 695.

21. There are six CWCs – each comprising of five social workers; and three JJBs – each having two social workers.

22. Figure 10.3, Crime in India 2010, National Crime Record Bureau, Government of India.

23. State of World's Children 2012, p. 109 (2012) UNICEF.

24. *Report of the Sub-Groups on Child Rights for 12th Five Year Plan (2012-2017)*Ministry of Women and Children, p. 1 (Undated). Available on www.wcd.nic.in. Accessed on 12 August 2012.

25. *Id.* at p.71.

26. *Id.* at p.128.

27. *Supra* n. 23 at p. 131.

Section 5

Social and Cultural Aspects

Socio-legal Measures for Protection of Child Rights in India: A Review

Sibnath Deb

Introduction

Violation of child rights in Indian society is very common and closely linked to socioeconomic, demographic and cultural beliefs and practices. Some forms of abuse and neglect are considered to be normal phenomenon like child marriage, children working as domestic assistant, in the agricultural field or in commercial establishments, using abusive wards against children for behavior modification, giving mental pressure for better academic performance, not giving immunization, not sending to school and corporal punishment. It is also true that Indian mind-set does not consider children as an independent person. Rather, parents and guardians try to have control over children regarding every aspect and disregard to the voices of children.

For normal physical, mental, social and career development of the children, they require adequate nutrition, medical care, education, love and affection, safety, security and a friendly environment. Unfortunately, a large number of the children do not receive adequate nutrition, education, safety, love, care and support. Statistically speaking, the children forms about 44.4% of the total population[1] but yet form a minority in terms of social protection, governmental policy and benefits as a citizen. They are almost always at the mercy of their immediate caregivers.[2] Moreover they experience violence in different forms. The Indian society can be divided into three broad groups in terms of income viz., low, middle and high-income groups. Each group has its unique beliefs regarding child rearing and parenting practices – converging on certain issues but divergent in case of most others.[5] Children experience

a range of major problems like malnutrition, corporal punishment, psychological abuse, sexual abuse, other maltreatment, exploitation, living on street children, child trafficking and prostitution, abandonment, problems while working as child labour, sex selection and female feticide, gender discrimination, child marriage, deprivation from primary education and basic medical care, begging, working as domestic assistant, suicidal ideation because of traumatic experience because of academic failure, academic pressure, and finally they are affected by war, terrorism, substance abuse, HIV/AIDS and displacement. In the following section, nature of violence, abuse and/or neglect experienced by the children have been discussed.

About one-third of Indian population live below the poverty line. Extreme poverty has made malnutrition an issue of national importance. Around three in ten (28%) children are born with low birth weight (UNICEF 2008). According to the 2005-06 National Family Health Survey-3, more than 56.0% of adolescent girls in India are anemic (NFHS-3 2005-06). Street children, who endure a particularly serious experience of poverty, are especially vulnerable to multiple types of maltreatment and suffering including malnutrition, and to associated problems such as substance abuse, sexually transmitted infections and HIV (Mathur et al. 2009).

Lack of education

Not attending school and school dropout are an alarming problem in rural India. As per Census of India, 2011, there were 362 million children aged

0 to 14, representing 29.7% of the population. An informed estimate of one-quarter of those of primary school age not completing primary school therefore equates to 40 to 50 million children. In India, until recently there was no legal requirement to attend school (The Right of Children to Free and Compulsory Education Act 2009). Evidence indicates substantial nonattendance. Statistics indicate that nationwide, 73% of children attend school to the end of primary school (UNICEF 2008). If accurate, the nationwide estimate means that more than one-quarter of all primary school aged children do not complete primary school. Because of the vast population of India, this means tens of millions of young children are denied an opportunity to gain an education and skills, thus vastly limiting life chances and social mobility. However, the latest verdict of the Supreme Court is a very significant legal step which upheld the constitutional validity of the Right of Children to Free and Compulsory Education Act, 2009, which provides for free and compulsory education to children between the age of 6–14 years and mandates government/aided and non-minority unaided schools to reserve 25% of the seats for disadvantaged children.

Corporal punishment

Child abuse and neglect are serious problems in India, influenced by many factors including poverty, over-population, unemployment, illiteracy and lack of education, cultural beliefs and practices, gender bias, patriarchy, and ineffective implementation of legal protections. Several studies have indicated the nature and extent of child maltreatment in India. Most recently, the Indian National Commission for Protection of Child Rights study carried out a study during 2009-10 covering seven states in India. Findings revealed that 99.7% of the children reported one or more types of punishment. As many as 81.2% children were subject to outward rejection by being told that they were not capable of learning. Further the study revealed that 75% children reported that they had been hit with a cane and 69% had been slapped in the check which has been banned as per the Rights of Children to Free and Compulsory Education Act, 2009 (The Report of the National Commission for Protection of Child Rights 2010). Another national study on child abuse in India, although it had a number of limitations in terms

of data collection method, revealed widespread abuse of girls and boys (MWCD Report on Child Abuse and Neglect 2007). This study, published in 2007, obtained self-report data from children in 13 States from 12,447 children aged 5-18. Results showed that 69% of children reported being physically abused (slapped, kicked, beaten, pushed and shaken). In addition, 65% of children who attended school suffered corporal punishment. Regarding sexual abuse, 53% of children reported having been abused in some way. Of all respondents, 20.9% reported severe forms of abuse and 50.8% reported other forms of abuse. Unusually for child sexual abuse, boys were more likely than girls to be victimized. Regarding emotional abuse, 48.4% of children reported being victimized. The study also collected data on girl child neglect, and produced significant findings including that 70.6% of girls reported having been neglected by family members; and that almost half of the girls stated that they had at least sometimes wished they were boys. For all types of maltreatment, the majority of children had not reported the abuse to anyone.

In a Kolkata-based study, Deb (2004) found that 30.0% of the male and 16.7% of the female teachers still believe in applying physical punishment to discipline the students in school. On the contrary, when it comes to practice, 33.3% of male and 40.0% of female teachers reportedly confessed that they punished students physically, although a good number of them did condemn this practice. Findings also revealed that 60.0% of the male teachers and 53.4% of the female teachers had been physically punished during their childhood. In another study, Deb (2004) revealed that 4.6% of the mothers openly stated that it is necessary to use physical punishment to discipline children or to make them obedient.

In another article on ethics in research on child abuse, the authors reviewed the national level study on child abuse carried out by Prayas Institute of Juvenile Justice and recognized the need for conducting an ethical inquiry in this area. Certain concerns about the conduct of the study were raised. Core ethical issues pertaining to consent and refusal, risk and benefit, effects of the study process on the researcher and the researched and the reporting of adverse events were discussed. The ethical implications of the study and ethical responsibilities of the researcher were emphasized (Veena and Chandra Prabha 2007). The worst form of violence against children in India is the killing of a child guided by religious and cultural beliefs (Deb 2006).

In the recent past, the media has reported a number of cases related to violence against children. The latest incidence in the village of Nithari, Noida, UP, revealed a horrifying picture of death of many children after they have been sexually abused. Perhaps the media coverage brought such practices to the attention of the public and that might have made them alert to the possibility of such horrible crime taking place in their backyard.

Girl child marriage is highly practiced in some of the communities in India and it is strongly associated with cultural practices, absence of educational facilities in rural areas, wrong perceived notion about value of education and/ or treating girl child as burden for a family. Child marriage is also often linked to good crop preceded by a good monsoon. When farmers make money in a prosperous season, they marry off children irrespective of their age (The Hindu, Chennai, April 22, 2012, p.18). Analysis of data from the 2005-06 National Family Health Survey-3 shows that among women aged 20-24, more than two-fifths had been married before age 18 (Raj et al. 2009). The fixing of the legal age of marriage at 18 years for girls and 21 years for boys has not prevented the continuation of early marriages. Nor has the Child Marriages Restraint Act, legally in force since 1929, been effective in restraining the practice. The Government's new National Plan of Action for Children 2005 flags complete abolition of child marriages as one of 12 key national priorities (National Plan of Action for Children 2005). Further the Prohibition of Child Marriage Act, 2006 (Jan 10, 2007) was passed towards this end.

Gender discrimination and child marriage

Gender discrimination in Indian society is an age-old practice. In general, boys are given better facilities in terms nutrition, social status, education and even love and affection compared to girls. Protection measures must address social, psychological, physical, mental, emotional and material risk, danger and damage. Protection must also safeguard and defend children against discrimination of all kinds, including neglect. In societies and communities where women are not respected, the girl child is not valued. In many parts of India, she is in danger of being unwelcome even before birth – and is denied fair care and treatment throughout childhood (Child Protection in the Eleventh Five Year Plan, 2007-2012, Sub Group Report). Parents have a notion that during their old age girl child will give them more support compared to boy child (Deb and Chatterjee 2008).

Sex selective abortion is another threat to gender balance in Indian society. Failure to protect the girl child is no longer just a health issue but an important child protection issue, deserving immediate and utmost attention. As per 2001 Census data and other studies illustrate the terrible impact of sex selection in India over the last decade-and-a-half. The child sex ratio (0-6 years) declined from 945 girls to 1,000 boys in 1991 to 927 in the 2001 census.

Child trafficking and thereafter using the children for commercial sexual exploitation is issues that are overlooked in spite of border security and patrol. Some parents sell off their children for meagre sums of money - mostly daughters - who are then trafficked to cities or across the border as labours, domestic help, or for other commercial purposes. Lack of available modes of entertainment in the lower income groups, especially in the rural areas, increase the dependence of young males on pornography, the brunt of which is bore by young females who are taken advantage of. A prevalent belief among the men in the rural areas is that one may cure oneself of sexually transmitted diseases through intercourse with a minor. Disciplinary procedures in the rural areas are mostly through corporal punishment and girls are more likely to be verbally and psychologically abused than their male counterparts.

Child labor and child trafficking

Economic employment of children in India is a very old and common practice. Although Government of India has come out with child labour prevention legislation and even in the Indian constitution there was an article (Article 24), the situation has not changed. Several million of children work in various industries and are exposed to multiple forms of abuse and other dangers. The employment of children in urban families as domestic assistants against small salaries has become a major source of survival for poor children, where they experience exploitation and maltreatment (Deb 2011). This has become a growing phenomenon of systematic exploitation of children in domestic work in urban areas. In many cases, such children have been forced to work for long durations, without food, and/or have worked for very low wages. Many of the live-in domestic workers are in a situation of near slavery. With the violation of their human rights, not only are there sub-human living and working conditions but even blatant injustice of non-payment of wages as well as criminal acts of physical, sexual and psychological violence amounting to torture have been reported (Bajpai 2003).

A study covering a group of 120 migrant child laborers working in households, tea stalls, garages and shops in South Kolkata revealed that an overwhelming number of the children were abused (Deb 2005). A study of 35 trafficked children and young women found that trafficking is usually conducted through offers of false marriages and jobs, or through outright abduction and sale (Deb et al. 2005). In another study, the authors (Chatterjee et al. 2006) found that six out of 41 trafficked children were affected by HIV/AIDS.

Evidence suggests that a large of children especially from the lower social strata and orphan and destitute children have become victim of HIV/AIDS. Either they got the infection from their parents or through sexual abuse and/or trafficked and then used for commercial sexual exploitation. There is no exact estimation of actual number of HIV/AIDS infected people in India. According to UNAIDS, in India, 0.16 million children in 0-14 age group are infected with HIV (UNAIDS Report on the Global AIDS Epidemic, 2004).

A large number of children live on the street (Deb 2006). Children live on the railway platforms, old abundant building, on the streets, in pipes and under bridges. Children along with their families are often forcibly evicted from their homes in the name of development and urban beautification (HAQ Report on Status of Children in India 2005).

Knowledge and awareness among parents and teachers about child rights

Individuals' attitudes and knowledge influence their behavior towards children, including whether children's rights and welfare are promoted. The attitudes generally present in a society shape a culture of how children are perceived and treated. In an Indian study, perhaps first time in India, authors explored the attitudes and knowledge of 300 Indian parents and teachers regarding children's rights, and their perceptions about whether selected rights were secured in reality. Findings show that most parents and teachers had positive attitudes about whether children should have selected rights. However, about one quarter of participants had reservations about whether children should have the rights to freedom of expression and association. A similarly substantial proportion also held an attitude that corporal punishment and/or verbal abuse are sometimes essential to disciplining children. Knowledge among parents and teachers of both national and international laws about children's rights and protection from maltreatment and child protection was generally poor, and teachers were more knowledgeable than parents. Most parents and teachers perceived a lack of actual possession of seven key rights in Indian children's lived experience. Overall, the findings suggest a need to heighten awareness of fundamental children's rights. Efforts to enhance awareness of and sensitivity to children's rights and needs may enable societal progress in enhancing the lived experience of children through illuminating and facilitating reevaluation of existing harmful cultural practices (Deb and Mathews 2012).

Impact of abuse and maltreatment

Series of study revealed negative effects of child abuse and maltreatment on children mental and social adjustment (Deb and Mukherjee 2008). For example, Deb and Walsh (2012) sought to understand the pervasiveness and impact of psychological, physical and sexual violence on the social adjustment of grade VIII and IX school children in the state of Tripura, India.

The study participants, 160 boys and 160 girls, were randomly selected from Classes VIII and IX in eight English and Bengali medium schools in Agartala city, Tripura. Findings revealed that students experienced physical (21.9%), psychological (20.9%), and sexual (18.1%) violence at home, and 29.7% of the children had witnessed family violence. Boys were more often victims of physical and psychological violence while girls were more often victims of sexual violence. The social adjustment scores of school children who experienced violence, irrespective of the nature of the violence, was significantly lower when compared with scores of those who had not experienced violence (p<0.001). Social adjustment was poorer for girls than boys (p<0.001). The study speaks in favour of early detection and intervention for all maltreatment subtypes and for children exposed to intraparental violence.

In another study Deb and Mukherjee (2011) made an attempt to understand the adjustment capacity of sexually abused girls in the age group 13-18 years in Kolkata, India. The study also attempted to understand the perceptions of the sexually abused girls of psychological interventions i.e. individual and group counseling, which they had received. A group of 120 sexually abused Indian girls and 120 non-sexually abused Indian schoolgirls residing in Kolkata Metropolitan City and its suburbs were studied. Findings revealed that the majority of the sexually abused girls came from nuclear and poor families (93.3%) with a low educational background. More than two-thirds (73.3%) were lured with good job prospects, marriage and a better life and abused sexually afterwards. Emotional and social adjustment capacity of sexually abused and non-sexually abused girls differed significantly (p<0.05), irrespective of age group. Overall the perception of more than two-thirds of the sexually abused girls of the rehabilitation homes they lived in was found to be positive. It was also found that younger children (13-15 years age groups) suffered from more emotional and social adjustment problems as compared to their older counterparts (p<0.05). Further, the children who reported they gained considerably from counseling had a better adjustment capacity compared to those who reported they did not benefit from counseling. Another recent Kolkata based study indicates that the social adjustment scores of school children who experienced violence, irrespective of the nature of the violence, was significantly lower when compared with scores of those who had not experienced violence (p<0.001). Social adjustment was poorer for girls than boys (p<0.001) (Deb and Walsh 2012).

Legislations for protection of child rights in India

In order to address any social and health issue effectively, multiple strategies to be adopted. Among all strategies, legal measure is the first step as a yardstick followed by need-based social measures.

As stated earlier, rights of the children have been violated grossly in Indian Society despite of so many legal measures. For example, Articles 23 and 39 of the Constitution of India guarantee the Right to Freedom from all forms of Exploitation. Article 23 of the Constitution of India particularly prohibits trafficking in human beings and forced labour. The Constitution of India also directs all the States to provide free and compulsory education to all children of the age of six to fourteen years (article 21A). Through the National Policy for Children, 1974, the Government of India is committed to provide adequate services to children, both before and after birth, and throughout the period of growth, to ensure their full physical, mental and social development.

The Indian Penal Code (IPC), 1860, is meant for the victims of various kinds of crimes, including crimes committed in the course of trafficking a child. It provides for criminal liability and prosecution of offenders for simple and grievous hurt (sections 319 to 329); wrongful restraint and wrongful confinement (sections 339, 340-346); criminal force and criminal assault (sections 350 and 351); and import/export/removal/buying, selling/disposing/accepting/receiving/detaining of any person as a slave (section 370).

Section 372 and 373 of the IPC set punishment for selling and buying of minors for purposes of prostitution while section 376-2C spells out the punishment for rape.

The Juvenile Justice (Care and Protection of Children) Act, 2000 (amended in 2006) helps ensure care and protection for trafficked children and their restoration and reintegration with their families and the community. The law also recognizes certain offences against children as special offences and provides for punishment. These include cruelty against a juvenile (section 23), using a child for begging (section 24), giving liquor or drugs to a child (section 25), and procuring a child for employment (section 26).

The Immoral Traffic (Prevention) Act, 1956, has been passed by the Indian Parliament, for addressing the immoral trafficking of women and children. Section 6 of the Immoral Traffic (Prevention) Act, 1956, sets punishment for detaining a person (woman or girl) in premises where prostitution is carried on.

The Child Marriage Restraint Act 1929, prohibits marriage of a male child below twenty-one years of age, and that of a female child who is yet to reach eighteen years of age. Further, The Prohibition of Child Marriage Act, 2006 was passed by the parliament and implemented in 2007. As per the section 9 of the Prohibition of Child Marriage Act 2006, whoever, being a male adult above eighteen years of age, contracts a child marriage shall be punishable with rigorous imprisonment which may extend to two years or with fine which may extend to 100,000 Rupees or with both, while section 10 says that whoever performs, conducts, directs or abets any child marriage shall be punishable with rigorous imprisonment which may extend to two years and shall be liable to fine which may extend to 100,000 rupees. At the same time, section 11 of the same act punished a person for promoting or permitting child marriages.

The Child Labour (Prohibition and Regulation) Act 1986, defines the child as a person who has not completed his fourteenth year of age. This act prohibits employment of children in certain occupations and processes.

The National Charter for Children (2003) states (article 9) that all children have a right to be protected against neglect, maltreatment, injury, trafficking, sexual and physical abuse of all kinds, corporal punishment, torture, violence and degrading treatment. The National Institute for Public Cooperation and Child Development (NIPCCD, 1988) has come out with a definition towards this end. According to NIPCCD, child abuse and neglect is the intentional and non-accidental injury or maltreatment of children by parents/caretakers, employers or others, including those individuals representing Government/NGO bodies, which may lead to temporary or permanent impairment of their physical, mental, psycho-social development, disability or death.

The Commissions for Protection of Child Rights Act 2005 (implemented in 2006) is an act to provide for the constitution of a National Commission and State Commissions for Protection of Child Rights and Children's Courts for Providing speedy trial of offences against children or of violation of child Rights and for matters connected therewith or incidental thereto. This law came up after the Nithari serial killing incidents in Noida District, Uttar Pradesh. The Noida serial murders (also Nithari serial murders, Nithari Kand) took place in the house of businessman Moninder Singh Pandher in Nithari, India in 2005.

The Rights of Children to Free and Compulsory Education Act 2009 was passed by the parliament for ensuring free and compulsory education to all children of the age of six to fourteen years. Section 17 of the said act also prohibits physical punishment and mental harassment to child in the schools. It is relevant to mention here that corporal punishment in Indian schools is highly practiced in some schools in India across geographical locations.

State-wise conviction rate in India (*Source: NCRB, 2010*)

High conviction rate in some of the small and backward states in India is a good example before rest of the country. Although it is believed that community pressure on the Criminal Justice System helped to take rape cases seriously result into higher conviction rate, there is a need to carry out a study to find out the facilitating factors behind high conviction rate. In turn, this learning lesson will help other states to improve the situation.

States with high conviction rate

- Mizoram – 96.9%
- Nagaland – 73.7%
- Arunachal Pradesh -66.7%
- Sikkim -66.7%
- Meghalaya – 44.4%

Now the question arises why conviction rate in the major cities and states with reasonably better infrastructure and manpower is low. Perhaps poor investigation and delayed justice system are mainly responsible for poor conviction rate. In the given situation, it is important to think what needs to be done for higher conviction rate based on evidence.

States with low conviction rate

- Maharashtra – 13.9%
- Andhra Pradesh – 13.7%
- West Bengal -13.7%
- Karnataka – 15.4%
- Jammu & Kashmir – 2.6%

Strengths, Short-comings and/or Practical Constraints in Implementing Legal Measures

Need-based legal measures should be developed based on primary and secondary authentic evidences or data and it should be reviewed and amended from time to time based on the feedback from the field. For formulating new legislations, much importance is not given on research based evidence in India like developed countries. However, in the recent past, the Government of India has come out with various new legislations as mentioned earlier for protection of child rights. Definitely these new legislations will bring change in the life of thousands and thousands of children in the country.

Although there are a number of legislations for protection of rights of children in India, the main problem lies with its implementation across the country. For example, section 63 of the Juvenile Justice (Care and Protection) Act 2000 clearly states that every police station should have at least one 'juvenile or the child welfare officer' for handling with the juvenile cases and they should be properly trained. However, in reality, the same provision in law could not been implemented across the country. It is the responsibility of the different state governments to implement the laws and make needful arrangements in terms of manpower and infrastructure. Some state governments take up issues seriously while some neglect them. Therefore, if collective efforts are not made, situation does not improve much. At the same time, continuous follow up from the centre is required.

Legal measures are implemented by the law enforcement agencies like Police, Judiciary and rehabilitation organizations whether government or private welfare organizations. Personnel of law enforcement agencies including NGO people need to be oriented on new legal measures about various provisions so that they are able to interpret different provisions of law from right perspective and apply it as and when required. Unfortunately, in a country like India various legal and social measures are taken about any issue when it becomes very critical and/or pressure is created from various corners. From personal experience while conducting the training programs on child protection for the professionals of the law implementing agencies like police, judiciary, and medical personnel, it has been observed that a large of professionals do not have basic awareness about the legal measures related to child protection and various provisions in it. Even the higher authority was also not aware of the legal measures like JJ Act 2006 and provision of recruitment of female officer for dealing with sexual abuse cases in the police stations. Therefore, the question of implementation of those legal measures did not arise. This was the situation since no orientation program was organized for making law enforcement agencies aware about the upcoming legal measures. Although, there are Police Training School and Police Academy for training of the law enforcement agencies, in reality, perhaps people of law enforcement agencies attend some training at the time of induction in the service and one/or twice in their long career for further promotion. There is a need to organize regular orientation training for the law enforcement agencies on new laws passed by the parliament so that they can apply the same. It is also necessary to update the curricula of the Police Training Schools and Police Academy not for the sake of doing it, but with serious thought reviewing the latest situation. Even, there is no provision of sending a bare act to each and every Police Station about a new law, which might be beneficial to some extent.

For reporting of child abuse and neglect cases, new legislation or amendment of some of the existing laws are required for mandatory reporting of child abuse and neglect cases by teachers, doctors, other health and social welfare service providers.

Social measures for child protection in India

The Government of India (GOI) acceded to the UN Convention on the Rights of the Child on Dec.11, 1992, which reflects the seriousness of the government in addressing the CAN within the broad framework. The Ministry of Women and Child Development and the Ministry of Social Justice and Empowerment, GOI, are mainly responsible for ushering and implementation of the prevention and intervention program for protection of child rights.

The Child Protection Programs of the two aforesaid Ministries focus on the group namely, children in crisis situation such as streetchildren, children who have been abused, abandoned children, orphaned children, and children in conflict with the law, and children affected by conflict or disasters, etc. Some of the programs of the government include An Integrated Program for Street Children, Chidline Services, and Government of India – UNICEF Work Plan on Child Protection, Central Adoption Resource Agency, The National Institute of Public Cooperation and Child Development and so on.

The National Charter for Children (2003) states: The State shall take legal action against those committing such violations against children even if they be legal guardians of such children; (c) The State shall, in partnership with the community, set up mechanisms for identification, reporting, referral, investigation and follow-up of such acts, while respecting the dignity and privacy of the child; (d) The State shall, in partnership with the community, take up steps to draw up plans for the identification, care, protection, counseling and rehabilitation of child victims and ensure that they are able to recover, physically, socially and psychologically, and re-integrate into society.

The Government of India passed a new legislation i.e., the Commissions for Protection of the Child Rights Act 2005. Therefore, the National Commission for Protection of Child Rights has been established in 2006 and all the States and the Union Territories are in the process of setting up State Commissions for Protection of Child Rights. The objective of these National and State Commissions is to ensure proper enforcement of children's rights and effective implementation of laws and programs relating to children.

With the alleviation of the status of Department of Women and Child Development to an independent Ministry headed by the Minister of State having independent charge, it was necessary to change the above provision to make the Minister in charge of the Ministry of Women and Child Development as the Chairperson of the Selection Committee for the selection of the Chairperson of the National Commission for Protection of Child Rights. The Commissions for Protection of Child Rights (Amendment) Bill 2006 have been passed by both the Houses of Parliament for the same.

The Juvenile Justice (Care and Protection of Children) Act 2000 (amended in 2006) is an Act to consolidate and amend the law relating to juveniles in conflict with law and children in need of care and protection, by providing for proper care, protection and treatment by catering to their development needs, and by adopting a child-friendly approach in the adjudication and disposition of matters in the best interest of children and for their ultimate rehabilitation through various institutions established under the enactment. Under this Act, two committees are supposed to be established, the Juvenile Justice Board and Child Welfare Committee in each district or for a group of districts for dealing with juvenile cases in conflict with the law.

The Juvenile Justice Board shall consist of a Metropolitan Magistrate or a Judicial Magistrate of the first class and two social workers of which at least one shall be a woman. The Magistrate should have clear knowledge or training in child psychology or child welfare while social workers should at least seven years working experience in the field of health, education and/or child welfare activities. This board is empowered to deal exclusively with all proceedings under this Act relating to juvenile in conflict with law.

The Child Welfare Committee under the Juvenile Justice (Care and Protection) Act 2006 is empowered to ensure care and protection to children in need. The Committee shall consist of a Chairperson and four other members. At least, one of the members of the committee shall be a women and an expert on matters concerning children. A non-judicial person can become a Chairperson of the Child Welfare Committee. A child in need of care and protection may be produced before an individual member for being placed in safe custody or otherwise when the Committee is not in session. The Committee shall have the final authority to dispose of cases for the care, protection, treatment, development and rehabilitation of the children as well as to provide for their basic needs and protection of human rights. The Committee has the power to deal exclusively with all proceedings under this Act relating to children in need of care and protection.

So far as social measure is concerned, the recent initiative of the Ministry of Women and Child Development, Government of India for protection of children is called "Integrated Child Protection Scheme (ICPS)". This scheme concretizes the

Government/State responsibility for creating a system to protect children in the country. ICPS is based on the cardinal principles of 'protection of child rights' and 'best interests of the child'. It aims to promote the best interests of the child and prevent violations of child rights through appropriate punitive measure against perpetrators of abuse and crimes against children and to ensure rehabilitation for all children in need of care and protection.

It aims to create a protective environment by improving regulatory frameworks, strengthening structures and professional capacities at national, state and district levels so as to cover all child protection issues and provide child friendly services at all levels. The following key principles underlie the ICPS approach:

Child protection – a shared responsibility

The responsibility for child protection is a shared responsibility of government, family, community, professionals, and civil society. It is important that each role is articulated clearly and understood by all engaged in the effort to protect children. Government has an obligation to ensure a range of services at all levels.

Reducing child vulnerability

There is a need for a focus on systematic preventive measures not just programmes and schemes to address protection failures at various levels. A strong element of prevention will be integrated into programmes, converging the provisions and services of various sectors on the vulnerable families, like livelihood support (NREGS), SHGs, PDS, health, child day care, education, to strengthen families and reduce the likelihood of child neglect, abuse and vulnerability.

Strengthen family

Children are best cared for in their own families and have a right to family care and parenting by both parents. Therefore a major thrust will be to strengthen the family capabilities to care for and protect the child by capacity building, family counselling and support services and linking to development and community support services.

Promote non-institutional care

There is a need to shift the focus of interventions from an over reliance on institutionalization of children and move towards more family and community –based alternatives for care. Institutionalization should be used as a measure of last resort after all other options have been explored.

Intersectoral linkages and responsibilities

Child protection needs dedicated sectoral focus as well as strengthening protection awareness and protection response from other sectors outside the traditional protection sector including in emergencies and HIV/AIDS programming.

Create a network of services at community level

An appropriate network of essential protection services is required at all levels for supporting children and communities.

Establishing standards for care and protection

All protection services should have prescribed standards, protocols for key actions and should be monitored regularly. Institutionalization should be for the shortest period of time with strict criteria being established for residential placement and all cases of institutionalization reviewed periodically.

Building capacities

Protection services require skilled, sensitive staff, equipped with knowledge of child rights and standards of care and protection. Capacities of all those in contact with children require strengthening on a continuing basis, including families and communities.

Providing child protection professional services at all levels

There is a need for varied special services for the many situations of child neglect, exploitation and abuse, including for shelter, care, psychological recovery, social reintegration, legal services etc., which have to be professional and child-focused.

Strengthening crisis management system at all levels

First response and coordinated intersectoral actions for responding to crisis need to be established and institutionalized.

Reintegration with family and community

Systems to be put in place for efforts to reintegrate children with their families and community and regular review of efforts instituted.

Addressing protection of children in urban poverty

Children in urban poverty are at high risk, constantly under threat of eviction, denial or exclusion from basic services and social turmoil. Poverty and ignorance stretch the capacity of the adults to function as adequate caretakers. This indicates the need for developing a strong social support and service system.

Child impact monitoring

All policies, initiatives and services will be monitored.

Following are some of the other social programs for addressing the specific needs of the disadvantaged children:

1. An Integrated Program for Street Children
2. Childline Services
3. A Program for Juvenile Justice
4. Central Adoption Resource Agency (CARA)
5. National Institute of Public Cooperation and Child Development (NIPCCD)
6. Integrated Child Development Scheme (ICDS)
7. National Council of Child Welfare
8. Childline Foundation
9. Rajiv Gandhi National Creche Scheme for the Children of Working Mothers
10. UJJAWALA: A Comprehensive Scheme for Prevention of trafficking and Rescue, Rehabilitation and Re-integration of Victims of Trafficking and Commercial Sexual Exploitation
11. Scheme for welfare of Working Children in need of Care and Protection

Indian Council for Child Welfare (ICCW) (born on 31st day of December 1974) a trust has been working for child protection for a long period. The objectives of the ICCW are (i) initiating, undertaking or giving aid directly or through its State/Union Territory Councils or affiliated bodies, schemes for furtherance of child welfare/development in India; (ii) supporting wherever possible, and guide the progress of any approved schemes of child welfare/development which may already exist; (iii) supporting wherever possible, and guide the progress of any approved schemes of child welfare/development which may already exist; and (iv) promoting generally the welfare of children in India having regard to their social, economic and other needs.

The specific activities of ICCW include advocating children's rights, creches for children of working and ailing mothers, training programmes for child care workers, sponsorship for school education of under-privileged children, projects for street and working children, scrutiny of adoption cases, rehabilitation of abandoned children, institutional and day care services for differently abled children, programmes for children in difficult circumstances, programmes with special focus on the girl child, education centres and support services, honouring children for bravery, honouring child artists, national integration camps/ adventure camps.

Strengths and weaknesses of social measures

A range of social measures have been adopted by different Ministry of the Government of India for addressing the needs of the disadvantaged children. Undoubted all these measures benefitted a large number of children across the country especially disadvantaged children who live in and around urban areas. Still a large number of children across the country are out of reach. Therefore, there is a need to think of how to reach the unreached children population.

Social measures are implemented through NGOs across the country. Since there is no evidence regarding efficacy of all the social measures for protection of child rights, it is very difficult to comment whether disadvantaged, abused and neglected children have access to all these social measures and they are benefitted. Ideally, in any intervention program baseline study should be carried out to determine the existing situation and based on that prepare need-based intervention programs and develop strategies. Another lacuna of all social measures is the centralised system, which often fails to deliver the benefits of various programs to the disadvantaged children of interior rural areas.

As per the National Commission for Protection of Child Rights Act 2006, every state should establish State Commission for Protection of Child Rights. The progress of establishment of State Commission for Protection of Child Rights is very slow in some states. Likewise, as per the Integrated Child Protection Scheme (ICPS), every district should have a child protection officer. In some districts of some states Child Protection Officers have been recruited on a contract basis (for a temporary assignment), which discourages motivation and leads to negligence in delivering services. Thus despite good policies and programs, the commitment toward implementation is inadequate.

During six years of working with an international NGO, particularly in the field of child protection, I had the opportunity to observe the functioning of other NGOs and international funding agencies. My experience suggests that whereas some NGOs implement the programs religiously and utilise the fund properly, others often misuse and are wasteful. This matter requires careful attention of funding agencies. Another problem is that after some years of extending services to the community, some NGOs phase out from the field without making any alternative arrangements for sustainability of the program. Therefore, the issue of sustainability of any social welfare program is always questionable. A lack of commitment on the part of persons working in different projects is a big challenge in delivering quality services to the children. Since documentation of most NGOs about different activities is very poor, one cannot be sure about the success of the program. Thus it is essential to rigorously monitor and document the outcomes of various programs. At the same time, the funding agency should carry out mid-term and end-term evaluation all programs through external professional agency, which would help to identify the lacunas in the program and take course corrective measures for maximum utilisation of resources. The evaluator for evaluation of any

intervention program should be identified from a credible academic and research institution, otherwise the actual situation may not be revealed

My own evaluation of a number of social and health related programs for different national and international funding agencies showed varying results. For example, in some districts of West Bengal ICDS programs funded by UNICEF were functioning very well with local community support while in others the implementation was poor. The chief factor for the success appeared to be the enthusiasm and caring attitude of the Anganwadi Worker and her helper, who were instrumental in mobilizing the community that resulted in a good attendance of children at the ICDS centre her helper, food, Timely supply of food materials from the district office and proper distribution of good quality distribution of good quality food also encouraged community support.

Lack of allocation of funds for delivering need-based services to the disadvantaged, neglected and maltreated children through NGOs and lack of trained professional manpower for dealing with abused and maltreated children, lack of coordination among the NGOs and between government and NGOs especially in the rural areas are some of the major weaknesses of the system in addition to lack of government accommodation facilities for safe custody of the rescued children from the red light areas and for the children in need of care especially orphan and destitute children.

Since there is no provision for systematic documentation of reported cases of abuse in the police stations and in the hospitals, organizations find it difficult to develop evidence-based comprehensive intervention programme for child protection. On the other hand, there are no family-based services to identify the high-risk families for prevention of child abuse and neglect. Most of the educational institutions especially the primary schools do not have child protection policy. As compared to need, very few workshops, orientation and/or sensitization programmes have been undertaken in the community for creating awareness among the parents on the issue.

Overpopulation resulting in poor service delivery, poverty, illiteracy, abandonment of children, cultural beliefs, poor reporting and practices pertaining to parenting style and child development are some of the biggest challenges in addressing the child abuse and neglect issue in India. For example, corporal punishment, early girl child marriage, gender discrimination, not giving colostrums to a new-born out of a feeling that it might upset the stomach of the infant are some of the common cultural beliefs and practices prevalent in some communities in India. Child trafficking is another problem increasing alarmingly, since India shares its border with Bangladesh, Pakistan, Nepal, Myanmar and Bhutan. Another major challenge is to locate the biological parents in case of trafficked children and merge them with their own families. A good number of children from the said countries cross the border and finally land up in commercial sex trade. Even, within the country, a good number of girl children from poor families are becoming the victim of child trafficking.

Mental health of the abused and traumatic children did not receive much importance in most of the social measures. In reality, there is hardly any psychologist in the social programs and in the hospitals for addressing mental health needs of traumatic children.

Media and sociolegal measures

Print as well as electronic media can be instrumental in creating social awareness about different sociolegal measures. A recent TV program (*Satyamave Jayate*) focusing on child abuse was widely viewed and appreciated. It highlighted several sensitive social issues prevailing in India such as female feticide, child sexual abuse, dowry, honour killings, physical disabilities and domestic violence. It would be useful to examine the impact of such programs and consider expanding their scope and reach.

Mental health of caregivers and child abuse and neglect

Child abuse and neglect has a direct relation with the mental health problems of the parents. Children from disturbed family or broken families, or where the parents indulge in substance abuse, are particularly affected by neglect and abuse. There is often a stigma attached to mental health problems (as also with some other diseases, such as HIV infection, tuberculosis) in countries like India, professional psychiatric help may not be sought. A child with a mental health problem is often subjected to early marriage.

Legal measures should be instituted to penalise the guardians who arrange marriage of their children having mental health problems or some other problem such as substance abuse without disclosing such information.

Conclusion

The available evidence clearly indicates that a large number of Indian children are not protected and their rights are grossly violated. They experience neglect, abuse, maltreatment and exploitation in different forms. Social and legal measures instituted by the Government are poorly implemented and there is a lack of coordination, poor documentation, and little lack of accountability. A paucity of trained workers, absence of quality monitoring and evaluation of different programs, and failure to take timely corrective measures for effective implementation of different programs are major constraints for protection of child rights in India. Judicial measures should be adequate and prompt. Free social-legal aid services need to be strengthened in every district of every state of India.

It is crucial to address the core issues such as overpopulation, poverty, illiteracy, unemployment and primary health care, sanitation which are directly linked with child abuse and neglect. The Integrated Child Protection Scheme (ICPS), a recent initiative should be effectively undertaken. The issues of child neglect and abuse and child protection need to be prioritize in the national policies (Table 1).

Table 1 Measures to comprehensively address the problems of child abuse and neglect and child protection

- Ensure implementation of policies and programs in truest with more allocation of fund and infrastructure development across the country.
- Improve documentation system for reporting cases of child abuse and neglect in hospitals and other medical facilities.
- Sensitize politicians and policy makers about the need for child protection.
- Inform and educate teachers, NGO personnel, judiciary, doctors other professionals, parent about child rights child neglect and exploitation.
- Make child development and protection including their rights a compulsory subject at the school and college level and in medical curriculum.
- Train law enforcement personnels including child protection officers, and doctors to apprise them about socio-legal measures.
- Have well defined protocols and manuals for all stakeholders involved in child protection.
- Make reporting of child abuse and neglect mandatory by doctors, teachers, and others.
- Employ print and electronic media to create awareness through culturally sensitive programs.
- Involve community leaders and corporate sectors in addressing the issues of child abuse and neglect.

References

1. Bajpai AB (2003) Child rights in India- law, policy and practice, Oxford University Press, New Delhi.

2. Census of India (2001) Office of the Registrar General, India, Ministry of Home Affairs, Government of India, New Delhi.

3. Chatterjee P, Chakraborty T, Srivastava N, Deb S (2006) Short and long-term problems faced by the trafficked children: a qualitative study. Social Science International, 22(1):167–182.

4. Child Protection in the Eleventh Five Year Plan, 2007-2012, Sub Group Report.

5. Deb S (2011) Exploitation and harassment of migrant women and girl children working as domestic assistant. In: Sarkar S and Srivastava M (ed) Globalization and gender, New Delhi, Rowat Publication.

6. Deb S, Srivastava N, Chatterjee P, and Chakraborty T Processes of Child Trafficking in West Bengal: A Qualitative Study. Social Change, 2005; 35(2):112–123.

7. Deb S and Chatterjee P (2008) *Styles of Parenting Adolescents: The Indian Scenario*. New Delhi, Akansha Publising House.

8. Deb S (2006) *Chidlren in agony*. New Delhi, Concept Publishing Company.

9. Deb S (2004) Defining child maltreatment in India. *World Perspectives on Child Abuse, Sixth Edition*, an Official Publication of the ISPCAN, USA, 63–67.

10. Deb S Child abuse and neglect in a metropolitan city: a qualitative study of migrant child labour in south Kolkata. Social Change, 2005; 35(3):56–67.

12. Deb S and Mukherjee A (2008) *Impact of Sexual Abuse on Mental Health of Children*. New Delhi, Concept Publishing Company.

13. Deb S and Walsh K (2012) Impact of physical, psychological, and sexual violence on social adjustment of school children in India. School Psychology International, *1-25 (published online)*.

14. Deb S and Modak S Prevalence of violence against children in families in tripura and its relationship with socioeconomic, cultural and other factors. Journal of Injury and Violence Research, 2010; 2(1): 5–18.

15. Deb S and Mukherjee A Background and adjustment capacity of sexually abused girls and their perceptions of intervention. Child Abuse Review, 2011; 20:213–230.

16. Deb S. Child protection: scenario in India. Child Health and Human Development, 2009; 2(3):339–348.

17. Deb S and Mathews B. Children's rights in India: parents' and teachers' attitudes, knowledge and perception. Children's Rights, 2012; 20:1–24.

18. HAQ: Centre for child rights. Status of children in India Inc., 2005. p. 169.

19. Raj A, Saggurti N, Balaiah D and Silverman J. Prevalence of child marriage and its effect on fertility and fertility-control outcomes of young women in India: a cross-sectional, observational study. Lancet, 2009; 373:1883–1889.

20. Report of the National Commission for Protection of Child Rights, 2010.

21. Report on child abuse and neglect. Ministry of Women and Child Development, Government of India, 2007.

22. Veena AS and Chandra PS. A Review of the ethics on research on child abuse, *Indian JME*. 2007; 3:25–34.

23. Mathur M, Rathore P and Mathur M. Incidence, type and intensity of abuse in street children in India. *Child Abuse & Neglect*, 2009; 33:907–913.

24. National plan of action for children 2005 Ministry of Women and Child Development, Government of India.: (adopted 20, Aug. 2005): Pt 13, p. 3).

25. National Family Health Survey (NFHS-3) 2005-06, IIPS and Macro International: India, Mumbai, International Institute for Population Sciences and Macro International, 2007.

26. National Crime Records Bureau 2010, Ministry of Home Affairs, Government of India.

27. The Hindu, Chennai (April 13, 2012) *Court Upholds RTE*, p.1.

28. The Hindu, Chennai (April 22, 2012) *Prevent Child Marriages on Akshya Tritiya, States Told*, p.18.

29. The Indian Constitution, Nov. 26, 1949.

30. The Rights of Children to Free and Compulsory Education Act, 2000.

31. The Commissions for Protection of the Child Rights Act, 2005.

32. The Juvenile Justice (Care and Protection of Children) Act, 2000 (amended in 2006, India).

33. The Child Marriage Restraint Act, 1929.

34. The Prohibition of Child Marriage Act, 2006 (Jan 10, 2007).

35. The Child Labour (Prohibition and Regulation) Act, 1986.

36. The Immoral Traffic (Prevention) Act, 1956.

37. The Indian Penal Code, 1860.

38. The National Crime Records Bureau, 2010.

39. UNAIDS, Report on the global AIDS epidemic 2004, Geneva.

40. UNICEF. (2008). *India: maternal, newborn and child survival*. Retrieved March 8, 2010, from http://www.childinfo.org/profiles.html.

24

Cultural Issues and Child Maltreatment: Challenges in the Asia-Pacific Region

Shanti Raman, Mary J Marret,
Chhaya S Prasad

Introduction

The children of today live in a vastly different world from that of two decades ago when the United Nations Convention on the Rights of the Child (CRC) was enshrined internationally. Migration and globalization have increased the 'culturally plural' nature of modern societies and created rapid economic, organizational, health and social-psychological change. Amidst these waves of migration, are humanitarian migrants, fleeing from persecution both internally and externally. Nowhere has this pace of change been as marked as in the Asia-Pacific region, where most of the world's children and young people live and grow up.

Interest in the influence of culture specifically on children's health and development extends across a range of disciplines, including anthropology, sociology, philosophy, and psychology. [1-2] While the influence of culture on child rearing and child development is acknowledged, the nexus between children at risk of maltreatment and dealing appropriately with culturally diverse populations is more challenging. This nexus is movingly portrayed in Fadiman's account of a Hmong child with intractable seizures growing up in California. [3] Her parents believed that her seizures were caused by the flight of her soul from her body, calling her condition by its Hmong name: *qaug dab peg*. Complex interactions between medical services, community services, child protection services and a cultural broker were required before the child returned to her family after a prolonged stint in foster care. In the UK, the Laming Inquiry, [4] highlighted the cultural issues that contributed to the fatal abuse of Victoria Climbié, a black African girl. Challenges such as these are almost every day affairs in the Asia-Pacific region, where traditional beliefs and strong religious and cultural practices jostle with modernisation, economic growth and the reality of the largest child and youth population, many of whom are just surviving. Practices that are threatening, dangerous and harmful to children seem to co-exist within pro-child societies. Child health/welfare professionals and advocates working with children within the region often find themselves faced with the challenge of identifying if children have been maltreated as defined in child protection practice, or whether cultural/traditional practices and/or broader societal pressures are the cause. We will unpack this challenge.

Conceptualizing culture

Is there an 'Asian' view of the world, a 'Pacific' way to do things; as opposed to the 'western' way? To get a handle on what is happening to children in our diverse and changing world, we need to look at how we conceptualise 'culture'. In particular, we need to examine how culture shapes our understanding of childhood problems and how to deal with them. There has been a trend in social welfare in the west to subsume 'culture' within the concept of ethnicity and racism has often been regarded as a more significant issue than culture. Cultural heritage of children and their families at the pointy end of the child protection system, has sometimes been perceived as oppressive, and culture has been misinterpreted to explain and to tolerate unacceptable behavior.[5] We need to put culture at the heart of our thinking; to be clear about definitions and understand some of the elements of cultural identity formation and influences on child wellbeing.

'Culture' as a concept and term in itself has been discussed and debated about for over a century. It is often defined simply as a 'set of beliefs, attitudes, values, and standards of behavior that are passed from one generation to the next'.[6] The intergenerational idea is an important element here, as is the understanding that it relates to some shared elements which connect people in a common way.[7] While human migration has been happening for a very long time indeed, migration today needs to be understood as a highly heterogeneous phenomenon, involving push and pull factors; not all migrants are likely to face similar experiences before or after migration.[8]

Culture, race, ethnicity, cultural identity, acculturation and a myriad other terms may have overlapping boundaries and are often used interchangeably. Helms defined ethnicity as a "social identity based on the culture of one's ancestors' national or tribal groups and modified by the demands of the larger culture or society in which one currently resides."[9] As an all encompassing term, one that deals with today's changing world, 'cultural identity' incorporates diversity and pluralism; an implication is that there are a number of different 'selves' at different levels and their true psychological integration will lead to better psychological functioning.[10] Bhabha suggests that the negotiation of cultural identity involves the continual interface and exchange of cultural ideas and practice that in turn produces mutual recognition of cultural difference.[11] The United Nations Educational, Scientific and Cultural Organization (UNESCO) supports a new approach to cultural diversity acknowledging that a wide range of distinct cultures are living together; this approach takes account of its *dynamic* nature and the challenges of identity associated with the permanence of cultural change.[12]

Defining child maltreatment in a cross cultural context

How 'child maltreatment' is defined critically informs how and when professionals working in the field respond. While there is a tacit understanding that child abuse occurs everywhere, much of the published research is from Western countries although there is now an emerging literature from non-western countries. There is considerable variation over time and between cultures about what is deemed abusive to children. In the 2006 survey involving 72 countries across major regions of the world, there was strong agreement that sexual or physical abuse of a child by a caretaker constitutes child maltreatment.[13] Other behaviors frequently mentioned as being abusive to children included children living on the street, child prostitution and abandonment by parents or caregivers. There was wide regional variation however in acknowledging other behaviors such as physical discipline as abusive. In a survey of teachers in a Pacific Island nation about what constitutes CM, sexual abuse was rated as the most serious type of abuse, interventions were recommended for serious forms of CM, but some traditional parenting practices that might be considered maltreatment by other cultures were not considered abusive.[14] A recent study in Hong Kong eliciting primary school children's views found that children did not have a homogeneous view on issues about CM, and their awareness and sensitivity to different kinds of maltreatment were different. While they shared some ideas about CM with adults, some ideas were uniquely their own; most importantly children's disclosure of abuse was strongly affected by the Chinese notions of filial piety and loyalty to parents.[15]

There is no universality regarding child rearing standards, nor the definition of CM,[16] and the cultural perspective of maltreatment can present something of a dilemma. On the one hand, lack of a cultural perspective in defining abuse can promote the professional's own cultural values and worldview as the guiding force in making decisions. Conversely, when definitions of CM are totally guided by that cultural group's norms, the outcome may result in children receiving a lesser standard of care and protection. Korbin identified the following three aspects which may be useful in developing culturally responsive definitions of child maltreatment:[16]

- *Acknowledgement of cultural differences in child rearing practices*
- *Recognition that deviations from the culturally appropriate child-rearing practices of any specific cultural group are considered by that cultural group to be abusive.*

- *Knowledge of the circumstances that exist where societal harm undermines children's well-being beyond the control of the parent* (e.g. poverty).

Korbin suggests that while the behavioral components of the abusive 'act' itself are important, the contextual factors must be taken into account for the act to be meaningful. Cultural acceptance of an act and rules about its occurrence can provide a means for assessing what is abusive. The intent of the adults involved is an important factor and the child's perceptions of the incident must be considered. The age of the child and cultural standards for physical and psychological development of children of differing ages must be taken into account.[17] Korbin argues strongly that incorporating a cultural component in child protection, prevention and intervention is a necessity rather than an optional extra.[18] Where would child labour or children/families living on the streets fit into this conceptualization? We would therefore suggest adding the protective framework of the United Nations Convention on the Rights of the Child (CRC); supporting the child-centred approach that any potential violence or harm to children and young people cannot be tolerated.[19]

Child rights and specific challenges in the Asia-Pacific

In western countries child protection work is often seen as 'uninvited intervention within the sphere of 'private' family life' due to the contested nature of some of the fundamental rights-based concepts of 'best interests', 'welfare' and 'good enough parenting'.[20] It is likely that concepts such as these would be even more contested and problematic across the Asia-Pacific, which lacks the same level of child welfare and social service involvement in most of the region. The United Nations CRC provides a framework for good child protection practice and most nation states have signed up to it. The right of children to protection from harm is set out in Article 19 of the CRC:

'States Parties shall take all appropriate legislative, administrative, social and educational measures to protect the child from all forms of physical and mental violence, injury or abuse, neglect or violent treatment or exploitation, including sexual abuse, while in the care of parent(s), legal guardian(s) or any other person who has care of the child.'

Several of the articles of the CRC pertain to child protection work. Article 24 specifically states - "parties shall take all effective and appropriate measures to abolish traditional practices prejudicial to the health of children". However, more than 15 years ago Kiwie and Dibbie argued that children in developing countries were not being protected despite the progressive covenants of human rights law, due to a 'failure to challenge harmful fundamental cultural values and practices that promote (certain) child-rearing practices and endanger the world's children and young women'.[21] They were strongly critical of the ideological position that family privacy must be protected, which then provided "blanket protection' for abusive practices that take place within the family setting.[21]

Human rights are universal, but in many parts of the world children have not to date received the full protection of human rights legislation. A survey of 42 developing and developed countries, which rated country effectiveness in implementation of CRC, and the current level of effectiveness of child protection systems, found that Malaysia and South Korea were among the top ranked countries.[22] These countries were judged as having well developed child protection legislation, child welfare services and at least one information-based intervention support program. Most other countries in the region do not have all three of the essential components of a working child protection system. In addition, there are particular challenges for children and young people, which are more commonplace, although not unique to the region. These include widespread acceptance of corporal punishment in schools and in homes, [23-24], [25], [26] child prostitution,[27] child slavery,[28] gender-based violence and related feticide/infanticide,[29-31] as well as the seemingly inescapable juggernaut of child labor.[32], [33], [34]

Pemberton *et al* suggest that a rights-based strategy is necessary to the development not only of international and national jurisprudence but to a global civil society that challenges the structures of global poverty. However, they argue possibly contentiously, that for developing countries it is appropriate to move away from an approach that gives all rights equal weight, to prioritising the CRC rights relating to child survival and non-discrimination.[35] While the CRC might provide an international framework for addressing children's rights, there are vast differences in legislation and child welfare practice across the Asia-Pacific. It may be difficult to achieve a consensus within a country on issues as germane as the definition of a child, age of consent and age of marriage, leave alone regionally. For example, a child is defined under the United Nations CRC as 'below the age of eighteen years unless, under the law applicable to the child, majority is attained earlier', the International Labour Organization definition recognizes a child to be below fifteen years of age; in India various legal instruments define the child as anyone below 12 years, 14 years or 18 years.

Cultural issues in parenting/child development

There is widespread understanding that parenting is a universal but 'cultural' activity. Cultural models of parenting comprise shared practices and shared ideas that are oriented toward broader socialization goals.[36] To understand childhood deviance or problems in childhood we must also understand what is considered a 'normal' childhood, as Timimi would argue.[37] Every culture defines what it is to be a normal child within their context. We know that childrearing practices influence the rate and expression of children's development. Different ethnic groups have wide variations as to how they view their child's development; their emphasis is influenced by their view of the child and the value they place on him/her. There is a wealth of cross-disciplinary literature on children's development and behavior across cultures that can be incorporated into CM practice.[1-2 17 38] Parenting practices such as breastfeeding, infant feeding, co-sleeping, toilet training and disciplining need to be understood in their cultural context.[39-42]

Cultural differences can be explored by comparing two diverse ways of bringing up children, well described in the hallmark text on child development across cultures by LeVine and others.[1] Although appearing an over simplification of the diversity in child rearing practices and parental goals for child development, exploring 'pedagogic' versus 'child-centred' styles of parenting illustrates different approaches well (Table 1). In the pedagogic style the major parental goals for children are to learn to feel emotionally independent from their parents and to develop interactive and language skills, whereas, in the child-centered style of child rearing, the major parental goal is to protect the health and survival of the infant. A similar conceptualization of these two extremes of cultural paradigms is to consider 'individualistic' versus 'collectivistic' cultures.[43] Timimi suggests that the dominant western (market economy) ideology of 'freedom' and 'individualism' gives rise to a societal ambivalence towards children. In contrast to this ambivalence, children of many non-western societies are welcomed into nurturing extended family structures where duty and responsibility over-ride individualism as the dominant value system.[44] In practice, most families today may adopt most aspects of one parenting style or borrow elements from a variety of parenting styles rather than fit neatly into either end of the spectrum. We also have to acknowledge the paradox of societies that are nurturing and celebratory of children and childhoods while tacitly accepting or ignoring practices that are cruel or harmful to children. A particular challenge today is unprecedented migration and mobility; creating circumstances for CM to occur.[45-46] Families are often moving from traditional and/or close knit communities; they may struggle to maintain cultural practices in a context where they have lost the traditional support system but do not have a new support system to replace it or may be reluctant to accept support systems from other cultures (Table 1).

Table 1 Contrasting Parental Goals in Child Rearing Practices	
Pedagogic	**Child-centred**
Lack of co-sleeping	Co-sleeping and breastfeeding on demand
Relatively tolerant of other separations	Respond rapidly to infant crying
Inceased emphasis on verbal interaction	Decreased verbal interaction
Decreased emphasis on physical contact	Increased physical contact
Modified from LeVine et al[1]	

Koramoa suggests a useful way of understanding cultural differences in beneficial and harmful child rearing (Table 2) with some scenarios unacceptable at one end for example extreme neglect compared with those that enrich the child's cultural development and individuality.[47] Although helpful, there is little guidance on how to deal with families from different cultures having different attitudes to physical discipline, which is probably the most common cause of cross-cultural clashes in the child protection field in the Western world. Many cultures traditionally accept physical punishment of children. Studies in diverse populations including Chinese,[24] Latinos,[48] and South Koreans[49] have explored the issue of physical discipline and its continuum of physical abuse. Belonging to an ethnic group does not necessarily mean that all aspects of that group are embraced, but research suggests that levels of verbal and physical punishment do vary in different ethnic groups.[50] In a similar way, levels of nurturing are also linked with cultural background and the negative effects of abuse on the child may be countered by a strong, positive, nurturing

element.[51] Koramoa's continuum categorises female genital mutilation,[52] also known as female genital cutting or circumcision as "harmful" whilst circumcision referring to the male ritual as "potentially harmful". Labelling FGM as "tradition", cannot justify this practice, which is recognized as a human rights violation and is well-documented to result in severe physical and psychological complications affecting 100 - 140 million girls and women mainly in parts of Africa and Asia.[53, 54-56] However, dealing with this practice sensitively in a rapidly changing world is still a challenge.

Child maltreatment in the Asia-Pacific region: what the literature tells us

Does the published literature provide an accurate guide to the epidemiology and burden of CM in the region and is cultural identity and ethnicity recorded adequately? In 2001, Behl *et al* published their results on the exploration of ethnicity in content analysis of CM literature between the

Table 2 Cultural practices in child rearing in Asia-Pacific: A continuum.[1,47]		
Practice	**Professional Response**	**Example**
Beneficial	Promote	Breast feeding Infant massage Showing respect Child celebratory Culture
Neutral	Respect	Threaded beads Toilet training at one year Rites of passage rituals Traditional 'healing' practices
Potentially harmful	Educate	Inner cleansing Co-sleeping* Circumcision Moxibustion, cupping coining Traditional 'healing' practices
Harmful	Prevent	Chilli in vagina Female foeticie/infanticide Neglect of girl child Child marriage Female genital mutilation Honour killings Forced marriage Child trafficking

*If there are risk factors such as cigarette smoking, drug misuse and overweight parents Breast feeding, infant massage, showing respect, child celebratory culture

1970s to 1990s finding that only seven percent of the studies focussed on ethnic or cultural issues while half reported on ethnicity of participants.[57] Miller *et al,*[58] found an improvement between 1999 and 2005, as 13% of studies focussed specifically on ethnocultural issues, whilst three-quarters reported on ethnicity of participants. In western countries, comparative studies on CM in different groups is often marred by what Fontes terms "ethnic lumping",[59] where "Asian Americans" or "Asian Pacific Islander", and "Black and ethnic minority" (UK terminology) can lump together cultural groups from very diverse backgrounds, with striking differences in other social and environmental indices.

Arriving at the burden of CM accurately is difficult due to the wide range of definitions, legislative frameworks, workforce availability in health and welfare systems and societal concern about the issue. In the surveys of child abuse in 28 developing and transitional countries, the highest prevalence of abuse was in African countries; however even for children in transitional countries (many Asian countries) the prevalence of psychological, moderate, and severe physical abuse for the preceding month was 56%, 46% and 9%, respectively. The risk of all forms of abuse was higher for male children, those living with many household members and in poorer families.[60] A meta analysis of all published studies on child sexual abuse prevalence,[61] found lowest rates for both girls (113/1000) and boys (41/1000) in Asia, and highest rates for girls in Australia (215/1000) and for boys in Africa (193/1000). A recent study from Taiwan documented the incidence of hospitalization due to CM in the decade 1996-2007 and found that it varied from 13.2/100,000 for infants, 3.5/100,000 for children aged 1-3 years, 2.1/100,000 for children aged 4-6 years and 3.3/100,000 for children aged 7-12 years.[62]

A high school survey from southern China in 2005 revealed very high reported levels of parental psychological aggression (78%), corporal punishment (23%), severe physical maltreatment (18%), but low prevalence of sexual abuse (0.6%).[63] Even more troubling figures from the Indian Government sanctioned CM survey in 2007 revealed that two thirds of children surveyed were physically maltreated (overwhelmingly by their parents), 65% of school going children faced corporal punishment, half of the children surveyed worked every day of the week and 22% reported

facing severe forms of sexual abuse.[64] A Malaysian study of adolescents in high school exploring the types of childhood victimization experiences young people reported found that emotional and physical types of victimization were most common, with 22% exposed to more than one type and males reported more physical, emotional, and sexual victimization.[65] A survey of urban middle-class professions in India found that over 40% admitted to using "abusive" violence towards their children in routine child rearing.[66] The particularly heinous crime of female infanticide and feticide that is well documented in India and China, receives global media attention, but child welfare professionals have been powerless to tackle this issue.[30-31 67] On the other hand, there are parts of Asia-Pacific, where CM rates may well be significantly lower than reported in western countries. Graham in the paper comparing the United Kingdom and Japan in various social indices, suggests that the rate of CM and criminality is much lower in Japan due to lower rates of family breakdown, greater respect for authority and emphasis on discipline in Japan.[68] A recent study investigating multiple types of CM in Vietnam, found that the combined influence of adverse individual and family factors and of CM upon mental health in adolescents in Vietnam was consistent with research in western countries. The authors highlighted the pernicious effects of emotional maltreatment which was widespread in this survey, on the wellbeing of adolescents, given that CM in Asian communities is often construed as severe physical violence alone.[69] There is a clear need for a more rigorous research base as well as a more nuanced cultural understanding of the research base, from which to base our advocacy efforts in this region.

What do we know about harmful practices in Asia-Pacific region?

Harmful and cruel practices against children unfortunately are far too prevalent in the Asia-Pacific region. Large-scale societal scourges such as child labour are widespread despite most countries adhering to International Labour Organization guidelines, such that the numbers of working children in countries in South Asia number in the millions.[32-34,70] Vast numbers of children also end up as street children and are particularly vulnerable to all forms of maltreatment as well as health

Case Example 1

The greater role of the extended family in child rearing (Malaysia)

A seven-year-old boy presented with multiple injuries characteristic of physical abuse including bruises/lacerations from being beaten, and multiple burns from being branded with heated kitchen utensils. This child was the only one of his siblings who was placed in the care of his grandmother from early infancy, because he was regarded as bringing "bad luck" to the family. As a result, his attachment figure was his grandmother. The child was sent back to live with his parents when he started school. He was not allowed to see his grandmother, who tried to meet him when he was at school. His parents said that he was naughty and that he had been spoiled by his grandmother who was too indulgent.

Case formulation

The involvement of the extended family in child rearing is very common in the region. It is useful when it complements the role of the parents by filling gaps in the provision of care to the child and guiding young, inexperienced parents. However, conflicts and problems may arise when such involvement interferes with the establishment and maintenance of the parent-child relationship and parents feel excluded from making decisions regarding the upbringing of their child. Urbanisation and economic migration have changed the context in which the traditional support network of the family functions and creates gaps in support as nuclear families move away from their place of origin. Children may live with grandparents and extended family in rural areas during infancy and early childhood while parents work in urban centres. Tensions and conflicts may arise when children experience adjustment problems upon reuniting with their parents and other siblings as they start schooling. A combination of factors such as failure to establish attachment with parents, differing parenting styles, superstitious beliefs, the acceptance of corporal punishment to enforce discipline and the isolation from the extended family and community that may modulate the use of excessively harsh punishment may interact to increase the potential for maltreatment.

Case Example 2

Child Sexual abuse in a joint family situation (India)

An 11-year-old girl presented with recurrent abdominal pain occurring many times a day for the last 18 months. She avoided her friends, withdrew from normal activities and engaged in school refusal. She was shown to multiple doctors for these complaints, was extensively investigated to no avail. Physical examination was normal. She was treated with heavy painkillers; sometimes the pain was so unbearable, the girl would pass out. The mother suffered from severe depression following the death of a younger sibling. After multiple sessions of interviewing, the girl confided in the paediatrician that she had been sexually assaulted by her older male cousin on many occasions, while her mother slept in the same room. When the girl disclosed the abuse to her mother, she was warned that she would be thrown out of the house if she disclosed it to anyone else. The family had to keep it a secret so as not to bring shame upon them. Her cousin also threatened to kill her if she disclosed the abuse.

Case formulation

In this case, the paediatrician obtained a detailed behavioural and psychosocial history, appropriately situated the pain in the abdomen within the family and cultural context. The paediatrician developed a relationship with both the child and family, and was able to elicit details of the history that was not available to the many others involved in the assessment and investigation of this child. Co-sleeping and bed sharing with extended family members is not uncommon in Asia, and cousins are often given a similar status to siblings. Preserving family honour by maintaining family secrecy at the expense of children's wellbeing is also not uncommon. In this instance, it took protracted culturally oriented counselling sessions provided both to the girl and her family in a safe setting to improve outcomes for the girl.

problems.[71-74] Child trafficking, another crime against children, occurs in the context of poverty, gender inequality and discrimination, however demand factors play a significant role.[75-77] Korbin in her hallmark anthropological explorations of CM in traditional cultures, discussed the vastly different parenting practices of indigenous groups in the Pacific from the Polynesians noted for high indulgence of children to the Enga of Papua New Guinea who subject their children to severe physical punishments for seemingly trivial offenses.[17] Table 2 lists potentially harmful child rearing practices in the Asia-Pacific, using Koramoa's continuum concept. Some traditional healing practices such as coining, cupping and moxibustion are particularly common in Asia. These practices may cause pain and result in bruising and burns, which may be regarded as maltreatment by health professionals.[39,78] Approaching these situations with sensitivity and educating the community to opt for alternatives that are more effective requires the recognition that the primary motivation of families who seek these treatments is to heal and not intentionally harm the child, as well as the acknowledgement that many beneficial treatments in modern medicine are also painful and unpleasant.

Towards a culturally competent response to CM in the Asia-Pacific region

There is no simple answer to the relationship between diverse cultures and CM. Taking into account the child in the context of the family, the culture and an adequate assessment of 'risk', we propose a philosophical and practical move towards a culturally competent response to CM. Cultural competence is a set of congruent behaviors, attitudes, and policies that come together in a system, agency or among professionals and enable that system, agency or those professions to work effectively in cross-cultural situations.[79] Cultural competence is much more than awareness of cultural differences; the focus is on the capacity of our systems to improve health and wellbeing by integrating culture into every aspect of delivery of our services. At its core, cultural competency for the individual practitioner is about self-reflexive practice, and not about assumptions or generalizations. It is the misperception of some

cultural knowledge, believing that 'I know about this custom', that often leads to false assumptions and stereotyping.[80]

We believe there are many examples of positive and child affirming strategies and interventions that are culturally congruent if not competent within the Asia-Pacific region. For example, in the 1960s, neonatal jaundice in glucose-6-phosphate-dehydrogenase (G6PD) deficient infants and consequent severe disease created a major public health problem in Singapore.[81] A combination of factors accounted for this: a significant proportion of G6PDdeficiency in the population, increased vulnerability of Asian neonates to non-haemolytic jaundice compared to Caucasians, and the practice of consumption of traditional herbs by the mother that could increase biological vulnerability. A multipronged approach has virtually eliminated the occurrence of the severe complication (kernicterus) in the local population in Singapore and Malaysia. This includes universal screening for G6PD deficiency at birth to identify vulnerable infants, surveillance for neonatal jaundice through improved maternal and child health services, the provision of these services at relatively low cost by government, education of the population through the media and the availability of phototherapy as an effective treatment for neonatal jaundice. The move towards culturally competent care for the child and the family is best realized when all the components of the care continuum work together, i.e. the individual (i.e. health worker, welfare professional, child advocate), the professional body (e.g. Indian Academy of Pediatrics)[82], the organization (health service, government or non-governmental organization) and the systems within which all this occurs.

Clearly, the Asia-Pacific region with its large and growing child and youth population faces particular challenges in this arena as already outlined. The recently held Asia Pacific Child Abuse & Neglect conference in New Delhi in 2011 brought together over 600 health, welfare, policy and legal advocates for children from governments and non-governmental organizations across the Asia-Pacific region. Many of the presentations dealt with the unique or commonplace child rights violations in the region, such as trafficking, neglect of the girl child, street children; however, there were a few significant culturally competent success stories that ameliorated risks and enhanced child safety. The historic 'Delhi Declaration' made at the conference urged state parties to make the "recognition of child abuse, neglect, exploitation and all forms of violence against children a critical issue of justice and development in the Asia-Pacific region; as well as work for the ratification and implementation of relevant international and regional conventions, strengthening regional commitment to protecting children".[83]

Acknowledging the role of culture and the child's cultural identity can have health enhancing effects and is strongly promoted in the CRC.[20,84-85] As Korbin eloquently states, a cross-cultural perspective on CM challenges complacency about what is good or bad for children and forces a re-examination of commonly held definitions of and causal explanations for

CM.[18] Children, young people and their advocates in this dynamic region in the 21st century face these challenges everyday. We need relevant cross-disciplinary research and practice on child rights and CM from the Asia-Pacific to be made more visible as well as more rigorous. Korbin suggests a three-pronged approach to dealing with this complex area: efforts need to be made to "unpack" culture, to promote the understanding of culture in context, and to enhance research on CM and culture.[18] To this, we can only echo the pledge from the Delhi Declaration: 'strive for achievement of child rights and the building of a caring community for every child, free of violence and discrimination,'[83] in the best interests of the child.

References

1. LeVine RA, LeVine S, Dixon S, Richman A, Leiderman PH, Keefer CH, et al. *Child Care and Culture: Lessons from Africa* Cambridge, UK Cambridge University Press, 1994.

2. LeVine RA, New RS, editors. *Anthropology and child development: A cross-cultural reader*. Malden, MA: Blackwell Publishing, 2008.

3. Fadiman A. *The Spirit Catches You and You Fall Down: A Hmong Child, Her American Doctors, and the Collision of Two Cultures.*. New York, NY: Farrar, Straus, and Giroux, 1997.

4. HMSO. The Victoria Climbié inquiry. Report of an inquiry by Lord Laming. In: Office TS, editor. London, 2003.

5. O'Hagan. Culture, cultural identity, and cultural sensitivity in child and family social work. *Child & Family Social Work* 1999; 4(4):269–81.

6. Abney V. Cultural competency in the field of child maltreatment. In: JEB Myers LB, J Briere, C Terry Hendrix, C Jenny & TA Reid, editor. *The APSAC handbook on child maltreatment*. Thousand Oaks, CA: Sage, 2002.

7. Connolly M, Crichton-Hill Y, Y W. *Culture and child protection: reflexive responses.* London: Jessica Kingsley Publishers, 2006.

8. Bhugra D. Migration and mental health. *Acta Psychiatr Scand* 2004; 109(4):243–58.

9. Helms JE. *Black and White racial identity: Theory, research, and practice.* NY, England Greenwood Press, 1990.

10. Bhugra D, Bhui K, Mallett R, Desai M, Singh J, Leff J. Cultural identity and its measurement:

A questionnaire for Asians. *International Review of Psychiatry* 1999; 11(2–3):244-49.

11. Bhabha HK. *The Location of Culture*. London and New York: Routledge Classics, 2004.

12. UNESCO World Report. Investing in cultural diversity and intercultural dialogue. In: Georges Kutukdjian JC, editor. Paris: United Nations Educational, Cultural and Scientific Organization, 2009.

13. Daro D, editor. *World Perspectives on Child Abuse: Seventh Edition*. West Chicago, Illinois: ISPCAN, 2006.

14. Collier AF, McClure FH, Collier J, Otto C, Polloi A. Culture-specific views of child maltreatment and parenting styles in a Pacific-Island community. *Child Abuse & Neglect* 1999; 23(3):229–44.

15. Chan YC, Lam GLT, Shae WC. Children's views on child abuse and neglect: Findings from an exploratory study with Chinese children in Hong Kong. *Child Abuse and Neglect* 2011; 35(3):162–72.

16. Korbin JE. Cross-Cultural perspectives and research directions for the 21st century. *Child Abuse & Neglect* 1991; 15(Sup1):67–77.

17. Korbin J. Anthropological contributions to the study of child abuse. *Child Abuse & Neglect* 1977; 1(1):7–24.

18. Korbin JE. Culture and child maltreatment: cultural competence and beyond. *Child Abuse & Neglect* 2002; 26(6–7):637–44.

19. Waterston T, Goldhagen J. Why children's rights are central to international child health. *Arch Dis Child* 2007; 92(2):176–80.

20. Welbourne P. Culture, Children's Rights and Child Protection. *Child Abuse Review* 2002; 11:345–58.

21. Kawewe S, Dibie R. United Nations and the problem of women and children abuse in the Third World nations. *Social Justice* 1997; 26:78–98.

22. Svevo-Cianci KA, Hart SN, Rubinson C. Protecting children from violence and maltreatment: A qualitative comparative analysis assessing the implementation of U.N. CRC Article 19. *Child Abuse and Neglect* 2010; 34(1):45–56.

23. Lau JT, Liu JL, Cheung JC, Yu A, Wong CK. Prevalence and correlates of physical abuse in Hong Kong Chinese adolescents: a population-based approach. *Child Abuse & Neglect* 1999; 23(6):549–57.

24. Tang CS-k. Corporal punishment and physical maltreatment against children: A community study on Chinese parents in Hong Kong. *Child Abuse & Neglect* 2006; 30:893–907.

25. Kim DH, Kim KI, Park YC, Zhang LD, Lu MK, Li D. Children's experience of violence in China and Korea: a transcultural study. *Child Abuse & Neglect* 2000; 24(9):1163–73.

26. Mishra N, Thakur KK, Koirala R, Shrestha D, Poudel R, Jha R. Corporal punishment in Nepalese school children: Facts, legalities and implications. *Journal of Nepal Paediatric Society* 2010; 30(2):98–109.

27. Lau C. Child prostitution in Thailand. *Journal of Child Health Care* 2008; 12(2):144–55.

28. Lee ACW, So KT. Child slavery in Hong Kong: case report and historical review. *Hong Kong Medical Journal* 2006; 12(6):463–6.

29. Premi MK. Female infanticide and child neglect as possible reasons for low sex ratio in the Punjab, 1881-1931. *Population Geography* 1994; 16(1–2):33–48.

30. Sahni M, Verma N, Narula D, Varghese RM, Sreenivas V, Puliyel JM. Missing girls in India: Infanticide, feticide and made-to-order pregnancies? Insights from hospital-based sex-ratio-at-birth over the last century. *PLoS ONE* 2008;3(5).

31. Bandyopadhyay M. Missing girls and son preference in rural India: looking beyond popular myth. *Health Care for Women International* 2003; 24(10):910–26.

32. Gulzar SA, Vertejee S, Pirani L. Child labour: a public health issue. *JPMA - Journal of the Pakistan Medical Association* 2009; 59(11):778–81.

33. Dalal K, Rahman F, Jansson B. The origin of violent behavior among child labourers in India. *Global Public Health* 2008; 3(1):77–92.

34. Hadi A. Child abuse among working children in rural Bangladesh: prevalence and determinants. *Public Health* 2000; 114(5):380–4.

35. Pemberton S, Gordon D, Nandy S, Pantazis C, 3 6 . Townsend P. Child rights and child poverty: can the international framework of children's rights be used to improve child survival rates? *PLoS Medicine* 2007; 4(10):1567–70.

37. Lamm B, Keller H. Understanding cultural models of parenting: the role of intracultural variation and response style. *Journal of Cross-Cultural Psychology* 2007; 38:50–57.

38. Timimi S. *Naughty boys: anti-social behavior, 39.ADHD and the role of culture*. Hampshire: Palgrave Macmillan, 2005.

40. Hackett L, Hackett R. Parental ideas of normal and deviant child behavior. A comparison of two ethnic groups. *British Journal of Psychiatry* 1993; 162:353–7.

41. Boon WH. Child health in Singapore: traditional practices and their effects. *Clinical Pediatrics* 1969; 8(10):611–16.

42. Ramamurthy MB, Sekartini R, Ruangdaraganon N, Huynh DHT, Sadeh A, Mindell JA. Effect of current breastfeeding on sleep patterns in infants from Asia-Pacific region. *Journal of Paediatrics and Child Health* 2012:no-no.

43. Koc I, Camurdan AD, Beyazova U, Ilhan MN, Sahin F. Toilet training in Turkey: the factors that affect timing and duration in different sociocultural groups. *Child: Care, Health and Development* 2008; 34(4):475–81.

44. Bandyopadhyay M. Impact of ritual pollution on lactation and breastfeeding practices in rural West Bengal, India. *International Breastfeeding Journal* 2009; 4(2):8.

45. Triandis HC, Suh EM. Cultural influences on personality. *Annual Review of Psychology* 2002; 53(1):133–60.

46. Timimi S. Effect of globalization on children's mental health. *BMJ* 2005; 331:37–39.

47. Wong WCW, Chen WQ, Goggins WB, Tang CS, Leung PW. Individual, familial and community determinants of child physical abuse among high-school students in China. *Social Science & Medicine* 2009; 68(10):1819–25.

48. Jirapramukpitak T, Abas M, Harpham T, Prince M. Rural-urban migration and experience of childhood abuse in the young Thai population. *Journal of Family Violence* 2011; 26(8):607–15.

49. Koramoa J, Lynch MA, Kinnair D. A Continuum of Child-Rearing: Responding to Traditional Practices. *Child Abuse Review Vol.* 2002; 11:415–21.

50. Fontes LA. Child discipline and physical abuse in immigrant Latino families: reducing violence and misunderstandings. *Journal of Counseling and Development* 2002; 80(1):31–40.

51. Park MS. The factors of child physical abuse in Korean immigrant families. *Child Abuse & Neglect* 2001; 25(7):945–58.

52. Runyan DK, Shankar V, Hassan F, Hunter WM, Jain D, Paula CS, et al. International Variations in Harsh Child Discipline. *Pediatrics* 2010:peds.2008-374.

53. Ferrari AM. The impact of culture upon child rearing practices and definitions of maltreatment. *Child Abuse & Neglect* 2002; 26(8):793–813.

54. Adam T, Bathija H, Bishai D, Bonnenfant Y-T, Darwish M, Huntington D, et al. Estimating the obstetric costs of female genital mutilation in six African countries. *Bulletin of the World Health Organization* 2010; 88:281–88.

55. Walder R. Why the problem continues in Britain. *BMJ* 1995; 310(6994):1593–94.

56. Black JA, Debelle GD. Female genital mutilation in Britain. *BMJ* 1995; 310(6994):1590–92.

57. Gallard C. Female genital mutilation in France. *BMJ* 1995; 310(6994):1592–93.

58. Almroth L, Elmusharaf S. Genital mutilation of girls. *Women's Health* 2007; 3(4):475–85.

59. Behl LE, Crouch JL, May PF, Valente AL, Conyngham HA. Ethnicity in child maltreatment research: A content analysis. *Child Maltreatment* 2001; 6(2):143–47.

60. Miller AB, Cross T. Ethnicity in child Maltreatment research: A replication of Behl et al.'s content analysis. *Child Maltreatment* 2006; 11(1):16–26.

61. Fontes LA. *Child abuse and culture: Working with diverse families*. New York: The Guildford Press, 2005.

62. Akmatov MK. Child abuse in 28 developing and transitional countries-results from the multiple indicator cluster surveys. *International Journal of Epidemiology* 2011; 40(1):219–27.

63. Stoltenborgh M, van Ijzendoorn MH, Euser EM, Bakermans-Kranenburg MJ. A global perspective on child sexual abuse: Meta-analysis of prevalence around the world. *Child Maltreatment* 2011; 16(2):79–101.

64. Chiang WL, Huang YT, Feng JY, Lu TH. Incidence of hospitalization due to child maltreatment in Taiwan, 1996-2007: A nationwide population-based study. *Child Abuse and Neglect* 2012; 36(2):135–41.

65. Leung PWS, Wong WCW, Chen WQ, Tang CSK. Prevalence and determinants of child maltreatment among high school students in Southern China: A large scale school based survey. *Child and Adolescent Psychiatry and Mental Health* 2008; 2(27).

66. Kacker L, Varadan S, Kumar P. Study on child abuse India 2007. New Delhi, India: Ministry of Women and Child Development - Government of India, 2007.

67. Choo W-Y, Dunne MP, Marret MJ, Fleming M, Wong Y-L. Victimization experiences of adolescents in Malaysia. *Journal of Adolescent Health* 2011; 49: 627–34.

68. Segal UA. Child abuse by the middle class? A study of professionals in India. *Child Abuse & Neglect* 1995; 19(2):217–31.

69. van Balen F, Inhorn MC. Son preference, sex selection, and the "new" new reproductive technologies. *International Journal of Health Services* 2003; 33(2):235–52.

70. Graham P. Child rearing and child outcomes in Japan and the UK. *Acta Paediatrica Japonica* 1998; 40(2): 164–7.

71. Nguyen HT, Dunne MP, Le AV. Multiple types of child maltreatment and adolescent mental health in Viet Nam.[Erratum appears in Bull World Health Organ. 2010 Mar; 88(3):236]. *Bulletin of the World Health Organization* 2010; 88(1):22–30.

72. Saddik B, Nuwayhid I. Child labour in Arab countries: Call for action [7]. *British Medical Journal* 2006; 333(7573):861–62.

73. Pagare D, Meena GS, Jiloha RC, Singh MM. Sexual abuse of street children brought to an observation home. *Indian Pediatrics* 2005; 42(2):134–1139.

74. Mathur M, Rathore P, Mathur M. Incidence, type and intensity of abuse in street children in India. *Child Abuse & Neglect* 2009; 33(12):907–13.

75. Navipour R, Mohebbi MR. Street children and runaway adolescents in Iran [9]. *Indian Pediatrics* 2004; 41(12):1283–84.

76. Njord L, Merrill RM, Njord R, Pachano JDR, Hackett A. Characterizing health behaviors and infectious disease prevalence among Filipino street children. *International Journal of Adolescent Medicine and Health* 2008; 20(3):367–74.

77. Rafferty Y. Children for sale: Child trafficking in Southeast Asia. *Child Abuse Review* 2007; 16(6):401–22.

78. Busza J, Castle S, Diarra A. Trafficking and health. *BMJ* 2004; 328(7452):1369–71.

79. McCauley HL, Decker MR, Silverman JG. Trafficking experiences and violence victimization of sex-trafficked young women in Cambodia. *International Journal of Gynaecology & Obstetrics* 2010; 110(3):266–7.

80. Ravanfar P, Dinulos JG. Cultural practices affecting the skin of children. *Current Opinion in Pediatrics* 2010;22:10.1097/MOP.0b013e32833bc352.

81. Cross TL BB, Dennis KW, Isaacs MR *Towards a Culturally Competent System of Care*. Washington, DC: Georgetown University Child Development Center, 1989.

82. Webb E, Maddocks A, Bongilli J. Effectively protecting Black and minority ethnic children from harm: Overcoming barriers to the child protection process. *Child Abuse Review* 2002; 11:394–410.

83. Brown WR, Boon WH. Hyperbilirubinemia and kernicterus in glucose-6-phosphate dehydrogenase-deficient infants in Singapore. *Clinical Pediatrics* 1968; 41(6):1055–68.

84. Aggarwal K, Dalwai S, Galagali P, Mishra D, Prasad C, Thadhani A. Recommendations on recognition and response to child abuse and neglect in the Indian setting. *Indian Pediatrics* 2010; 47(6):493–504.

85. Delhi declaration: Outcome document of 9th Asia Pacific Conference on Child Abuse and Neglect, (APCCAN 2011) New Delhi, India. 9th Asia Pacific Conference on Child Abuse and Neglect; 2011; New Delhi, India.

86. Raman S. Cultural Identity and Child Health. *J Trop Pediatr* 2006; 52(4):231–34.

87. Raman S, Hodes D. Cultural issues in child maltreatment. *Journal of Paediatrics and Child Health* 2012; 48:30–37.

25

Media and Child Protection

Devendra Sareen

Introduction

Media is one of the 4 pillars of democracy besides the Legislature, Judiciary, and the Executive. The existence of an independent judiciary, independent executive and a free media is essential for a healthy Constitutional democracy. Media plays a vital role in dissemination of information to the people at large and in raising public awareness of children's rights. However media freedom also entails a certain degree of responsibility. Journalists need to be aware of the consequences of their reporting. The way the media portrays children has a very profound impact on society's attitude towards them. Sensationalism is a great problem. Some journalists feel that if news is presented in a sensational manner, it would catch the attention of a larger group. Commercial competition leads to exploitation. In the rat race to garner more fame and money, journalists sometimes forget the essence of news reporting, and adopt unfair measures of collection of information and its publication. Media cannot make themselves the exploiters. Journalists can create sexually provocative images of children, which in turn may be used for pornography. A problem can be presented in such a way that certain aspects of the reality are highlighted and others downplayed. This directly and profoundly affects people's attitude and behavior in response to the news and to the child concerned. If a simple problem is presented in a more than required sensational manner, it can do more harm than good. Therefore journalists must be careful that a correct and precise report is given.

A free media is very important and freedom of expression is right of journalists. However,

that freedom must be balanced against other important rights, particularly the right of children freedom from fear and exploitation. Journalists should maintain high ethical standards especially in the news pertaining to children.

How does media influence the rights of a child?[1]

Children have the same human rights as adults but many children do not achieve their rights. The United Nations Convention on the Rights of the Child (UN-CRC) came into force in 1990. A lot of campaigns for child rights are based on the Convention. Human rights are commonly understood as "inalienable fundamental rights to which a person is inherently entitled, simply because she or he is a human being." Human rights are thus conceived as universal (applicable everywhere) and egalitarian (the same for everyone). Human rights belong to the people, they are intrinsic. They are inalienable, interdependent and indivisible. They are also equal and non discriminatory. Now if we discuss about childhood, we would see that children do not have full power to execute their rights. They are dependent on adults, and must depend on the support of adults to exercise their rights.

The rights of the children worth mentioning in this context are:[2]

The right to privacy

As per Article 8 of CRC:

1. States Parties undertake to respect the right of the child to preserve his or her identity,

including nationality, name and family relations as recognized by law without unlawful interference.

2. Where a child is illegally deprived of some or all of the elements of his or her identity, States Parties shall provide appropriate assistance and protection, with a view to re-establishing speedily his or her identity

The right to have views and express them

As per Article 12 of CRC:

1. States Parties shall assure to the child who is capable of forming his or her own views the right to express those views freely in all matters affecting the child, the views of the child being given due weight in accordance with the age and maturity of the child.
2. For this purpose, the child shall in particular be provided the opportunity to be heard in any judicial and administrative proceedings affecting the child, either directly, or through a representative or an appropriate body, in a manner consistent with the procedural rules of national law.

Freedom of expression and access to the media

As per Article 13 of CRC:

1. The child shall have the right to freedom of expression; this right shall include freedom to seek, receive and impart information and ideas of all kinds, regardless of frontiers, either orally, in writing or in print, in the form of art, or through any other media of the child›s choice.
2. The exercise of this right may be subject to certain restrictions, but these shall only be such as are provided by law and are necessary:
   a. For respect of the rights or reputations of others; or
   b. For the protection of national security or of public order (order public), or of public health or morals.

Journalists must know about such legislation and must have very clear policies for interviewing young children.

Recently the National Commission for the Protection of Child Rights has received complaints on the use of the name and photographs of an 8 year old boy in Begusarai, Bihar. The boy who is alleged to have killed three children was tagged a "serial killer" in the media reports.[3]

No child who is in conflict with law should be named or his photograph published.

The child acts without experience or knowledge of what he or she is doing.

Media: Its positive impact on the overall development of a child

Media can have a positive influence in the development of a child. But those positive aspects need to be highlighted and followed.

Article 17 recognizes the positive role of the mass media on the development of the children. It says:

States Parties recognize the important function performed by the mass media and shall ensure that the child has access to information and material from a diversity of national and international sources, especially those aimed at the promotion of his or her social, spiritual and moral well-being and physical and mental health.

To this end, States Parties shall:[1]

a. Encourage the mass media to disseminate information and material of social and cultural benefit to the child and in accordance with the spirit of article 29;
b. Encourage international co-operation in the production, exchange and dissemination of such information and material from a diversity of cultural, national and international sources;
c. Encourage the production and dissemination of children's books;
d. Encourage the mass media to have particular regard to the linguistic needs of the child who belongs to a minority group or who is indigenous;
e. Encourage the development of appropriate guidelines for the protection of the child from information and material injurious to his or her well-being, bearing in mind the provisions of articles 13 and 18.

Juvenile Justice: A burning problem and the role of media in it

"Young people today are unbearable, without moderation... Our world is reaching a critical stage. Children no longer listen to their parents. More and more children are committing crimes and if urgent steps are not taken, the end of the world as we know it, is fast approaching." These words sound familiar but are from the Greek poet Hesiod writing in the 8th Century BC.

"Juvenile in conflict with law" would mean a juvenile alleged to have committed an offence and not completed 18 years of age on the date of commission of such an offence.[1.]

However, only if the enquiring authority, in the interest of the juvenile, permits such a disclosure in writing, can we justify the publication of such news by the press.

Sometimes sensationalism can lead to grave problems. Media can at times distort the reality of a crime by very selective reporting. This can encourage anti-social behavior in young people by portraying a more glamorous picture of crime.. Privacy of the minor deserves special attention. Any damage to the environment of the minor must be taken seriously. No action of the journalist must cause any trouble for the future of the minor.

Usually the courts give privacy orders, in which, the identity of the accused cannot be disclosed if he submits a request stating that it would harm his privacy.

Section 83 of the Indian Penal Code (IPC), states that nothing is an offence which is done by a child above 7 years of age and under 12 years, who has not attained sufficient maturity of understanding to judge the nature and consequences of his conduct on that occasion. It should also be noted that children below the age of 7 years are deemed to be incapable of criminal offence as per section 82 of the IPC.

The Juvenile Justice (Care and Protection of Children) Act 2000 [Further referred to as JJ Act] clearly lays down: "No report in any newspaper, magazine or news-sheet or visual media of any enquiry regarding a juvenile in conflict with law (under an amendment proposed and now under consideration by the Standing Committee of Parliament, the words or 'a child in need of care and protection' are to be added here) under this

Act shall disclose the names, address or school or any other particulars calculated to lead to the identification of the juvenile."

So the following points must be kept in mind by media personnel while reporting the cases pertaining to juveniles:,[4, 4]

1. Privacy of a child is of utmost importance, and should be respected at all stages. Media must never publish anything that would lead to the identification of the victim. The Juvenile Justice Board can initiate action against journalists who violate this principle.
2. The records of juveniles must be kept strictly confidential, and should not be disclosed to any third party.
3. The media must always remember that they can cause harm to the juvenile, who might get labeled as an "offender". Their irresponsible actions of publicizing juvenile crimes can jeopardize the future life and job opportunities for such juveniles. The past of such children will always haunt them and they will never be able to lead a happy and stress free life.

Hence, juvenile legislation protects the juvenile's **right to privacy** by restricting media reportage.[5, 6]

If such laws and guidelines for juveniles are followed by media personnel, and prompt and adequate action is taken against the offending journalists, it would certainly help the cause of juvenile justice and would make life easier for these children.

Ethical guidelines for interviewing a child

It is not important to set a rulebook which says "what to do and what not to do" Rather journalists must develop moral and ethical thinking. Guidelines given to journalists should help them to think rationally, and give them extra confidence to bring forth problems and their solutions. Journalists who think through ethical issues are more liberated in their opinions and more confident that they can apply principles in a consistent way.

First of all we should know the basic things a journalist should follow while interviewing children.

1. Interviews with children should, except in exceptional circumstances, always take place in the presence of someone acting in the best interests of the child.

2. The interviewer should sit or stand at the same height as the child.
3. The child should be comfortable and relaxed and not under any kind of pressure.
4. The interviewer should adopt very calm tone so that the child feels relaxed and comfortable.
5. The interviewer should ask open ended rather than leading questions. Leading questions might lead to eliciting of wrong information. Open ended questions give a better opportunity to the child to bring across the exact story.
6. Questions should be directed to the child, not to the adult; the adult should observe and not intervene, unless absolutely necessary.
7. The story can be verified from the guardians, principal, other children etc.
8. If the help of a translator is being taken, the journalists must make sure that they translate the exact words of the child and not distort the information.

Journalist offer ask unreasonable question and are not very familiar with the actual content. They are more interested in gathering sensational and bad news and may project the information in a distorted manner. More over mostly fresh news is reported and there is very either subsequent follow up.

Journalists needs to build trust amongst the official sources and the best interest of the child must guide their actions. They must show their credibility by preparing themselves beforehand. They should ask questions intelligently and provide a broader context of the issue. All journalists and media professionals have a duty to maintain the highest ethical and professional standards and should promote the Rights of the Child. Media organisations should regard violation of the rights of children as important situations question for investigation.

Guidelines while photographing a child

Certain guidelines should be followed while photographing a child:

1. Gaining consent to photograph or interview- Children should never be photographed without their specific consent.
2. They should use long shots.
3. Shoot from behind.
4. Use the child's environment.

5. Shoot hands, legs etc. Sometimes these can tell a powerful story.
6. It should be confirmed that journalists, photographers, camera operators and other media professionals do not violate children's rights.
7. A child is likely to be excited or get afraid at the sight of the cameras or TV crews, depending on its age and experience.

For example, an international NGO had organized a media visit to a refugee camp where photographers took pictures of weeping children. Their pictures stormed the newspapers across the world the following day. Later the press officers were startled to discover why the children were crying. They thought the long lens cameras were guns and that the photographers were soldiers who had come to kill them.[1]

One important point here is that photographers who take pictures in one country for use in another often feel that the pictures are not intrusive because they will not be seen by anyone who knows or can identify the child. Not every picture becomes famous and not everyone grows up as Kim did to become a UNESCO Ambassador. However, this is not always true, and explicit consent is needed form the child and responsible adults for any additional use.

Also, the picture of a child taken "innocently" may be later used by a pedophile for sexual gratification. But if used properly, it may convey the story of a child in difficult circumstances.

So **to summarize**, while obtaining information, the following should be kept in mind:

1. Get consent
2. Look for red flags
3. Prepare/ brief the child
4. Prepare yourself
5. Choose an appropriate location.
6. Set guidelines for the photographer.

Reporting child abuse[1,10]

Abuse has a very profound effect on the mindset of a child. It leaves a child worried, stressed and traumatized[11]. Along with the physical trauma due to injury,[12] it involves emotional trauma as well. The child is not able to exactly articulate what happened, is not able to talk about it openly due to social stigmas and fear of people not believing him/ her. Also, there is a guilt of other people knowing about it.

So it is very important for the journalists to pay special attention to the reporting of stories of child abuse.

They should also remember that children are not homogenous. All of them do not respond in the same way. There can be issues like gender issues. Always remember, journalists can give voice to children. It is their duty to throw light on those being mistreated, forced to work, and pushed into the sex trade. They must make the people aware of what is happening around them. The myth that children are protected from HIV and other STD's must be aggressively countered.

The following should be kept in mind while reporting the cases of child abuse:

1. Always remember, journalists can give voice to children.
2. It is their duty to draw light on these maltreatments. They must make the people aware of what is happening around them.
3. While it is important for the journalists to make sure that they do not reveal the identity of the child, at the same time they must report their story in a compelling way. A definite balance must be struck.
4. Some special points must be kept in mind while reporting about child labor. They must make sure that the intervention of media does not create problems for the child later.
5. They should talk to children involved and should also follow up what happens to the children afterwards.
6. A lot of figures are given, telling the number of children who are recruited in sex trade. Journalists must throw a light on the facts and bring the correct numbers in front of the people.
7. Journalists should always be clear in their reporting that the young people being exploited are children.
8. They must use the appropriate language.
9. They must reveal as to how the children come to be put on sale?
10. There are a lot of myths that children are protected from HIV and other STD's. Journalists must counter these myths.
11. Sensationalism must be avoided.
12. Consider carefully the consequences of publication of any material concerning children.
13. Avoid the use of sexualized images of children.
14. Journalists must try to preserve the identity of the child, unless it is in public interest and in the interest of the child.
15. They should avoid the use of words like traumatized (can use distressed instead), child sex workers (can use children forced into prostitution) etc.
1. While it is important for the journalists to make sure that they do not reveal the identity of the child, at the same time they must report their story in a compelling way. A definite balance must be struck.
2. When reporting about child labor, they must make sure that the intervention of media does not create problems for the child later.
3. When reporting on child labor, they should not just talk to children involved, but should also follow up what happens to the children afterwards.
4. Journalists reporting on exploited children must use appropriate language. They should avoid the use of words like traumatized (can use distressed instead), child sex workers (can use children forced into prostitution) etc.
5. When reporting on children being exploited sexually, they must reveal how the children come to be put on sale.
6. They must conceal the identity of the child, unless it is essential in public interest and in the interest of the child.
7. They must consider carefully the consequences of publication of any material concerning children.
8. They must avoid the use of sexualized images of children.
9. Above all, sensationalism must be scrupulously avoided.

Irresponsible reporting can lead to stigmatization, reprisal, distress, negative publicity and victimization of the child. So media persons have to be very careful about what they publish and how they publish.

Informed, sensitive and professional journalism is a key element in any media strategy. While reporting, journalists must move beyond the typical story to focusing on the circumstances surrounding the abuse, and also focus on what makes children in certain circumstances more vulnerable.

Journalists must be provided training to achieve high ethical standards. Media organizations should regard violation of the rights of children and issues related to children's safety, privacy, security, their education, health and social welfare and all forms of exploitation as important questions for investigation, internal action, as well as public debate.[13]

What do the media professionals need to know?

It is very important for the journalists to have proper knowledge of child abuse and other problems faced by the children. They must know why abuse occurs and how can it be prevented. be aware of the social, legal, economic causes and consequences of abuse.

Recommendations[1,6]

Media professionals need to develop strategies that strengthen the role of media in providing information on all aspects of children's rights

1. Journalists must be offered proper training to ensure proper reporting. They must be well acquainted with the Convention on The Rights of the Child and must follow ethical guidelines pertaining to the reporting of issues concerning children. In fact, media organisations should consider appointing specialist children's correspondents for covering all aspects of child abuse.

2. Journalists must be given special training to be able to understand the point of view of children. They must understand that all children are not same and different children have different requirements. They must handle each case at an individual level and should try to understand the psychology of the child.

3. All journalists must be very cautious in dealing with children, following certain codes of conduct. These include taking consent of the child for reporting, interviewing and photographing the child appropriately, not intimidating the child, etc.

4. Journalists must provide confidence to the child, that whatever they tell will be kept confidential. Only then will children, especially victims of abuse, open up to them fully.

5. They must publish the story in such a way that the children's rights are highlighted and they are protected/ rescued from abusive situations, yet they must make sure the children concerned are not victimized in the process.

6. Society and government bodies must respect the need for independent journalism. But journalists must recognize the fact that although freedom of expression is important, but they must strike a balance between this and protection of child rights.[14]

7. Children must undergo Media Literacy. They should be well aware of what is happening around and should be the well informed "media consumers".

Children are the mirrors of our society. It is very important to safeguard their rights. The child of today is the citizen of tomorrow. If a child is being abused somewhere, it is the moral duty of the journalist to bring a clear picture in front of the society and also do the needful to protect the child.[16] Media is a very powerful tool and if used properly, it can do wonders.[15]

Conversely, if a child is oppressed, wrong portrayal might further add to his or her dismay. A balance must be struck between the independence of journalism and the privacy of a child. Sometimes a child may commit some crime, even without knowing its gravity. Such cases have to handled delicately. Improper reporting by the media on such issues can completely destroy the child's future. It must be born in mind that the same issue, pertaining to a child and an adult, has to handled differently.[17] We must try to preserve their innocence and not crumple it underneath sensationalism and petty gains. Together we must make this world a better place to live for them.

Acknowledgement

I am grateful to Dr Abhishek Ojha, Dr Srishti Sareen and Manasvin Sarin for their help in preparation of this chapter.

References

1. Child Rights and The Media : Putting Children in the Right: Guidelines for journalists and media professionals: Peter McIntyre, Oxford UK

2. Convention on the Rights of the Child. 1989. Adopted by the General Assembly of the United Nations on 20th November

3. Media and child protection: Indian Scenario; Namita Anne Minj

4. Children, rights and the Law: Philip Alston; Stephen Parker, John Seymour.

5. Implementing the UN Convention on the Rights of the Child: A Standard of Living adequate for Development; Arlene Bowers Andrews; Natalie Hevener Kaufman

6. Child Rights and the Media: The Nigerian Experience Rasaq Kayode Awosola* and Osakue Stevenson Omoera

7. Andrews, A.B., McLeese, D.G. and Curran, S., 'The impact of a media campaign on public action to help maltreated children in addictive families', Child Abuse and Neglect, 1995; 19(8):921–932.

8. Franklin, B. and Horwath, J., 'The media abuse of children: Jake's progress from demonic icon to restored childhood', Child Abuse Review, 1996; 15:310–318.

9. Krugman, R.D., 'The media and public awareness of child abuse and neglect: It's time for a change', Child Abuse and Neglect, 1996; 20(4):259–260.

10. McDevitt, S., 'The impact of news media on child abuse reporting', Child Abuse and Neglect, 1996; 20(4):261–274.

11. Saunders, B.J. and Goddard, C.R. (1999a), Why do we condone the physical assault of children by their parents and caregivers?, Child Abuse and Family Violence Research Unit, Monash University, Melbourne, and Australians Against Child Abuse, Melbourne.

12. Saunders, B.J. and Goddard, C.R., 'Why do we condone the 'physical punishment' of children?', Children Australia, 1998; 23(3):23–28.

13. Vinson, T. (1987), 'Child abuse and the media', Paper presented to Institute of Criminology Seminar, Sydney University.

14. Wellings, K. & Macdowell, W., 'Evaluating mass media approaches to health promotion: A review of methods', Health Education, 2000; 100(1):23–32.

15. Garbarino, J. (1992), 'Preventing adolescent child maltreatment' in D. Willis, E. Holden, and M. Rosenberg (eds) Prevention of child maltreatment: Developmental and ecological perspectives, John Wiley and Sons, New York.

16. Goddard, C. (1996), Child abuse and child protection: A guide for health, education and welfare professionals, Churchill Livingstone, South Melbourne.

17. Wurtele, S. & Miller-Perrin, C. (1993), Preventing child sexual abuse: Sharing the responsibility, University of Nebraska Press, Lincoln.

26

Involving Children in Policy Making: The Norwegian Experience

Anne Lindboe, Reidar Hjermann

Norway was the first country to establish an ombudsman with statutory rights to protect children and their rights. Since 1981, the Ombudsman for Children has been working to protect and promote children's rights and interests in the country. The office is official, but still independent from the authorities, and the Ombudsman has the power to define his or her own agenda. There are about eighty ombudsmen for children in the world today, and several governments consider establishing an office in their country. In India, Shanta Sinha is heading the National Commission for Protection of Child Rights (NCPCR), which resembles an Ombudsman for Children's office.

Dr Anne Lindboe is appointed by the Government, succeeding Reidar Hjermann who stepped down after eight years as an Ombudsman for Children in June, 2012. Dr. Lindboe is today the head of an office of 20 professionals. We have both extensive experiences with child participation in our work, and we have chosen to join efforts in order to bring out the best of our common and sincere enthusiasm for children, their views, their experience and their knowledge.

In the first part of this essay we will explain our use of children and young people as experts. Here we will also share some examples and some valuable tools for creating successful expert meetings and expert groups. In the second part of this essay we will share some ideas and examples on how children and young people can and should be involved in matters affecting them. Firstly, we will discuss how professionals like the police and judges can work more directly with children, secondly how lowering the voting age can have

real benefits for young people, and thirdly how young people should have a larger role when employing staff. In the appendix we have shared some checklists for organising successful expert meetings and groups.

When we talk about the concepts *children* and *young people* in this article, we always refer to the group of people under the age of 18 years, according to the Convention of The Rights of the Child.

Why should children participate?

Almost all countries in the world have ratified the Convention of the Rights of the child. The convention states that all children shall have a say in everything concerning them:

Article 12.1: States Parties shall assure to the child who is capable of forming his or her own views the right to express those views freely in all matters affecting the child, the views of the child being given due weight in accordance with the age and maturity of the child.

Children should be involved not only because they have the right to be involved, but also because decisions are better made on their behalf if they had the chance to voice their opinions. Even though children have the right to participate, we must also remember that most decisions made are adult's responsibility. Children have the privilege of participating without having the responsibility for decisions made on their behalf.[1]

The national and local policy in a country affects children in various ways. As long as only adults have the right to vote at political elections, children do not have as much political influence as them. One major problem that comes along with this, is that children's experiences, views and opinions are too easily ignored or forgotten when political decisions are made, thus leaving out important information from those with first-hand experience in being children of today.

All of the examples we offer will show that participation of the young is a responsibility for adults. Adults must facilitate participation for children and young people, otherwise it will most often not happen. The examples you will see come from various participation projects in relation to the Ombudsman for Children. We would, however, underline that adults in all professional relations to children can involve them in similar ways.

Children as experts

The Ombudsman for Children has through the years been holding expert meetings and met expert groups of children and young people with a range of different experiences. This way they can be heard, and their opinions and experiences can be forwarded by the Ombudsman and taken into consideration when the authorities make decisions that are relevant for children with similar experiences.

The experts' primary task is to advise the Ombudsman, based on their experiences, on the kind of recommendations the Ombudsman should make to better help children and young people who find themselves in a similar situation as the children the children we consult.

Children are experts at being children

Children and young people are the experts on being children and young people. At the same time, adults make decisions on their behalf. It is therefore all too easy for adults to overlook a range of factors in the process of designing services for children; this applies particularly to services for vulnerable groups.

In the following you will see two concepts discussed: *expert meetings* and *expert groups*. The first refers to one-off meetings and the latter to groups of children that meet with us again and again over a longer period.

The expert consultations have been extremely useful for the Ombudsman for Children, and we see changes in national policy as a result of expert activities. We believe that anyone making decisions on behalf of children and young people will find this kind of consultation extremely productive. This applies particularly to central and local government levels, but also to health and social workers, and to school personnel.

The Ombudsman has experienced that the recommendations given by the experts are often straightforward and feasible. At the same time, adults rarely consult young people, despite the fact that the children may have a wealth of experience in their fields. Information from children and young people can be of great help to municipalities and other public authorities providing services to children.

Meetings or groups?

As mentioned, we distinguish between *expert meetings* and *expert groups*. When we talk about expert meetings, we mean relatively short, one-off meetings with a group of children and young people. A meeting could centre on an issue we are currently concerned about. We frequently hold these expert meetings prior to a conference; they can take the form of a meeting at a school, a visit to a youth club etc. Such meetings normally last between one and four hours.

The size of groups varies from three to fifteen. Our experience is that expert groups and expert meetings work best with five to eight children and two adult leaders.

Meetings with young people in Norway have been focusing on topics such as:

- Child welfare services
- Psychological health and therapy
- Circumcision of boys
- Belonging to an ethnic minority
- Domestic violence

Expert meetings have also been carried out on the Ombudsman's international missions. In **India**, there was a meeting with children with very difficult life situation, such as poverty and lack of housing.

- In **Georgia,** an expert meeting focused on being internally displaced after armed conflict.
- In **Nepal**, several meetings were carried out with focus on the need for an Ombudsman for Children in Nepal

- In the **Chech Republic** an expert meeting was held with children living in institutions
- In **Hong Kong** meetings were held with groups of children in disadvantaged economical life situation.

Expert groups are made up of children and young people with experiences in a particular area who work for a period of time on important issues together with us. Expert groups meet approximately every six weeks, and the duration of the group vary from some months up to more than a year, depending on how much there is to be discussed, the availability of the young experts and budget.

Examples of expert groups at the Ombudsman for Children:

- Experts on incest (Fig. 1)
- Experts on domestic violence

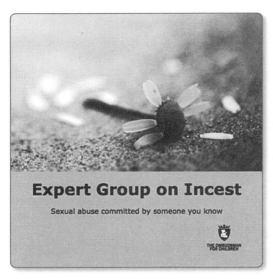

Fig. 1 Introductory poster

- Experts on having parents in prison
- Experts on surviving terrorist attack
- Experts on dropping out of school
- Experts on living in institution
- Experts on hospitalization
- Experts on being children in conflict-ridden divorces

The majority of our experience is with children between the ages of nine and 17 in expert meetings and expert groups. Still, we have not set an age requirement for participation, and we believe that children of most ages can participate, as long as they are able to voice their concerns, and the situation is attuned to them.

Examples of what and how we learn from the experts

Expert meeting, New Delhi, 2011

Reidar Hjermann and adviser Tone Viljugrein were in New Delhi in for the Asia-Pacific Conference on Child Abuse and Neglect (APCCAN) in November 2011.

The children were asked to participate in an expert meeting to teach us as visitors what it is like for them to live disadvantaged lives in New Delhi, and what suggestions they had for improvement for lives of children in India. We met them together with an interpreter (Fig. 2). First we greet them, saying:

I am not here to help you with anything. You are invited to help me to understand what is most important for children who live lives like you do. You are here to advise me, so I can be a better Ombudsman for Children, and give a better lecture tomorrow.

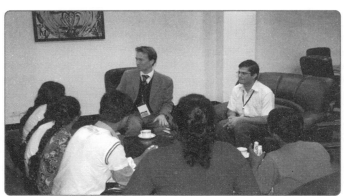

Fig. 2 Reidar Hjermann meeting with children.

Other adults in the room were kindly asked to leave, and the children were promised total confidentiality. They were told that their messages would be brought forward in a lecture the following day, but that their anonymity was absolute.

When asked about what was the most important thing to do to stop violence against children in India, one boy replied:

They have to start valuing boys and girls equally.

When he elaborated further he could tell us:

More girls than boys are abused because they lack education. The parents say: What is the use of educating the girl child? She will be married away anyway.

A girl filled in:

If girls get education, they will also know their rights after they are married. Some girls are not allowed to go out of the house. This nurtures violence.

Another girl commented:

If girls get education, they will also know their rights after they are married.

Some of the children could tell us about violence and abuse of children's rights in school:

One child does something wrong, the rest has to suffer. Sometimes all children must stand in the sun as punishment.

When asked why many parents still believe in physical punishment, one girl reply:

They carry the mindset of their grandparents.

Furthermore, she had her views on how awareness raising amongst parents should happen:

Temple priests, the family priests must bring the message to the parents.

These messages were brought forward in two lectures at the University of New Delhi the following days, and this way their voice were heard amongst people with power to push change.

Experts on incest

The office of the Ombudsman for Children established an expert group of young, female incest victims in order to give a voice to children who have been subjected to this kind of experience, and so that their opinions and experiences may be taken into consideration when politicians

and others make decisions which impact on this group of children. The expert group made recommendations to us in relation to how the community can help and take care of children and young people who have experienced incest.

Mum asked me if there was something wrong with Dad. I lost the plot: 'How can you think that about Dad, he's my DAD for God's sake!' I have often wondered what was going on in my head when Mum asked what was happening.

This quote tells us something about how difficult it is for a young person to disclose abuse. The expert group discussed and developed recommendations to the child welfare service, police, dental health service, mental health service and school. The expert group also met with cabinet ministers and they were also received at the Royal Palace to meet the King and the Queen.

Their recommendations were all compiled in a report. Since the expert group delivered their report we have seen a development of the policy, resulting in better information to children about child abuse and neglect, and about their right to physical and psychological integrity. There are developed official programs for information about child abuse for use in schools and there are awareness raising plans for the public to better know their local child welfare services.

"It took two years from reporting the abuse to going to court. As well as that, the trial was postponed and then the ruling was appealed against. It feels like my life is on hold."

Our experience is that when politicians make decisions on children's behalf, messages directly from those affected tend have a strong impact. Even though stories from real life might seem anecdotal, every child who experiences such severe violations of his or her rights, is an evidence that the system is not working sufficiently, and that changes have to be made.

Step-by-step on expert consultations

In this section we will go more detailed into how expert meetings and –groups can be carried through. These guidelines are partly extracted from a handbook, developed through the last couple of years at the office of the Ombudsman for Children.

It is important that you are fully aware of what you want to achieve by holding expert meetings with children and young people. You have to communicate to the participants what you hope to achieve by holding the meetings and follow up on this.

Before starting the consultation, you must ensure that the participants:

- *understand* the intention of the project
- *know* who wants them to participate and why
- *have a meaningful* (not decorative) task
- *participate* voluntarily after having the project explained to them

We will now provide a more in-depth discussion of the kind of issues it is important to remember when involving children as experts.

Expert meetings and expert groups

Whether you are arranging a short expert meeting or a more protracted expert group, it is wise to keep certain points in mind. In the appendix, you will find some advice that can be helpful in planning your meetings with children and young people.

The lists of advice applies to expert consultations that address issues of varying seriousness; those that demand a great deal and those that are less demanding in nature.

You might not have to jump in at the deep end right away, but even when dealing with typically "light" subjects such as the kind of leisure services that should be developed, it may be wise to consider factors that make it easier for young people to share their experiences.

Expert meetings

An expert meeting is, as earlier mentioned, a one-off meeting with a group of children and young people that provides us with information in relation to a meeting, a lecture we are planning to give or an issue that we want to investigate more closely.

How long can meetings last?

There are no rules for how short or how long a meeting should be. In general, the time you have at your disposal will dictate the length of the meeting. In addition, children and young people often have limited time, especially if the meeting is arranged during school hours.

In any case, you should use between five and ten minutes at the end of the meeting for evaluation. This allows participants to get feedback on their contributions and gives you the chance to hone your skills in terms of holding expert meetings.

How to use the information

It is important to plan the goal of the expert meeting. The information gained from the meeting should be used actively. You must always assess what can be used from consultations with children in lectures or other subsequent conversations. This is vitally important in order to maintain the integrity and anonymity of the experts.

Difficult, controversial and/or sensitive subjects will be talked about sometimes. Remember that experts who live in small communities will have a greater need for anonymity.

This means that you should make time to go through the material at a later point to familiarize yourself with the parts of the information you can use. For example, you should identify any quotes you are going to use. It is also important to view the information through the filter of any duty of confidentiality you may be subject to.

Ideally, the children/young people should be given the chance to work towards some universally agreed upon conclusions that you can subsequently use. Here are some suggestions:

- Do the participants agree on anything or do you just have a lot of quotes from them?
- Spend time on cultivating a few themes
- Make a list of priorities (3 tips from young people on...)

All participants should be notified of the results of the expert meeting, whether this is notification of improvements to the municipal system based on the information they provided, publications or other relevant outcome.

Expert groups

Expert groups are expanded expert meetings. Some key issues require more in-depth investigation. It can therefore be useful to hold several meetings. It is more resource demanding, both for us as professionals, but also for the children. The advantages, however, are many. More information and more child participation is provided. In addition, the children in the group will get to know each other. This way they feel safer, they get support from the other participants, and they develop ideas together.

The composition of the group may depend on age and theme. You should discuss group size and optimal methods with an adult who knows the children/young people as well as whether the children/young people are used to using any particular methods.

The Ombudsman has a few ground rules for expert groups:

- Special advisors should be the main points of contact and be reachable via email and telephone.
- Parental approval must be sought where appropriate.
- Minutes of every meeting should be taken and sent to all participants for their comments.
- Anyone in the group can ask anybody about anything, also private issues, as long as it is done in a nice way. Everyone is free not to answer questions.

How long can meetings last?

The group should hold between four and six meetings, sometimes longer. This should be agreed at the first meeting. Again, it is important to emphasize the importance of not trying to achieve too much too quickly. Let each meeting last two hours, for example, and inform the participants of how much time you think you are going to spend. This will make it easier for them to relate to the programme.

Below we show how a four-meeting programme can be put together. Here, the idea is for each meeting to last two hours with a 15-minute break.

Suggestions for a four-meeting programme

Meeting 1 – Get to know each other and define main issues

At the first meeting, you can define the main issues for the group the young people are representing in their role as participants. Agree to focus on (e.g.) three issues, which will form the basis of future meetings.

Meeting 2 – Focus and expand on the main issues

Present the key issues again and continue to work on them.

You can, for instance, divide the children into groups of two to four children, sitting at separate tables. At each table, the participants are allocated a challenge/main issue that was hammered out at the previous meeting.

You will now investigate the issues in even more depth, and participants will get the chance to expand on their contributions from the last time. Look upon this as a "yes! phase" during which everything is on the up.

Meeting 3 – How to resolve the main issues defined in the previous meeting

Use a simple group assignment: Divide the participants into (new) groups and use the main points you identified in the previous meetings to find solutions for overcoming the obstacles. Be creative, and believe that everything is possible. The adults can provide advice and tips, and contribute with access to the media, politicians, ministries etc.

Each group makes a note of the main points on the flip-over for in plenum discussion.

The groups make three-minute presentations of their suggestions. There is opportunity for brief questions and input.

Meeting 4 – Further work and summarizing

At the last meeting, you have the opportunity to tie up, unravel any loose or knotted ends, but more importantly you have the chance to sum up. Make certificates for the participants and hand them out formally.

Meet the decision makers

It is usually be a good idea to have a meeting with the relevant authorities in attendance who are in a position to make the kind of changes that you have arrived at. Invite them or visit them. This can be done as part of an extra meeting.

How to use the information

Information from the flip-over and notes now has to be systematized. It is usually wise to compile a short report that includes the following:

- Presentation of the expert group and the goal of holding this kind of consultation.
- Participants – age, gender, relevant experience.

- The methods used.
- Main conclusions/results. These may be placed alongside relevant figures and research.
- Proposed action.

A clear report with pictures, quotations, research and proposals can make a significant impact. But there are other ways of presenting the material, for instance using media. Involve the children and young people and agree on how the information may be used.

How speaking with children on children's terms can help police, judges and child protection services to make right decisions

In all the Nordic countries the governments have developed a concept termed *Children's houses*, multidisciplinary competence centers for children that have been exposed to violence and abuse. In these countries all forms of corporal punishment as well as physical and psychological abuse of children is strictly forbidden, also in the home. The Norwegian code on criminal procedure, section 239, dictates that children up to the age of 16 should be interviewed in a neutral (out-of-court) setting. When a suspicion that a child (3–18 years old) has witnessed or been victim of violence or sexual abuse is present, the child can come to a *Children's house* for judicial interviews, medical examinations, guidance and treatment. The child is interviewed and examined by qualified police personnel and pediatricians that are specially trained in interviewing children.

The child usually feels very safe in such a child-friendly environment and gets the opportunity to play, eat and relax between the sessions. Before becoming the Ombudsman for Children, Dr. Lindboe, a pediatrician and forensic physician, worked a lot with children exposed to abuse. We see a big difference in what children dear to tell when they are interviewed this way compared to a traditional setting where interviews are conducted by ordinary police investigators in the hospital or at the police station. In the old, traditional setting a child was often too scared to open up and tell its story, and often the interviewing adult — whose role was more of an interrogator's — did not listen patiently and carefully enough to what the child had to say.

By interviewing children in an environment where they can feel safe, and by letting them be interviewed by a trained person with good communication skills, children open up and speak more freely. Under such conditions a child can provide much more detailed descriptions of the violence or abuse it may have been exposed to. It is, of course, of crucial importance that the child feels safe, and in order to ensure this, the child is not exposed to possible further traumatization by being forced to talk about difficult matters in ways that are too disturbing.

Listening to the children's stories can also help the child protection services (CPS) to make a better decision on whether a child should be moved from its family or not. The detailed stories, sometimes combined with findings from the medical examination, will also often make the police's job easier. The increased level of information and evidence provided by the children themselves has led to more cases of violence and abuse against children being brought to court. In court, we see a tendency that the judges emphasize children's explanations more than before.

Finally, listening to the children gives us information on what they want and need to feel safe. Surprisingly often, it is not the same as the adults in Child Welfare Service or police initially believed was in the best interest of the child. The child's own voice helps them to make better judgments.

Right to vote

Having the right to vote is both an access to real influence and an important symbol of being a part of a democracy. Several countries in the world consider lowering the age for voting, and some countries already allow sixteen year olds to the polling station. Moreover, Council of Europe has in their Resolution 1826 (2011) suggested that member states consider lowering the voting age to 16 years.[2] Many countries in Europe have lowered the voting age already in municipal and local elections. Most noteworthy is perhaps Austria where 16 year olds have gained the right to vote in not only local elections but also in national and European elections.[3]

Through the years the Ombudsman for Children has had many encounters with young people who feel that their voice is not properly heard in the local democracy. The Ombudsman lobbied the government together with organizations for young people, convincing the government to pilot a project of lowering the voting age from 18 to 16 years at municipal elections.[4] The government accepted and in November 2011 Norway carried through local elections. The age of voting was lowered to 16 years in 20 municipalities.

The test election has been deemed a success after the 16 and 17 year olds had a 58 percent turnout.[5] This is below the national average of 64,5 percent but considerably higher than the 46 per cent turnout among the 18 to 21 year olds.

The main arguments for lowering the voting age were the following:

- When we have voting age at 18 years, the *average* first time voter will be 20. In Norway, high school ends the year we turn 19, and then many of the first time voters have left home and the municipality where they have lived many years, maybe their whole life. The community needs their vote before they leave.
- Young people have a lot of experience with municipal services, such as school and health system.
- Having age of voting at 16 forces the politicians to care more about what is important for young people.

There was a lot of controversy around this issue before the pilot project. The independent evaluation report after the pilot is still to be finalized, but the minister of internal affairs has already voiced that she supports a permanent voting age at 16 in all local elections, as a result of the pilot.

We can already conclude that the right to vote evoke a political curiosity amongst the young people. It also made politicians more aware of what is important for the young generation. The Ombudsman at that time, Mr Hjermann, was present at political meetings in most of the pilot municipalities prior to the election, and could easily see that young people understood how politics influence their lives, and why they should care.

Children participating in recruitment

In 2012 in Norway children were involved in the recruitment of the new Ombudsman for Children. This happened after pressure from Mr. Reidar Hjermann, the Ombudsman for Children at that time. The rationale behind the idea was that *if you to become a good ombudsman for children you*

must be able to communicate and connect with them. The only way to really find out about this is to observe the candidates in action with children.

The recruitment process drew inspiration from Ireland where the Ombudsman for Children was recruited by a youth panel. Their experiences were thoroughly recorded in a recruitment report which offers excellent guidelines.[6]

Ten children aged 12 years through 17 years were recruited from different youth organizations to form a *youth panel*. They helped decide the formal qualifications necessary to hold the position, and contributed in making the ad for the position. A professional recruitment agency picked the four more qualified candidates. These candidates were then interviewed again, first by the youth panel, and finally by the Norwegian ministry of children.

Dr. Lindboe was interviewed by the children for more than an hour. She says:

The connection between the youth panel and me was instant, but that did not mean that they went easy with me. They asked all kinds of questions, not letting me of the hook every time I gave a vague or bad answer. The questions where intelligent, sharp and open, like 'How will you manage the press and media, just being a doctor? How will you be able to lead an office that must be very different from being in charge in the medical emergency room?'

The dialogue was tough but the tone was positive and cheerful. After the interview I was totally exhausted. In my opinion, this interview was the most important of all the ones I went through because the children gave me the opportunity to show them who I really am, my personality and my communication skills.

The youth panel finished by making an evaluation report for each of the four candidates. The candidate's communication skills with the members of the panel were mentioned as one crucial component of the candidate's competence. The children wanted candidates who talk *with* them and not only *to* them. They preferred candidates with a sense of humor, and they wanted to feel safe and respected in the dialogue. It was later confirmed by the Ministry that this interview changed the ranking of the remaining candidates, and that they actually listened to the children's opinion.

The recruitment of the Ombudsman for Children should serve as an example on how the society can use children in recruiting other professionals working with children, such as teachers, pediatricians and people working in Child Welfare Services. Involving young people in recruitment is possible and the right thing to do.[7] It is the safest way to make sure that you get the best possible candidate, one that has got the right formal qualifications *and* a talent for communicating with children.

Let the children in

Too often adults, and in particular decision makers, use children as decoration. Not seldom we see children stand in a supportive and cheering circle around a politician launching a new policy concerning children. Other times you will see them as members of a choir opening a great conference on issues relevant to children. Still, they hardly ever contribute with their expertise in being children. Luckily, there is a growing awareness about the need for real participation and we are glad to see that more adults now feel more competent in how to involve children and young people in policy making and governance of a society.

For adults who want to involve children and young people in a serious and inclusive way it is — unfortunately — often a struggle to convince other people that children are real stakeholders that should be heard and that their experiences and opinions actually can make decision-making both easier and better. For all of you who consider having children influencing how you work, we can assure you that it makes both your work and your life better and more joyful.

Decision making authorities in a society will always be dependent on professional advice. These advices can come from you, being a professional working on issues concerning children. You can write columns in the newspapers, approach media with your views, and you can ask for meetings with politicians or other people in power. The decision makers will surely receive better advice when children also have influence on how you bring your professional input into the corridors of power. And remember, as a professional it is actually your responsibility to lobby on children's behalf. We cannot expect the children to lobby for themselves.

Conclusion

Norway is a small and wealthy nation with a relatively homogenous population. It may be easy to jump to the conclusion that this little place cannot serve as an example for emerging countries, many times as big and much more diverse. We, however, strongly believe that children's involvement is even more important in countries with more challenges. Societies that have a wider range of people and cultures will also have a greater field of children's experience to harvest. And, according to the Convention of the Rights of the Child, it is every state's responsibility to ensure protection of and necessary provisions for children. These responsibilities can only be fully accomplished if the state acknowledges it's duty to ensure participation of all children in everything concerning to them.

List of issues to be considered before child expert consultations

The following are not exhaustive lists. They are result of our experiences with child participation at the office of the Ombudsman for Children. You will have your own experiences. Add them on, use them and circulate them to others working with experts.

Before the meeting

- How many participants, and of what age, is optimal?
- Will you have to order refreshments? Talk to the young people or the adults around them about the kind of food that would be appropriate. Food is important for sustaining concentration levels throughout the entire meeting.
- Assess whether the participants are eligible for living expenses/travel expenses. Clarify where participants will be refunded travel related expenses. A lack of funds may result in some young people not being able to take part.
- Do the participants have to travel far? Assess whether they need supervision on journeys to and from the meeting.
- Stipulate who has responsibility for the meeting. It is wise to allocate responsibility to at least two people in the event one chairperson is sick or otherwise unable to attend.
- Recruit children and/or young people who are directly/indirectly connected to the issue. Inform them and ask them if this is something they would like to be involved in. Do you need parental consent?

- Do you need to get consent to make a media appearance?
- All participants must be informed about the purpose of holding the meeting, what you will discuss and how you will go about it. Where possible, this can be done in advance by sending a letter to the school, to a contact person or directly to the children/young people. Remember to keep the language age-appropriate.
- Specify the role to be played by the adults accompanying the participants. Will they attend the meeting or wait outside?
- Where particularly difficult issues, such as poverty, violence and abuse, are going to be addressed, you should determine whether an adult with a connection to the experts should take responsibility for subsequently following up the children and young people.
- Investigate available equipment/visual aids. Flip-overs are helpful and should always be in place. Remember felt-tip pens and post-its too!
- Make sure you have contact details, e.g. business cards, available at the start of the meeting. Show that you are taking the meeting seriously.

During the meeting

- Work out some ground rules for the meeting together with the participants.
- Make sure that no other adults than those with a defined role are present in the room. Be aware, but don't let it stop you, that some adults might feel offended when asked to leave the room.
- Allocate a chairperson and a minutes-taker.
- Introduce yourselves if not you have not already done so.
- Set a time to take a break. We recommend a maximum session length of 45 minutes, regardless of time constraints.
- Provide information about your duty of confidentiality.
- Provide information about your obligation to report to child welfare services. In Norway, all government employees are obligated to report to child welfare services where there are grounds to suspect that a child is being subjected to abuse or other serious failures of care, and the children must be informed of this.
- Inform participants that they can choose to leave the room/group if they need to and that an adult or one of the other children will be on-hand where required.

- Can participants be quoted? Inform the participants that what they say may be presented anonymously on request.
- You can circulate a register so that you can get in touch with the participants later to give them feedback on what they said. Important information may otherwise be rendered useless.
- Ask if it is all right to take pictures, and clarify how they may be subsequently used.
- Where possible, take a note of the names and ages of the participants on the flip-over so that they can get to know each other's names. Frequent use of the participants' names is also friendly and inclusive.
- Always take notes during the meeting and include quotations that illustrate the situation. It is a good idea to use a flip-over because it makes what is being said visible and enables participants to follow up.
- Go through the main points in your notes with the participants so that they get the chance to add or take away their views.

You can read more about the use of experts as well as tips and tools in the Ombudsman for Childrens Expert group handbook available online.[2]

Suggested Reading regarding the involvement of children and young people in recruitment processes.

Save the Children and The Scottish Alliance for Children's Rights (2005) "The Recruitment Pack: Involving Children and Young People in the recruitment of staff"

Participation works, "Involving Children and Young People in Recruitment and Selection", http://www.participationworks.org.uk/

Butler Scally, D. (2004), "Report on the Selection Processes for the Appointment of the Irish Ombudsman for Children", Public Appointments service.

Action for Children: "The Right Choice: Involving Children and Young People in Recruitment and Selection", http://www.actionforchildren.org.uk/

Michel, E. and Hart, D. (2002) "Involving Young People in the Recruitment of Staff, Volunteers and Mentors." National Children's Bureau.

References

1. United Nations, Committee on the Rights of the Child,General Comment no 12 (2009), "The Right of the Child to be Heard" CRC/C/GC/12.

2. http://assembly.coe.int/Mainf.asp?link=/ Documents/AdoptedText/ta11/ERES1826.htm and http://assembly.coe.int/Documents/WorkingDocs/ Doc11/EDOC12546.pdf

3. European Election Database (EED): http://www. nsd.uib.no/european_election_database/country/ austria/parliamentary_elections.html

4. The Ombudsman for Chuildren (2007), Booklet: "What's the point? – a booklet on the right to vote for 16-year –olds: http://barneombudet.no/vote16/

5. http://www.regjeringen.no/en/dep/krd/press/ press-releases/2012/higher-turnout-among-first-time-voters.html?id=670637

6. Butler Scally, D. (2004), "Report on the Selection Processes for the Appointment of the Irish Ombudsman for Children", Public Appointments service.

7. Save the Children and The Scottish Alliance for Children's Rights (2005), "The Recruitment Pack: Involving Children and Young People in the recruitment of staff"

8. http://barneombudet.no/young-experts

9. Agrudic, Milos, "Expansion of democracy by lowering the voting age to 16", Report, Political Affairs Committee, Council of Europe.

10. Council of Europe (2011), "Expansion of democracy by lowering the voting age to 16", Resolution 1826, Parliamentary Assembly

11. The Ministry of Local Government and Regional Development (2012), Press release: "Higher turnout among first-time voters", http://www.regjeringen. no/en/dep/krd/press/press-releases/2012/higher-turnout-among-first-time-voters.html?id=670637

12. The Ombudsman for Children (2012), Handbook: "Young Experts, http://barneombudet.no/young-experts

Asia-Pacific Conference on Child Abuse and Neglect 2011 for the Safety of Childhoods

Razia Ismail Abbasi

The children of Asia and the Pacific are the largest child numbers in the world population. They are also among those most vulnerable to neglect and deprivation. Proportionate to the whole population of the combined Asia-Pacific region, the child percentage may lag several points behind that of Africa. But the absolute numbers are far higher, with India the uneasy home of the world's largest population of children.

How safe and secure are the children of the Pacific and Asia? The pressures of tradition and custom vie with newer contemporary pressures of market, migration, social distance and jobless growth, and millions of children struggle through undefended childhoods. Many things, including policies and programmes and their promotion not specifically aimed at children, do affect them and their prospects, often adversely.

The sites of abuse and neglect abound in both the so-called 'developed' and 'developing' world. Children suffer emotional and psychological risk and damage everywhere. Even where economic growth is said to be on an upward curve, and even where governments are not engaged in declared or undeclared war within or across their borders, risks remain and children suffer. Where the battles and tensions and shortages are inside the borders of a household, childhoods are in jeopardy right at home.

Across virtually the whole of the Asia-Pacific expanse, and especially where the numbers of people and thus the numbers of the disadvantaged are large, poverty is a reality for the majority of communities, sites and settings, and thus for the children in them. Essential development services are inadequate and poorly resourced in most of these countries, and children are adversely affected. The identity and category into which people are 'classified' influence their access to a fair share of support and opportunity. Is this abuse? It often amounts to that. Is it neglect? Very often.

What qualifies a child to expect a caring justice? Just being a child should be qualification enough. But it does not seem to be.

Whose responsibility is it to address these risks and abuses? The ISPCAN initiative raises the question again and again, in both regional and international settings, in a resolute progression of conferences. Declarations and pledges have emerged from each, over the years. APCCAN in 2011 brought forward the Delhi Declaration. It calls upon the entire Asia-Pacific region to act effectively against child abuse and neglect. Many of the participating countries were involved in the UN Secretary-General's worldwide Study on Violence Against Children in 2005-2007, and all of them had received the UN's directive to make country plans – and implement them. Not many have actually done so.

The Delhi Declaration evolved out of the proceedings and deliberations of APCCAN-2011 – the 9th Asia Pacific Conference on Child Abuse and Neglect. Experts and participants from 40 countries met in New Delhi to offer their knowledge and insights, to debate priorities, and argue for what they collectively identified as 'non-negotiables.' As with all such pledges, and all such meetings, the challenge is one of collective ownership. In drafting the declaration, a special effort to involve delegates in the actual formulation of the declaration was made at many of the workshops, working hours, but bore fruit in a final document that people could feel they owned. It was adopted unanimously in the final plenary. A representative from the Government of India assured national attention. He obviously could not speak for all the countries present, but he did express a positive resolve. This brought the conference to a successful conclusion – but it was actually the beginning of the hard task of pushing for real action. The question of how to negotiate for attention to the 'non-negotiables' – and with whom – was everyone's take-away package.

A year on from the Asia Pacific experience, there is no dramatic change in children's status and condition in any of the countries. Positive steps have been taken by some, but no one can at all claim that every childhood in every country is safeguarded. Does this mean failure? No, but it signifies a heightening of the challenges, and thus an underlining of the need to act.

In the many years before the mandate of human rights was internationally invoked for children in the UN Convention on the Rights of the Child (UN CRC), welfare was an acceptable term and concept, and 'universalization' was equated with '80 per cent.' From the standpoint of rights, there is no universalization until and unless the 20 per cent have also been reached. Is it neglect to leave the 20 per cent waiting? It is. Is it abuse? In many instances, it is.

This becomes clear when the comprehensive definition of violence is used to assess and judge what is happening to countless children. The UN CRC offers this definition of violence, and of every country's obligation to eradicate it: "all forms of physical or mental violence, injury or abuse, neglect or negligent treatment, maltreatment or exploitation, including sexual abuse..."[1]

The UN General Comment against All Forms of Violence Against Children[2] has used and reaffirmed this comprehensive definition.

What are the implications of such a definition for both advocacy and action? This is in fact the question posed by the Delhi Declaration. How does a country, or a society, actually clarify what it means to act against violence? It is useful to place the elements in the context of UN CRC provision on the adequacy of living standards: "States Parties recognise the right of every child to a standard of living adequate for the child's physical, mental,

spiritual, moral and social development."[3] Most countries assessing and reporting child rights action tend to see this provision as related to questions of housing, water supply, etc., and even the UN CRC reporting handbook tends to do that. But that is no real measure of the adequacy of living standards.

What then is? A violence-free world for children then infers a living environment in which the treatment of a child – and thus the child's expectations – will be not only kind and caring, but also fair and just, above neglectfulness and negligence, safeguarded against maltreatment, free of doubt and fear, confident of benevolence. The slap or the blow, and the hurtful word, are a sign of violence and abuse; the rebuff and the forgotten duty are a sign of neglect – but neither is the whole of it.

The Delhi Declaration draws upon this wider view, and calls for the countries of the region to broaden their own vision and to act upon it.

- Physical or mental violence
- Injury or abuse
- Neglect or negligent treatment
- Maltreatment or exploitation
- Sexual abuse

'All appropriate legislative, administrative, social and educational measures to protect the child' do not exist anywhere. Perhaps the least addressed challenge is the one of mental and emotional health and well-being. Children are not damaged only on the surface; the emotional, psychological and 'inner' hurts run deep. In many situations, nothing is done. Where a parent or household member is an offender against the child, it is often the abused child – whatever the form of abuse – who has to adjust to what happens. In the case of neglect, at times this manifestation of violence is not even acknowledged for what it is.

What is 'injury,' what is 'maltreatment,' what is 'exploitation?' Every society or culture, every status setting, and every governance frame presents its own definitions. Many are unseeing of the child's reality, inattentive to the child's needs, and completely unfair to children. The Delhi Declaration invites closer attention to discovering what is often left between the lines.

The calls for action continue. The 2012 ISPCAN International Congress has already brought out the Istanbul Declaration. It is a renewed call for attention and action. Its opening words are a reaffirmation that "prevention of child abuse and neglect is the biggest responsibility of humankind to children." But violence still awaits prevention.

The Istanbul Congress has called on all States to establish and enforce child protection services that ensure identification, assessment and intervention to combat child abuse and neglect, and to make certain that provision of services result in improved outcomes for children. This only echoes and endorses the Delhi Declaration appeal for "national strategies and plans of action to address, punish and overcome violence against children, with measurable, specific and time-bound goals and commitments," and the allocation of due attention and resources – and a healing approach – for the child's recovery, and the restoration to an honourable place in the community and society.

It is difficult to judge what is really changing in children's favour, and whether the Asia Pacific deliberations have had an adequately encouraging impact. It is hard to say whether all or any of those who were moved by the conference have been good messengers.

In a political and economic scenario increasingly burdened by ideas of profit, the acknowledgement of human benefit and public good as the real indicators has weakened, and their leverage power is undercut. Across the world, development policies and programmes are now couched in the vocabulary of the market – and the issue of who is left unprotected is not being addressed. As long as children are in the front rank of those most vulnerable and worst affected by such skewed priorities, these policies remain questionable. The children of the poor are bypassed along with the under-served communities in whom they struggle to survive their childhoods. Such deep divides between the haves and have-not are increasingly questionable.

In drawing attention to these underlying factors the Delhi Declaration has done its duty to list genuine imperatives. Somewhere at mid-point in the text is the core responsibility, stated in clear and simple words: 'The conscious creation of a caring attitude and approach in both authorities and society in all dealings with children, to be manifest in all actions affecting children's lives.' This says it all. What remains is to do it all. And to keep a watch. And to report regularly.

This may take years. Governments that persist in providing children the very least service or support possible will resist persuasion, often claiming they do not have the resources required. Meanwhile, children will continue to be brutalized, and children will continue to perish.

It is true that many States do appear to lack one essential resource that children urgently deserve. This is the spirit of caring about children, and thus about what happens to them, which stands far above simply giving them some 'care.' It was the internationally respected public health expert Dr Eric Ram of India who coined and advocated the concept of a 'caring community' as the birthright of every child. This means that every sector and service and component of the State's encounter with children, and with State standards that safeguard the child's best interests in every connection and interaction with wider society, the spirit of 'caring about' must be present and manifest. In invoking this essential requirement, the Delhi Declaration has joined battle with all those who forget to care.

Almost all States have accepted the Universal Declaration of Human Rights. All but two countries have accepted the UN CRC. Many have human rights policies and laws of their own. The promotion of the Delhi Declaration is an important contribution to reminding all defaulters. Children's right to safe, secure and happy childhoods is reason enough to make it a clarion call.

References

1. UN Convention on the Rights of the Child: Article 19
2. UN Committee on the Rights of the Child: General Comment #13./2011
3. UN Convention on the Rights of the Child: Article 27.

Delhi Declaration 2011

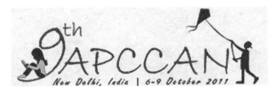

Preamble

We, the participants of the 9th ISPCAN Asia Pacific Regional Conference on Child Abuse & Neglect representing governments, non-governmental organizations, networks and institutions, including professionals from all sectors and disciplines, children and adolescents from 40 countries assembled in New Delhi, India, to review and assess the challenges posed by violence, neglect and abuse of children in our countries – such as the persistence of corporal punishment, to identify and determine the opportunities before us to address and overcome these violations of child rights, do hereby register our concern that neglect and abuse of children stand as a critical issue of development and justice across Asia and the Pacific, and believe that all our countries must act to secure for all children a protective and caring environment. In so doing, we ask for the commitment and leadership of our governments, legislatures and judiciaries, and of all those who determine or affect the status and condition of children.

We recognize that

Neglect is denial or deficiency of either the provision and delivery of services such as health care and education.

All Countries of our region are States-Parties to the UN Convention on the Rights of the Child and to the UN Declaration of Human Rights and its covenants and are thereby committed to securing these rights for all children in their jurisdiction;

The United Nations has, in its Special Study on Violence Against Children worldwide, mobilized all nations and their leadership to acknowledge the prevalence of neglect and abuse of children as a challenge of global proportions and of international and national concern.

The UN Committee on the Rights of the Child has issued a special General Comment[1] declaring the right of the child to freedom from all forms of violence and has set international standards to ensure the protection of children.

The International Society for the Prevention of Child Abuse and Neglect (ISPCAN) affirms that effective and sustainable prevention is achieved through education and professional cooperation "to promote opportunities, facilities and organizations which will enable the children of all nations to develop physically, mentally and socially, ensuring the protection of every child in every country, against all forms of cruelty and exploitation."

We express our concern at

The threats to children's right to life before and after birth and throughout the period of growth;

The violation of many children's right to a caring and protective environment and the unacceptable affront that this inflicts on children's dignity.

Denial of opportunities for all children to realize their full potential and enjoy all human rights of survival, development, protection and self-expression, with the security of nutrition, health care and education throughout childhood;

The suffering and damage that children experience because of the inadequacy and absence of protection in all settings;

The adverse and negative portrayal of children, the depiction of violence as acceptable and even attractive in both traditional and emerging media and channels of communication, entertainment and marketing, and the damage that this does to children's perceptions and values.

The absence or inadequacy of timely and appropriate preventive and remedial action against abuse, exploitation and violence or any kind of distress whenever children are affected by civil disturbances and armed conflict, natural disasters or situations of scarcity and/ or other conditions where security breaks down, or services and systems fail to operate.

The persistence of these risks and threats, despite the observance of a UN Decade for a Culture of Peace and Non-Violence against Children (2000-2010), and worldwide support for the child protection commitments made by the UN General Assembly Special Session on Children in adopting the declaration and action plan for 'a World fit for Children' (2002);

The insufficient action of governments and society to comprehensively protect children against all abuse and neglect, and failure to ensure that all services and settings safeguard children against any such affliction or even such risks.

The disrespect and damage done to children and childhood, in both governmental and social action, when access to rights and protection is undermined by factors of identity and not safeguarded by correctives.

The hurt and alienation that children suffer in cases where the State and society fail to ensure equal access to rights and protection regardless of a gender perspective.

We assert the urgent and immediate need to

Integrate principles, standards and measures in national planning processes to prevent and respond to violence against children;

Develop national strategies and plans of action to address, punish and overcome violence against children, with measurable, specific and time-bound goals and commitments.

Remove social and economic inequalities through sound policies and their execution;

Prohibit all forms of neglect, abuse and violence against children in all settings, through honest and accountable governance and by law and its enforcement;

Develop and establish reliable national data collection and responsible use of information on children; the lack of this results in insufficient knowledge or understanding of violence against children and its root causes.

Ensure comprehensive and restorative juvenile justice systems and mechanisms.

Set up independent commissions with authority to monitor, investigate and uphold child rights in all settings and to set standards in child protection.

Ensure the ratification and implementation of the Optional Protocol to the Convention on the Rights of the Child on the Involvement of Children in Armed Conflict and Optional Protocol to the Convention on the Rights of the Child on the sale of Children, Child Prostitution and Child Pornography

We welcome national, regional and international child protection initiatives and efforts of the past decade

The appointment of children's rights commissions and desks in several countries in the Region;

Child protection policies, laws, and schemes in response to Concluding Observations of the UN Committee on the Rights of the Child in several countries;

Setting up of juvenile justice systems in several countries;

Sensitisation of all service managers and providers and all those whose actions affect the security and well-being of children, to appreciate that each child and every childhood is special and worthy of respect and care.

We recognise that despite these advances

There is denial in some countries about the scale of violence against children and certain forms of violence have social sanction;

Certain conditions and circumstances increase the vulnerability of some children, with reasons such as disability, gender, race, culture, community, migration, social and economic marginalization.

Violence against children is hidden, unreported and under-recorded for many reasons including fear of ostracism and social acceptance of violence[2]

There is a need to reform the existing mechanisms for children to confidently report and raise issues of neglect and abuse.

Many countries are yet to frame and adopt national action plans on violence against children;

Laws and their enforcement are yet to be rights – based;

Some laws do not confirm to accepted international standards and commitments such as UNCRC.

Perpetrators of violence against children are not convicted;

Prevention strategies are not given priority;

There is a need to improve the attitudes and skills of professionals' working with children;

We therefore urge

Recognition of child abuse, neglect, exploitation and all forms of violence against children as a critical issue of justice and development in the Asia Pacific region;

That opportunity be ensured to all children to realise their full potential and enjoy the basic human rights of survival, development, protection and participation including nutrition, health care and education throughout childhood

The recognition and fulfillment by governments and all other stakeholders including parents,

of their key role and responsibility to prevent maltreatment of children and protect children from abuse, neglect, exploitation, violence and discrimination;

The conscious creation of a caring attitude and approach in both authorities and society in all dealings with children, to be manifest in all actions affecting children's lives;

Enforcement of existing laws in an efficient and timely manner, and review of all laws not in conformity with UNCRC and/or other international standards.

Generation of public support for respecting and protecting children's rights.[6]

The holding of a child in an institution must only be as a "last resort", with standards of safety and care ensured. Family-based alternative care should be consciously explored and its standard guaranteed.

Education to change public attitudes & develop an inclusive caring culture; and promote non violent values.

Child labour is to be abolished and eradicated.

Silence on all forms of abuse and neglect of children must be brought to an end;

Countries must implement all provisions and recommendations of UN general comment No. 13 (the Right of the Child to freedom from all forms of violence)

Ensure all organizations and institutions endorse the prevention of violence against children as a cross-cutting commitment.

Regard and respect the family as an institution and as the primary setting for the care and well-being of its children;

Establish a code of ethics to regulate and control adverse and negative portrayal of children and the depiction of violence as acceptable and even attractive in both traditional and emerging media and channels of communication, entertainment and marketing, and ensure required regulation and ethical standards.

We call upon all governments

To ensure the following policies and measures, and on all those whose policies, programmes and activities affect the lives, status and condition of children to support these policies.

Ensure that children affected by armed conflict, natural disasters and/ or any condition or situation of scarcity or of failure of services and systems, are protected through timely and appropriate preventive and remedial action against abuse, exploitation and violence or any kind of distress.

Develop integrated plans for cross-sectoral/ multi-sectoral action to address violence against children, as well as related conditions of risk of violence;

Strengthen national commitments and carry out time-bound and measurable strategies to prevent Violence against Children;

To accept and implement the concerns and recommendation of General Comment No. 13 issued by UN Committee on the Rights of the Child, calling for children's freedom from all forms of violence

Allocate adequate attention, resources and a healing approach for recovery and a restoration of an honourable place in the community and society;

Establish accessible mechanisms which are respectful of the child;

Define, prohibit and criminalise all acts of maltreatment of children in accord with internationally accepted principles and standards;

Recognise and address the harmful potential of certain social and cultural traditions and emerging values and practices and their influence on children. Identify address and correct forms of violence, which are socially accepted;

Set up juvenile justice systems and ensure that appropriate mechanisms are in place, operating and accountable;

Build community confidence in just governance by bringing all perpetrators of violence against children to justice;

Ensure that persons convicted of violent offences and sexual abuse of children are prevented from working with children;

Provide specialised training to investigative staff – police and the judiciary – and mandate this training under service rules for government employees and all service managers and providers whose work affects the child;

Evaluate all children's institutions at regular intervals, with children being involved and consulted in the evaluations;

Adapt and adopt "The international Guidelines for the Appropriate Use and Conditions of Alternative Care for Children" in all countries;

Progressively develop and establish children's participation in all measures and programs affecting their life and security and build the capacity and working approach of persons working with children;

Prioritize the prevention of Maltreatment of children by allocating adequate resources for awareness raising campaigns and mass education to change attitudes, of the public at large, on the perceptions of and the indifference to incidents of child abuse to build respect for children;

Ensure all children are registered immediately after their birth and take special measures to register all those up to the age of 18 years not yet registered;

Develop and implement systematic national data collection, analysis and monitoring, with due allocation of resources;

Work for the ratification and implementation of relevant international and regional conventions, statutes and rights standards; and strengthen regional and international commitment to protecting children.

Declaration and pledge

We, the participants at the 9th ISPCAN Asia Pacific Regional Conference on Child Abuse and Neglect, in New Delhi, representing the people of our many countries hereby declare our commitment to these aims and objectives, and pledge our resolve to stand against the neglect and abuse of children and to strive for achievement of child rights and the building of a caring community for every child, free of violence and discrimination.

New Delhi, 9th October 2011

Index

Page numbers followed by *f* for figure and *t* for table, respectively.